# But It Works

*An Alternative Doctor's Guide*

Dr. Rodney V. Holland, BS, DC, CCSP

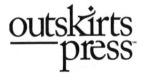

# Table of Contents

# Acknowledgements

My deepest appreciation goes to my lovely bride of almost 50 years, Linda. Thank you for giving me the time, encouragement, ideas, assistance in researching and putting on paper the thoughts that I wanted to convey. The idea for putting this together was to help those who wanted to take control and improve their health without relying on drugs or anything unnatural.

I would like to thank Hollie Hixson, my office manager, for giving me some free time during the day to write. Thank you to Joan Bostrom and Tom Huffman for "encouraging" me to finish the work and then editing the manuscript.

And most of all, I thank God for blessing me with wonderful patients and guiding me in my efforts to help them with their health concerns.

# Introduction

The concept of this book came from my patients. For years I've heard my patients tell horror stories about their experiences with the established healing arts. Common phrases they are told by their doctors include: "You're just going to have to live with it." "Let's try a different medication." "If you go to an alternative doctor you won't be seen in this office again." Common comments from patients include: "They've done a bazzilion tests and can't tell me what's wrong." "My doctor doesn't listen to me." "They just want to give me another pill."

The purpose of this book is to help those who are frustrated with the health care system and want to take control of their health. And also to those who want to stay healthy and can't afford to go to their doctor for every little bump and scratch. The following pages are not all encompassing for each topic, but rather gives the reader a glance at each area so that helpful decisions can be made.

The concepts in this book are presented, not to enlighten healthcare professionals, but rather to inform the reader so that good decisions concerning their health can be made. Therefore, long, impressive medical terms have been avoided and replaced with common vernacular.

Disclaimer: Nothing contained herein is meant to diagnose or take the place of a good holistic doctor. These are simply concepts, procedures and techniques that tend to work in my office that I would like to share. They were gathered together from years of classes, seminars, research, training and clinical experience. The ultimate decision for an individual's health care lies with the individual. Doctors can help based on their training. However, the ultimate decision rests with the individual.

An effort was made to keep the verbage to a minimum. The intent was to relate as much information as possible without going into great detail. Each topic addressed in this book could be elaborated on. If more information is desired on any subject, it's up to the reader to do further research. This book is not an end-all, it's a guide.

Sometimes when talking with people about their health and things they can do to improve how they feel and how they look I get this response, "Can't I just take a pill for that?" My response is generally, "God gave you a Farrari for a body. You don't put premium gas in it. You don't change the oil or filter. You don't change the tires. You don't wash or wax it. Yet you want it to run and look like a world class Farrari. It ain't going to happen." It takes effort. This book, hopefully, will help save some time in finding the answers the reader is looking for.

Holistic health care, in its strictest interpretation, infers a cooperative relationship between the patient and his/her doctors, regardless of philosophical background or training, progressing toward optimal health. That would include optimal physical, mental, emotional, spiritual and social aspects of life. The holistic practitioner looks at the whole person. He/she will evaluate the physical, mental, emotional, nutritional, spiritual and social aspects of the patient's environment to find the root cause of the condition. The doctor will then use any available resources (MRT, EAV, lab testing, x-rays, MRI's, CT scans, etc.) to arrive at an assessment or diagnosis of the patient's condition. A holistic doctor will generally work with the body by way of nutrition, exercise, diet, counseling, etc. to allow the body to repair, balance and rebuild itself. The last, but sometimes necessary, options are surgery and drugs.

Some terms that you will hear concerning healing are: **Con-**

**ventional Medicine, Alternative Healing, Complementary Healing and Natural Healing.** Conventional medicine, also referred to as allopathic medicine, refers to the mainstream, medical approach to health. This will incorporate the use of pharmaceutical drugs, surgery and physical therapy. Very often this approach is to alleviate symptoms but doesn't always address the cause of the condition. Complementary healing often refers to non-invasive, non-pharmaceutical techniques used as a complement to conventional, allopathic medicine. Alternative and natural healing terms are often used interchangeably. This form of healing usually refers to the use of non-invasive, non-pharmaceutical techniques to determine the cause of the condition and then treat the cause. By treating the cause, the symptoms will naturally be alleviated. Natural healing employs scientifically and clinically proven methods such as Chiropractic, Homeopathic, Acupuncture, herbal and supplemental nutrition, massage and many others.

For thousands of years, traditions in China and India stressed that living in harmony with nature led to a healthy lifestyle. Warning against treating only one part of the body, Socrates wrote "for the part can never be well unless the whole is well." It wasn't until the 1970's that the term "holistic" became a commonly used term describing the treatment of the whole person.

During the 20th century "scientific" medical advances caused holistic health care to fall out of favor with Western societies. Germs were identified as causative agents for disease. The spotlight shifted from treating the whole body to fighting bugs with new and ever advancing drugs. The public was taught that health could be attained by killing off tiny invaders with synthetic drugs created in a laboratory. We were led to believe that we could live unhealthy lifestyles and modern medicine could "fix" whatever popped up.

Unfortunately in many cases, the medical cure has proven more harmful than the disease. Television ads list side effects that, in many cases, are worse that the condition itself. Rarely do I find a patient who investigates the side effects and contraindications of the drug they're taking. And even more rare are those who research the effects of combining drugs either in a research facility or in the body.

Every day our environment changes, therefore, holistic health is an ongoing process. Basing one's life on one blood test or one diagnosis years ago can have devastating life-long effects. For example, if you had a doctor's appointment and you were running late, had a fight with the kids, drove quickly to get there, gulped a mocha, ran into the doctor's office, talked to the nurse or laughed at a joke she was telling while she placed the blood pressure cuff around your arm, your blood pressure would undoubtedly be high and you would be placed on blood pressure medications indefinitely. Any one of those factors could temporarily raise blood pressure above the normal level. A holistic practitioner will consider the circumstances and environment before taking the blood pressure and formulating a treatment.

Considering the whole person and the whole situation, the holistic doctor will recommend treatments, in office and at home, that support the body's natural healing system. The holistic doctor will most often look beyond the symptoms and search for the root cause.

# Chapter 1
## Natural Healing Through the Ages

Through the years, the healing arts have changed in many ways and yet remained the same in others. The exact origins of some cures remain a mystery. Archaeologistswho have excavated and explored ancient sites have revealed a world of healing much different than what we are accustomed to today. Cave paintings and symbolic artifacts indicate that early humans believed in spirits and supernatural forces. Special people, like Shaman or medicine men, were thought to be able to connect to these spirits and induce healing. Spiritual healers would cast spells or perform ceremonies to treat the sick. Special plants or herbs were used as a form of medicine.

Egyptian writings as far back as 2,000 BC indicate that herbal remedies were used extensively for healing. Symptoms and treatments for illnesses, as well as healing techniques, were detailed on papyrus (a type of paper). Compression to stop bleeding of a wound was described. Descriptions of healers specializing in obstetrics and gynecology were found during that time. Ointments, potions, inhalers and tinctures were used by the healers to treat specific illnesses. In 2,600 BC, Imhotep, an Egyptian healer, described the diagnosis and treatment of 200 diseases. He also diagnosed and treated 15 diseases of the abdomen, 11 of the bladder, 10 of the rectum, 29 of the eyes, and 18 of the skin, hair, nails and tongue. It is recorded that he performed surgery and dentistry and treated appendicitis, arthritis, gallstones, gout, and tuberculosis. Imhotep is the first physician known by name in written history.

Four hundred years before Christ, the Greek philosopher Hippocrates described the body as having a balance between four humors: blood, phlegm, black bile, and yellow bile. When a person became ill, there was an imbalance in their humors. His treatment focused on balancing the person's humors back to normal. He would use food, water, herbs, vomiting and bleeding. Ironically, Hippocrates is seen as the father of modern medicine although his methods were more equivalent to present day "alternative healing." Greek healers at this time recorded extensive interviews with their patients and developed extensive case histories. They would examine their patients and carefully diagnose the problem before recommending a course of treatment. This practice has survived through the ages. The Greek physician Galen imigrated to Rome and became the primary doctor for the gladiators. Although dissection of the human body was illegal, Galen dissected animal bodies to determine how the human body functioned. He shared his knowledge with Roman doctors to improve their surgical techniques. New instruments and military hospitals were developed to help treat wounded soldiers.

During the Middle Ages and with the fall of Rome, many of the health practices were lost. Included in the loss were public hygiene, access to clean drinking water, regular bathing, an efficient sewage system and a thirst for improving health care. Religion dominated the health care system. Illness was believed to be a punishment from God and therefore priests and religious scholars assumed the role of doctors. Hospitals commonly sprang up in monasteries and other religious establishments. Little was done to cure illnesses. Traditional cures, including herbs and potions, were regarded as witchcraft and outlawed by the church. Wealthy individuals were being trained in schools and universities in law, the arts, religion and medicine.

The Arabic world became the center of scientific and medical knowledge. Their physicians began to use diet, exercise and medicinal herbs in the treatment of their patients. Alcohol was used to clean wounds and prevent infection. Arabic doctors performed surgeries including the removal of varicose veins, kidney stones and the replacement of dislocated limbs. Narcotic drugs were used as anesthetics.

During the Renaissance age, physicians began to learn more about the human body. Translated texts from Arabic medicine enhanced their knowledge of human anatomy. Andreas Vesalius and Leonardo Da Vinci dissected human bodies and made anatomical drawings. During this period, the Greek view of the four humors prevailed. The four humors was a theory that held the human body is filled with four basic substances or liquids called humors. If in balance, the body will be healthy. It held that all diseases and disabilities resulted from excess or deficiency of theses humors. Sickness was due to an imbalance of these four humors and treatments were aimed at restoring balance to the body. During this period, hospitals and surgical procedures became more advanced and available.

By the end of the 19$^{th}$ century vaccines became more routine, the microscope was invented and advanced, and by 1895 Wilhelm Conrad Roentgen discovered a way of taking pictures of the body – inside and out. These pictures were called x-rays. In the late 1880's, Dr. Andrew Taylor Still rejected traditional medical treatment after losing three of his children to meningitis. He devoted ten years of his life to studying the human body and finding a better way to treat disease.

Through research and clinical observation, he concluded that 'bones out of place' could damage blood and nerve supply hence causing disease. By incorporating these concepts his fame in healing grew to the point that in 1892 he opened the first osteopathic medical school in Kirksville, Missouri. By the mid 1920's, the increasingly powerful AMA embraced osteopathy and began to help finance their schools and develop guidelines for osteopaths to follow. Osteopathy has been coolly embraced by the medical world since then.

## Naturopathy

Dr. Benedict Lust in the late 1800's combined several forms of natural medicines into one eclectic system. He called this system Naturopathy based on the healing power of nature. He had a deep confidence in the ability of the body/mind to heal itself given the opportunity. In 1902, he founded the American School of Naturopathy. During the next 20 years, Naturopathy grew in interest and public awareness. However, in the mid 1920s the editor of the Journal of the American Medical Association made a mission of attacking naturopathic physicians, accusing them of quackery. Fueled by the drug industry's financial backing, growing political and social dominance of allopathic medicine led to the legal and economic suppression of naturopathic healing. The AMA's political power was successful in getting many state naturopathic licensure laws repealed.

The past few decades have seen a growing interest in ecology and an awareness of the importance of nutrition. Along with this has come a disenchantment with organized, main-stream medicine with its dehumanization, unsympathetic interaction, reliance on drugs and prohibitive expense. More and more people are looking for a more natural and safer approach to healthcare.

## Homeopathy

In the late 1700's, Dr. Samuel Hahnemann became disillusioned with some of the common medical practices such as purging, bloodletting, and the use of toxic chemicals. While translating medical texts into German, Hahnemann began a quest for a better way of providing healthcare using the principles of "Similars." While doing his research he noted that the bark of the South American tree Cinchona caused symptoms similar to malaria. He continued his research into cures and "similar suffering" and began compiling his findings. He called this new science and practice Homeopathy.

Since that time, the primary principle of homeopathy has been "let likes be cured by likes." However, Hahnemann advocated a reduction in the dose to infinitesimal levels by diluting the solutions ten to one hundred times.

Homeopathy was introduced to the United States in 1825 by Hans Birch Gram, a student of Hahnemann. Hahnemann opened the first homeopathic medical school in the United States in the late 1835. In 1844, the first U.S. national medical association, the American Institute of Homeopathy was established. By 1900, there were 22 homeopathic colleges and 15,000 practitioners in the United States. Because of its success in treating epidemics rampant at that time, homeopathy became very popular in the early 1900's; by then there were 100 homeopathic hospitals and over 1,000 homeopathic pharmacies. However, by the mid 1920's, the AMA, lusting for full control of the American healthcare system, initiated a campaign against homeopathy that almost devastated the profession. At the same time, homeopathy was flourishing in Europe, Asia and South America. In recent times, homeopathy has made a slow recovery. Many chiropractors, medical doctors, and naturopaths have studied homeopathy and have incorporated that science into their practices much to the benefit of their patients.

## Chiropractic

On September 18, 1895, the first recorded chiropractic adjustment was performed by Dr. Daniel David Palmer, a Canadian born teacher and healer. While studying the cause and effect of disease, a janitor in the building, Harvey Lillard, complained of hearing problems for over 17 years. He allowed Dr. Palmer to examine his spine. A "lump" was found on Mr. Lillard's back and Dr. Palmer suspected that a vertebra might be out of place. A crude, but gentle, thrust was made and the vertebra was repositioned. After several such treatments, Mr. Lillard's hearing was restored.

Dr. Palmer believed he had found a cure for deafness. But as

5

more "adjustments" were made, "miracle" stories became more common place. In 1897, Dr. D.D. Palmer opened a chiropractic school in Davenport, Iowa. By 1902 the Palmer Infirmary and Chiropractic Institute was renamed Palmer School of Chiropractic. In 1908, after extensive travels in the west, D.D. Palmer College of Chiropractic opened in Portland, Oregon. The name would be changed later to Western States Chiropractic College. Dr. Palmer continued his research into the relationship between the vertebral system and the nervous system. Many diseases and conditions responded to Dr. Palmer's "Chiropractic" adjustments. As his fame grew, the medical community responded. He was criticized, threatened and even jailed for practicing medicine without a license. By the turn of the century traditional allopathic medicine was challenged by the rapidly changing and growing alternative - chiropractic. Allopathic medicine became licensed whereas chiropractic had not yet. Because of licensing and the threat to traditional allopathic medicine, hundreds of chiropractors were put in jail for practicing medicine without a license. In 1907 a landmark decision was made concerning one of Palmer's graduates in Wisconsin. While on trial for practicing medicine, surgery and osteopathy without a license, the judge and jury found that the doctor was not practicing medicine but something different – chiropractic.

On October 20, 1913, Dr. D.D. Palmer died. Shortly thereafter, B.J. Palmer, D.D.'s son, began promoting and advancing chiropractic. Beginning with a radio station in Davenport, Iowa, WOC (World of Chiropractic), B.J. Palmer began promoting the advantages of chiropractic. One of WOC's sports announcers would later become an actor and eventually President of the United States – Ronald Reagan. Palmer would later own several other radio stations and then became involved with television. He was one of the first to experiment with color television. From color television he progressed into film making. He owned a studio in California which pioneered in Technicolor and 3-D movies.

Chiropractic progressed and became a licensed profession in

every state. More chiropractic colleges were established as the popularity of chiropractic grew. However, as popularity grew for chiropractic, the traditional allopathic medicine community became more enraged. In the mid 1960's, the president of the AMA, in his speech at a national convention, vowed to discredit and destroy the profession of chiropractic. Periodically, inflammatory and derogatory "reports" were made attempting to display the dangers of chiropractic. Although no basis was given for their remarks, except they were made by the AMA, mainstream media picked up on these and flashed them in newspapers and magazines. To the medical world's dismay and frustration, chiropractic continued to flourish.

In 1976, four doctors of chiropractic filed suit against the American Medical Association and numerous medical co-conspirators for restricting cooperation between individual MDs and doctors of chiropractic. In 1987 the judge ruled that over the previous 25 years the actions of the AMA, its coconspirators, the American College of Radiology and the American college of Surgeons had resulted in serious damage to the cooperative process in health care, to the profession of chiropractic as a whole, to individual doctors of chiropractic, and to the patients they served. Studies introduced at trial showed that doctors of chiropractic were twice as effective as medical doctors in returning injured workers to their jobs. They further showed that orthopedic patients under chiropractic care in hospitals were discharged twice as fast as those without chiropractic care. But a greater point was made concerning organized medicine's attempt to eliminate chiropractic as a competitor in the U.S. health care system. The judge ruled that the AMA was guilty of engaging in a conspiracy "to contain and eliminate the chiropractic profession" and was in violation of the Sherman Antitrust Act.

Since that time, cooperation between the medical profession and the chiropractic profession has improved. Some major hospitals have added chiropractors as staff members. The military has opened doors to chiropractic in some areas. Integrative practices have begun throughout the United States merging medical and chiropractic practices. With these changes, the patients reap the largest benefits. There is a place for quality medical care just as there is a place for a natural approach to health care as an alternative to drugs and surgery.

# Chapter 2
## History of Electronic Testing

Over 5,000 years ago, the Egyptian physician and genius Imhotep used water, earth, herbs, plants, parts of animals, whole animals, and their discharges as medicine to relieve the maladies of the time. In 1872, the Ebers' Papyrus, dated 1550 B.C., was discovered. It described over 800 prescriptions. Some of these strange prescriptions were passed down to become "old wives' tales" and the source of research even today. About 400 B.C., Hippocrates, the Greek physician and renowned "Father of Modern Medicine," prescribed concoctions made from vegetables, spices, oils, and herbs. For centuries, healers and medicine men around the world used whatever was available to heal the sick.

The use of electricity in medicine is not new by any means. Egyptian tombs dating back over 2000 years B.C. recorded the use of a certain fish species, a type of electric eel, to heal a variety of disorders. The Greeks, following the example of the Egyptians, used electric eels to heal. Magnets and electricity were used as far back as the 1600's. Johann Schaeffer published a book called, "Electrical Medicine" in 1752, which described the use of electricity in "modern" medicine. By the mid 1800's, many doctors and dentists were using electricity for pain relief. However, this practice was not widely accepted by the general medical establishment.

In 1895, Wilhelm Conrad Roentgen, a German physicist at the University of Wurzburg, developed an electronic machine which could pass electrons through a body and produce a black and white picture of its contents on a special film. The picture was called a roentgenogram. We know it today as an x-ray.

Electronic devices were wide-spread promising all kinds of cures from cancer to lumbago. Many charlatans were making wild claims and fast money while praying on the fears and hopes of the unsuspecting public. So much fallacious information and claims made by unscrupulous peddlers were made that the Carnegie Foundation formed a commission to investigate the standards of medical education and practice. Because of their report in 1910, branding electrotherapy as unscientific, medical schools revised their education curriculums and the doctors using electrotherapy were labeled as quacks. Homeopathy was banned from medical schools. For all practical purposes, the use of electricity for diagnostics or therapeutics was lost for many years. The recovery has been very slow and guarded.

Fortunately there were 'rogues' who continued to investigate and advance the science of electrodiagnosis. Machines were devised to look at the blood and determine its contents. Normal values were assigned to various factors so that abnormal could be compared to the normals in different disease patterns. Laboratory diagnostics became a mainstay for the average doctor in the field. Along with x-rays, laboratory findings could help the practitioner determine what ailed the patient. Machines were developed to help neurologists find the sources of nerve interference. Emergency rooms and surgical rooms were made more efficient by allowing electronic devices to aid in saving lives.

Then came computers. With the rapid increase in technology, computers became a must for any respectable hospital or clinic. The vast amount of information that could be stored and retrieved saved time and money for the ever increasing demands on the medical world. Slow and laborious tests and trials were accelerated, saving many more lives than previously possible. As speed increased, size decreased. What once would fill a room with equipment could now fill a suitcase. Mobile testing and therapeutic facilities would become commonplace.

In the 1950's, Dr. Rhineholt Voll, physician and engineer in Germany, began studying the effects of electricity on the human body. He used electrical impedance or OHM metering to determine electrical conductivity and its effects on the body. Using the premise that some materials are more conductive or offer less resistance than others, i.e., certain metals are more conductive than wood, he used an OHM meter to measure conductivity in the body.

Dr. Voll found that generally the body was resistant to electrical conductivity. However, there were some points on the body that conducted electricity more readily than others. Those points coincided with points used in acupuncture. He used an OHM meter to repeatedly test his theory to determine if the results were repeatable. He then began his lifelong search to identify correlations between disease states and changes in certain acupuncture points associated with certain diseases. He felt he might be able to identify those diseases more easily or earlier and when treatment might be more effective. The results of his studies were termed EAV or Electroacupuncture According to Voll.

The way energy moves through the body has a great deal to do with the state of one's health. Acupuncture, homeopathy and other holistic health systems understand the biophysics of the body. An interruption or alteration of the energy flow can lead to symptoms and disease. They also understand that balancing the energy flow can relieve symptoms and help prevent many disorders. See the section on Meridians for more information.

After the political decisions of 1910, medicine was forced to take a path of diagnosis related pharmaceutical treatments. As one medical doctor said: "In the process of diagnosing, we put the patient into a pigeon hole. That pigeon hole has the medications for that condition. If the patient doesn't fit into that pigeon hole or the medications don't work, we move on to another pigeon hole and another set of medications. There is no in between." Medicine began to depart from the science that appreciated subtle energy. Thankfully, physicists continued to view and investigate the world as subtle energy. Advances in quantum physics and quantum mechanics continued to broaden their understanding of the world without and within.

With years of research and the increasing availability of computers, this technology became available for use in clinics and private practices to determine imbalances. Doctors not satisfied with the status quo of blood tests and x-ray studies found this non-invasive approach to body assessment a valuable tool in working with their patients. Voll's research influenced Dr. Helmut Schimmel, a medical and dental physician and clinical researcher from West Germany, to develop the Vegatest Method. Shortly thereafter James Hoyt Clarke introduced the Dermatron machine, the first computerized electro dermal screening system. Then in 1991 Clarke introduced the LISTEN (Life Information System Ten). In 1998 BioMeridian introduced its BEST System which improved the accuracy, convenience and scope of testing. It was replaced by the MSA 21 and later the MSA Pro. Joe Calloway, of G-Tech Engineering, developed the Asyra system to be quicker, more extensive, objective and reproducible.

EAV uses physics rather than chemistry to measure the body's energetic system. It does not measure physiology, biochemistry or pathology as with blood tests, however, it is a complement to those standard procedures. Although EAV testing has not been accepted by the traditional medical world or insurance companies, it has been used by thousands of doctors to find energetic imbalances and help determine preventative therapies for their patients. A great deal of time and money is saved in locating the root cause of a patient's condition.

EAV objectively monitors the energy status of the body by measuring electrical resistance. Different systems accomplish this in different ways. Some systems measure resistance at any of the over 800 acupuncture points on the body. Primarily these systems use the hands and feet to gain access into the organs and systems of the body. While the patient holds a brass handmass in one hand, the practitioner uses a pen-like probe to connect the patient to the computer at a specific acupuncture point. The results of the test can be immediately viewed on the computer screen - more about this later. Other systems use a pad for the hand to rest on. The system automatically scans the hand and uses the acupuncture points necessary for the specific test that's being performed. Yet other systems use brass handmasses to complete the connection between the body and the computer system. The computer system then automatically tests the body using predetermined tests which the operator selects. When there's a change in an organ or system, electrical resistance at the related acupuncture points change. These changes very often appear long before a disease process can be defined or symptoms appear. This is defined as functional testing.

Testing varies with each system. However, with all systems a low voltage is applied to acupuncture points with a small probe or handmass (brass bar) while the patient is holding another handmass. This completes the circuit between the patient and the computer. The computer will measure skin resistance and display the findings on a meter. The patient can, therefore, watch the test taking place and see the results immediately. The readings are recorded on a scale of 0 to 100. A range of 45 to 55 is generally considered the "normal range" or balanced area.

A plate or surface for testing and imprinting is normally attached to the computer and is in the circuit between the patient and the computer. A very complicated and sophisticated software program in the computer assists in recording measured readings and in finding balancing antidotes. Training is essential in the proper use of the systems and in finding and testing proper acupuncture points. The systems will not respond properly if the points are not addressed correctly.

With the Biomeridian's MSA system, as the patient holds the brass bar in one hand, the probe is applied to a specific acupuncture point or points to complete the circuit. On the screen, a line will appear to move up a scale until it levels out. When it has held a level line for two seconds, it is considered a good test. The line will level and hold between 45 and 55 if the organ or system is balanced. Should the line go above 55, according to Dr. Voll's research, the system or organ can be considered inflamed, irritated or in an acute state. However, if the line levels at a value below 45, the system or organ is considered to be weakened or in a chronic, deficient or degenerated state. After the initial reading is taken and the frequency is introduced into the system, the cells must work to maintain a natural, unpolarized state. Healthy cells can maintain a natural unpolarized state but weakened cells cannot. Weakened cells will cause what is called an indicator drop. The ascending line will level and then begin to drop (increased resistance). Dr. Voll considered this drop a very serious indicator of a dysfunction.

Testing with the MSA system generally utilizes acupuncture control points on the hands and feet. Each point represents a specific system or organ. The number of points tested depends on the focus of the examination. Once the points have been assessed, a report is printed and shared with the patient. Abnormalities found on the examination are evaluated by a qualified healthcare professional. A diagnosis is not made based on EAV findings alone. Patient's history, symptoms, laboratory tests, and any other tests along with EAV findings contribute to the proper diagnosis of a condition. By using the test plate, a practitioner can assess different substances to find one that balances the particular organ or system. Dr. Voll found that he could often predict how a substance would affect the subject clinically by testing in this manner.

When testing for allergies, we have found that by using the most excitable point on the hand, we can induce the frequencies of particular substances into the patient's body and observe the reaction. Again, if the indicator line goes above 55 (the red area), it indicates an acute reaction (possible allergy) to a particular substance. If the line stays below 45 (the yellow area), we generally determine that the substance has weakened an organ or system and we proceed accordingly.

The Asyra system, on the other hand, is similar in many ways yet different in many others. Instead of the practitioner probing specific acupuncture points, the patient holds two brass bars and the computer system reads the most suitable points to acquire the readings. The doctor or practitioner selects which systems or organs to be tested and the computer system does the rest. Tests are performed very quickly and both the patient and the practitioner can monitor the results. When the computer system finds an organ or system that is out of balance, it automatically retests with items that can balance the imbalance. The frequency of the balancing item is held in a holding area to be imprinted later. Once the test is complete, a report is printed and reviewed with the patient. A special bottle of distilled water and alcohol mixture is placed on the test plate and imprinted with the frequencies gathered to balance the unbalanced organs or systems. As with the MSA, the test plate can also be used to evaluate vitamins, minerals and other substances against the patient to determine if those items will be useful or not. After taking the frequency imprinted drops for a specified length of time, the patient is retested to determine the effectiveness of the drops. Again a report is printed so that the patient can follow his/her progress.

Since the time we were born we were taught that doctors were the gatekeepers of our health. We were indoctrinated in the mistaken idea that medical doctors held the secrets to staying healthy. That may have been the case in times past, however, the times have changed. There are still some very good and dedicated doctors but due to rising costs of doing business, high malpractice insurance rates, the AMA, FDA, pharmaceutical companies, HMO's and increasing demands from insurance companies, many have turned to treating symptoms only. Pharmaceutical companies invest heavily in the medical doctors' educational system as well as on-going seminars, conventions and advertisement. It is difficult to find a doctor who will investigate holistically into each individual patient. Because of this some doctors have turned from the ruling system to a more holistic approach to health care. Those same doctors therefore go under the microscope by their peers, their state medical associations and the AMA. Some lose their license to practice due to "practicing non-standard medicine" simply by prescribing alternative treatments.

As patients we rarely see the inner workings of the associations. We are led to believe that good health care is based on pills, shots and surgery. So, when something comes along outside of "the box," we become skeptical due to ignorance of a new paradigm or skewed information from the establishment. Such is the case with quantum medicine.

Quantum medicine as defined by the Oxford Pocket Dictionary of Current English is "a branch of complementary medicine that uses low-dosage electromagnetic radiation in the treatment, diagnosis, and prevention of disease." It is further defined by Dictionary.com's 21st Century Lexicon as a "multidisciplinary research using quantum physics to show that the human body is controlled and regulated by the human energy system; also, a branch of medicine that manipulates the body's energy to treat and prevent disease. Quantum medicine is a combination of German functional medicine, Oriental medicine, Herbal/Homeopathic, and Quantum Physics."

Our office utilizes two similar, yet different, systems; both were developed by Joe Galloway of G-Tech Corporation in Utah. Mr. Galloway has developed ten systems utilizing this technology since 1978. The MSA-21was developed in the 1990's for BioMeridian Corporation. Joe's latest system, the Asyra, has incorporated the best of all his designs as well as the latest technology. In the following paragraphs I will attempt to explain how these systems work. The general principles apply to both systems.

Because most are unfamiliar with this new paradigm, a little deeper explanation is due. As with wind or gravity, we believe in them even though we can't see them. However, we can see their effects. The Asyra and the MSA-21 are instruments for visualizing the biological patterns in the body. One definition of energy is the ability of a physical system to change. Energy can manifest in two different ways – force/movement and information. The following thoughts were gathered from an explanation of Asyra by G-Tech.

Energy can be visualized. Most of us, when we watch the nightly news or the Weather Channel, often see something called Doppler radar. Doppler radar scans an area and visualizes energy in the atmosphere. Through the use of computers we see areas of rain, snow, lightening or clear areas of no activity. In much the same way, instruments such as Gas Discharge Visualization (GDV) and Surface Scanning Electromyography (SSEMG) can create accurate visualizations of the human bioenergy field. GDV can give an accurate picture of how physical energy flows around the body.

Energetic frequencies are mysterious to most people. Cells, like a sponge, hold energy. Healthy cells, like a large sponge, hold more energy than unhealthy cells (small sponges). Stressed cells are already overloaded so they saturate more quickly. Visualize a Japanese bamboo water fountain. When we add water to an empty bamboo cup, it slowly fills until it tilts and dumps its contents into the next bamboo cup. When that cup is full, it tilts and dumps its contents into another cup or the pool below. Similarly, when we add extra energy into the body, there is a measurable time delay before the energy pours out again. By measuring this time delay, which is called the "Phase Angle," we can determine whether the cells are healthy, depleted, or stressed, that is, already overloaded. Numerous medical studies closely link general health and athletic performance to high phase angles. Some diseases are correlated with low phase angles indicating poor cellular energy capacity. Because the cells and tissues of the body are always engaged in energy exchange – releasing and recharging as they do biological work – they naturally create patterns of oscillation. Patterns of oscillation naturally set up because the body is always moving energy. Simple oscillations, like the filling and dumping of a Japanese water fountain where one stream of water dumps into a pool which, when full, dumps into another pool which, when full, dumps into another, and so on, can be compared to a single, simple frequency. Obviously, natural systems are far more complex in that their oscillating patterns have internal structure and are therefore characterized by waveforms rather than simple frequencies. The collection of all the body's possible modes of oscillation defines a set of vibrational "fingerprints" that can be analized, stored, compared and modified at will. He vibrational signatures can even be imprinted onto a physical carrier substance and function as a Homeopathic remedy, that can alter, modify and correct the vibrational patterns. The Asyra imprints test session data in just this way.

The sponges and bamboo fountain showed us that the body stores and releases energy as an organized set of signature waveforms. Each of the body's potential oscillations can be induced to reveal itself by resonance. Pushing a child in a swing is our most familiar example of resonance. When we time our push to the natural frequency of the swing, we can create a resonance that amplifies the swing's motion.

A tuning fork, even when it is resting without vibration, has a potential set of intrinsic resonant frequencies. When the fork is struck, it reorganizes random mechanical energy into well ordered ripples of resonant vibration. If a second, identical tuning fork is placed nearby, it will pick up the vibrations and begin to resonate in perfect synchrony. Asyra utilizes this effect. Many times each second, Asyra transmits specific waveforms associated with various organ systems and the body's response to toxins, pathogens, etc.

The probes in the subject's hands measure which of these many waveforms induce resonance in their body – just like the child's swing or the 2nd tuning fork. Asyra interjects questions to the body by way of energetic waveforms. Those "waveform questions" that resonate with the subject's field create measurable electrical changes recorded through Asyra's probes. While Asyra's measurements are more specific than those on a lie detector, it's basically the same concept. The Asyra will continually "ping" the body with waveforms associated with body function, organ function, emotional patterns and distress patterns, toxins, bacteria, viruses, etc. Some subset will "ping" when it recognizes the pattern and respond. Each time a disresonance is noted, Asyra will look into its repertoire of remedies. Asyra will look for patterns that will neutralize and balance and restore the proper waveforms. Asyra will take the waveforms of the remedies and test them against the disresonance and find the one that creates a balancing. It will then compare the findings to all remedies and make sure they all harmonize. The idea that our internal state can cause physically measurable reactions is not new.

One way Asyra dramatically improves its accuracy is something they call the "tin can telephone effect." Imagine two people talking over a tin can telephone. If the string isn't tight, then no sound is transmitted. But if the string is pulled tight, the sound energy vibrating the tin can makes the string vibrate in resonance, transmitting it to the other can. In the first few seconds of each test, Asyra does the same thing. It performs the bioelectric equivalent of tightening the tin can telephone string. When you send bioenergetic waveforms into the body, you need to know that they reach their targets and can successfully resonate with the necessary tissues and pathways. Because each person's electrical characteristics are somewhat different, a specific intensity is needed to ensure that you have a "tight string." Without this individual calibration, which no other system provides, you can't really know if the body's responses are accurate. Asyra's process is objective and 100% operator independent. Asyra provides consistent, reliable results every time.

# Chapter 3
## A Short Course in Physiology

Volumes can be, and have been, written about each of these systems. Presented here is merely a brief overview of each one. Hundreds, if not thousands, of details concerning each system have been omitted. This is presented to give you a greater appreciation of the miracles that take place in your body every second of your life.

## Digestive System

The digestive system is one of the most elaborate systems of the body. Greater detail could be devoted to each area but for now, a brief overview to give the reader a sense of the complexity of digestion should suffice. Remember, this is a very simplified version of the actual system.

Digestion begins in the brain. The very thought of food causes chemical reactions to occur in the body in preparation for the actual process of digestion, absorption and elimination. Saliva is often produced as a result of merely the thought process. From the time the food enters the mouth until the time it is eliminated is about 12 to 24 hours. From the mouth to the cardiac sphincter (opening to the stomach), it takes around 3 seconds. Within the first 1-5 minutes food moves to the pyloric sphincter between the stomach and the duodenum (small intestine). It takes 3-5 hours for the latter part of a meal to leave the stomach. In 4 ½ to 5 ½ hours the food begins to exit the small intestine to the large intestine through the ileocecal valve. It takes 6 to 10 hours to travel through the ascending colon, transverse colon and the descending colon. Because it takes 12-24 hours to complete the process, regular elimination is very important.

As the food is chewed in the **mouth** (mastication), the slightly acidic saliva from the salivary glands and the enzyme ptalin begin splitting the food particles into digestible components. The ground up contents (bolus) passes through the **esophagus** with the help of mucus and muscle contraction through the cardiac sphincter to the **stomach.** The stomach contains hydrochloric acid (HCl). This acid plus enzymes further emulsifies the food to a liquid state. As we get older (over 25), we produce less hydrochloric acid. Therefore we tend to have more "stomach issues." In this reservoir called the stomach, food is mixed with gastric juices and water, glucose and alcohol is absorbed into the bloodstream.

The **duodenum**, the first of the three stages of the **small intestine**, is an alkaline environment as opposed to the acid environment of the stomach. The **pancreas,** on the posterior abdominal wall inside the C of the duodenum, secretes enzymes into the initial section of the duodenum. These enzymes split fats, starches, proteins, sugars and amino acids. The hormones insulin and glucagon are secreted by the islets of Langerhans in the pancreas. On the opposite side of the duodenum the **liver and Gallbladder** secretes bile (slightly alkaline) to break down those ingredients even further for absorption into the blood and lymphatic vessels. Drainage from the liver through the bile duct merges with the drainage from the pancreas through the pancreatic duct and that combination drains into the duodenum. That drainage can then be used for digestion or eliminated as waste. The remainder of the small intestine, the jejunum and ileum, is alkaline and secretes more digestive enzymes. In total, the small intestine is 20+ feet long. It's divided into three parts: duodenum (10-12"), jejunum (8') and ileum (12').

The small intestine empties into the large intestine through a one-way valve called the **ileo-cecal valve**. This allows the watery contents to evacuate into the first of three parts of the large intestine to have the fluid extracted and to be compacted and eliminated. Occasionally that valve will lock open causing a diarrhea condition and conversely it can lock closed causing a constipation condition. Both conditions can be relieved by soft tissue manipulation.

The liquid enters the ascending colon on the right side of the abdomen,then to the transverse colon, then to the descending colon on the left, to the rectum and finally to the anal canal. The contents move along the colon by way of a progressive contraction/relaxation of the walls. This is called parastalsis. During this process, water and salts are removed firming the contents in preparation for elimination.

## Cardiovascular System

The cardiovascular system, also known as the circulatory system, is the chief transport system of the body. The heart pumps the blood to all parts of the body. The blood is a complex fluid that contains food materials, waste products, respiratory gases, and chemicals for protection and regulation. The blood is transported through a closed system of tubes called arteries that branch into capillaries where the interchange of gasses, food and waste substances takes place. The capillaries reunite to form veins to transport the blood back to the heart.

Blood returning to the heart enters the left atrium (left upper chamber) from the lungs where it has been oxygenated and then passes through the mitral valve into the lower left chamber called the ventricle. As the heart contracts blood is pushed through the aorta and on to arteries throughout the body. The arteries continue to flow and branch become arterioles and then capillaries at the end of the arterial flow. The blood is then sent back to the heart via venules and then veins. The returned blood enters the right atrium, through the tricuspid valve to the right ventricle. As the heart beats the blood in the right ventricle is pushed into the pulmonary artery and on to the lungs where the process is repeated many times a day.

The heart is actually a double pump. Each side is quite separate from the other. The left atrium receives the blood returning from the lungs with its oxygen supply increased. This blood passes into the left ventricle which pumps it around the body to supply the tissues with oxygen. The right atrium receives the blood returning from the body tissues with its oxygen supply diminished. This blood passes into the right ventricle which pumps it around the lungs for its fresh supply of oxygen.

In a normal cycle, blood enters the atria from the lungs (left side) and the body tissues(right side) during a period of relaxation. At this time the AV (atrio-ventriclur) nodes are closed. As the atria are filled the AV valves open and blood is pushed into the ventricles. As the valves close, the first heart sound (a LUBB sound) is produced. When the ventricles are full, they contract. The pressure forces the semilunar valves to push open. Blood is forced into the pulmonary artery on the right and the aorta on the left. As the valves close the second heart sound is made (DUBB). The pulmonary artery will take the blood to the lungs to be oxygenated while the aorta supplies the oxygen rich blood to the tissues of the body.

An area of great concern today is blood pressure. Increasingly, medical doctors are diagnosing their patients with high blood pressure, while prescribing expensive and potentially harmful medications. Pharmaceutical companies are producing more medications with serious side effects while the FDA turns a blind and prejudicial eye, and approves them. It's only until the lawsuits begin that the consumer is made aware of a problem. By then the pharmaceutical companies have made their billions and can afford to pay a few million out in claims.

Understanding blood pressure is not that difficult. With each heartbeat, each ventricle ejects forcibly about 70 ml. of blood into the blood vessels. ALL of this blood cannot pass through the arterioles into capillaries and veins during the heart's contraction. Therefore, slightly over 60% or roughly 5/8 of the cardiac output at each heart beat has to be stored during systole and passed on during diastole. The pressure is highest at the height of the heart's contraction, i.e. systolic blood pressure, and lowest when the heart is relaxing, i.e. diastolic blood pressure. The pressure is lowest as blood drains into the right atrium at the end of diastole and highest as blood leaves the left ventricle at the end of systole.

The normal range for blood pressure (based on an average American athletic teenager) is 120/80 or 120 mm Hg over 80 mm Hg. Many doctors are quick to give dangerous drugs whenever the patient's blood pressure is above 120/80. However, there are several things to consider prior to jumping in and popping pills. Blood pressure will rise and fall for many reasons. Because of that, several things should be considered when having your blood pressure taken.

- Relax. Tension and anxiety can elevate the reading several points. White coat syndrome (anxiety brought about by the presence of a doctor/nurse) is responsible for many people taking blood pressure medicine needlessly.
- Sit for at least 5 minutes before having the blood pressure taken. Sit with your back against the back of the chair and with your left arm elevated even with the heart.
- Sit quietly. Pain, a full bladder, talking, laughing, crying, anger and other emotions tend to elevate blood pressure.
- Make sure the pressure cuff is placed on skin (not over clothes) on your left arm. And again, don't talk, laugh, etc. before the pressure is fully taken.

An often overlooked organ along the circulatory route is the **spleen**. It is located in the left upper quadrant of the abdomen. An easy way to remember the dimensions of the spleen is the 1x3x5x7x9x11 rule. The spleen is 1" by 3" by 5", and weighs approximately 7 ounces. It lies between the 9th and 11th ribs on the left. Its primary function is as a blood filter. The spleen synthesizes antibodies, removes antibody-coated bacterial and red blood cells, and filters out foreign particles. It holds a reserve of blood to be used as needed, i.e., emergency situations.

## Respiratory System

Every cell in your body requires oxygen. The cells get the oxygen from the fluid around them and they release carbon dioxide to the same fluid. This is called internal respiration. External respiration is the exchange of oxygen and carbon dioxide between the body and the external environment.

The respiratory system is comprised of the oral and nasal passages, the larynx, trachea, bronchi, and lungs. Outside air enters the system via the mouth and/or the nose. The passages merge to form the trachea. At the upper end of the trachea lies the larynx (voice box). As air is expelled, ligaments in the larynx contract and relax causing sound.

In the trachea, the air is cleansed, moistened and warmed before it enters the lungs. As the air passes down the trachea it enters the main bronchi. The bronchi divide with the right main bronchi supplying air to the three lobes of the right lung and the left to the two lobes of the left lung. The bronchi further divide into smaller bronchioles. At the ends, the bronchial alveoli supplies oxygen to the capillaries of the pulmonary artery. The oxygenated blood is then taken to the heart where it is distributed to the body.

Inspiration and expiration involves a series of events. The closed cavity known as the thorax (or chest) is made up of ribs, sternum, intercostal muscles and diaphragm. It encloses the lungs, heart and great vessels. Muscular action brings about the rhythmical changes in the capacity of the thorax. During inspiration the external intercostals muscles contract moving the ribs and sternum upward and outward. This causes the width of the chest to increase. At the same time, the diaphragm contracts and descends increasing the depth of the chest. The lungs then expand to fill the thoracic cavity. Expiration is just the opposite in that the external intercostal muscles relax, the ribs and sternum move downward and inward and the width of the chest diminishes. The diaphragm relaxes and ascends. This action causes the internal pressure to become greater than the external atmospheric pressure. Air is therefore expelled.

## Excretory System

The kidneys, skin and respiratory system are the chief excretory organs of the body. Formation of urine begins in the kidneys. The urine passes from the kidneys through tubes called ureters. Urine is then stored in the bladder until such time as it is expelled through the urethra.

The kidneys keep body fluids relatively constant in amount and composition by excreting waste products of metabolism and by adjusting loss of water and electrolytes. About 25% of the left ventricle's output of blood in each cardiac cycle is distributed to the kidneys for filtration. Through a series of complicated processes, fluid and waste products are filtered from the blood and passed to the kidneys and then to the ureter.

Besides balancing the water and electrolytes, the kidneys also maintain the acid-base balance in the body. Large amounts of acids are produced in cells during metabolism. In spite of this the pH of the blood and body fluids is kept relatively constant (7.4).

Large amounts of acids are produced in cells during metabolism. These acids are first neutralized by buffering agents in the blood stream. The chief buffering substances of the blood which appear in the filtrate are phosphates and bicarbonates. The kidneys will conserve these during the filtration process so the body can maintain a neutral pH. If left alone, our bodies will maintain this neutral condition naturally. However, our diet and lifestyle tends to overpower this natural process. The American diet is more acidic than alkaline. This natural process cannot keep up with the increased acidity. Therefore, our bodies become acidic. Studies have shown that many disease processes, including cancer, love an acidic environment. Many therapies aimed at improving or eliminating chronic or "incurable" conditions begin by helping the body return to a neutral or slightly alkaline state.

Urine is ideally neutral to slightly acidic (pH 5.8-pH 7). Very acidic urine (below pH 5.5) encourages infections. An established infection gives rise to alkaline urine (pH 7.5 or higher) which causes stinging and burning. Test your urine with pH paper at any time except first thing in the morning. Cranberry juice lowers pH; vitamin C raises it.

The bladder is a hollow muscular organ that acts as a reservoir for urine. Urine, formed continually in the kidneys, enters the bladder in small spurts (1-5 per minute). It will expand to hold about 300 cc. of fluid. As the bladder fills, afferent and efferent nerves of the sympathetic and parasympathetic nervous systems monitor the distention and triggers the desire to void urine as it fills. Those same nerves assist in the voiding process.

## Endocrine System

The endocrine system is a system of ductless glands that produce hormones. The chemical messengers pass into the blood stream for general circulation to excite or inhibit activity of other organs or tissues. The primary organs that make up the endocrine system are: the hypothalamus, pituitary, thyroid, parathyroids, thymus, adrenal glands, pancreas, and testes in males and ovaries in females. Other organs that produce hormones, but to a lesser degree, are the stomach (gastrin), small intestine (enterogastrone, secretin, pancreozymin, cholecystokinin), and the kidneys (erythropoietin, rennin, DHCC). Although each endocrine gland has specific functions all are interdependent. Over activity or under activity of one tends to affect the whole system. The four primary glands of the endocrine system are the pituitary, thyroid, adrenal glands, and ovaries/testes.

## Pituitary Gland

The **pituitary gland** is divided into two parts – an anterior and a posterior. The anterior pituitary is considered the master gland of the entire endocrine system. It regulates the activity of all the other glands. All metabolic processes and growth are influenced by it. Hormones produced here travel through the blood to all other glands of the body. Under activity of the anterior pituitary can lead to under production of growth hormones. At the extreme, two major conditions can occur:

1. An alert, well proportioned, intelligent child with delayed skeletal growth and retarded sexual development.
2. A lethargic, somnolent, mentally subnormal child with arrested sexual development, stunted growth and obese.

Over activity of the pituitary causes an over production of growth hormone which leads to giantism in a child and acromegaly as an adult. Over production of the anterior pituitary can give rise to Cushing's Syndrome. Signs of this are: osteoporosis, muscle atrophy and weakness, high blood sugar, obesity, and suppression of the menstrual cycle in women.

The posterior pituitary helps reduce the output of urine, constricts blood vessels, contraction of the uterus after birth, and stimulates lactating mammary glands. Under activity of the posterior pituitary (by disease or trauma) causes diabetes insipidus characterized by excessive thirst and excessive production of urine.

## Thyroid Gland

One of the most misdiagnosed, yet one of the most important, organs of the endocrine system is the thyroid gland. Located in the lower throat area in front of the trachea (windpipe), the thyroid gland produces hormones that are essential for a well functioning body. It is made up of two parts called lobes. It extracts iodide from the blood stream to form iodine.

The thyroid releases active hormones to the circulatory system to distribute to the body to act as catalysts for oxidation processes in the tissue cells. It regulates the enzymes involved in energy production and metabolic processes.

The thyroid can become under active by stress, disease, or trauma. The condition is generally referred to as hypothyroidism. It occurs very commonly in people I call "pushers." They push themselves to work harder, do better, or to be the best at whatever they attempt. They put stress upon themselves and continually overtax the thyroid leading to a thyroid deficiency.

Symptoms of thyroid deficiency:

- Cold hands and feet
- Fatigue
- Hair loss
- Dry skin
- Mood swings
- Tendency to become depressed
- Loss of libido
- Anemia
- Slow pulse rate
- Low blood pressure
- Tendency towards obesity

Long term under activity can lead to increased weight, constipation, puffy, thickening skin and dry, brittle and sparse hair.

Over activity of the thyroid manifests as increased basal metabolic rate (BMR), elevated body temperature, profuse sweating, and depleted energy stores. Other symptoms may include: increased appetite, weight loss, increased movements in the digestive tract resulting in diarrhea, elevated heart rate, blood pressure and respiratory rate, muscular tremor, nervousness, excitability and apprehension. Protrusion of the eyeballs (exophthalamos) is characteristic of hyperthyroidism. However, it is probably due to an excess of a hormone from the pituitary gland.

Blood testing for the thyroid is not indicative of its state of health. The late Broda Barnes, M.D., the international thyroid expert, developed a simple at-home test that has proven more accurate in determining the state of the thyroid. See appendix four for the instructions.

Some symptoms of an over-active thyroid include:

- Increase in body temperature
- Profuse sweating
- Increased appetite
- Loss of weight
- Increased movements of the digestive tract
- Diarrhea
- Increased heart and respiratory rates
- Increased blood pressure
- Muscular tremor and nervousness
- Excitable and apprehensive
- Decreased energy
- Increased basal metabolic rate (BMI)

Natural, hormone-free, therapeutic grade thyroid tissue extract (taken orally) has been shown over the years to restore the function of an individual's thyroid. Overdose symptoms of natural thyroid include hyperactivity and hot flashes. By refraining from taking the supplementation for one day, the patient can resume taking it again at a reduced level and gradually increasing to the prescribed level.

Rather than relying on blood tests, which are notoriously inaccurate, we generally instruct the patient on the Barnes' temperature test (see Appendix 4). We have found that this has been more accurate in determining the actual function of the thyroid. After completing the test, if the patient's temperature is found to be below the normal range, the patient is given supplementation.

The procedure for taking the thyroid supplements is this:

Week 1   1 capsule (55 mg thyroid) in the morning
Week 2   2 capsules in the morning
Week 3   2 capsules in the morning and one capsule in the evening
Week 4   2 capsules in the morning and two capsules in the evening
Week 5   2 capsules in the morning and one capsule in the evening
Week 6   2 capsules in the morning

For most people, two capsules per day is a sufficient mainte-nance dose. However, with a natural thyroid supplement, some leeway can be taken. Rarely do we see overdose symptoms, but if they do occur, after clearing the system the patient can resume on a lesser dose.

Many of our patients have experienced "miracles" by taking thyroid supplementation. In fact, we have been jokingly threat-ened should we run short of natural thyroid supplements. The thyroid supplement that we have found to be the most beneficial through the years has been a supplement originating in New Zea-land. Dr. Barnes recommended it over 35 years ago and we have been using it since.

**Parathyroid Glands**

The **parathyroid glands** are four little glands situated behind the thyroid gland. They play an important role in the metabolism of calcium and phosphate. Under activity of the parathyroid glands, from atrophy or removal, will cause a decrease in the blood calcium level. This can lead to a severe convulsive disorder called tetany.

Symptoms of under activity include:
Twitching
Nervousness
Intermittent muscle spasms
Over activity of the parathyroid glands causes a rise in blood

calcium levels and can lead to osteitis fibrosa cystica. Excessive amounts of calcium are lost in the urine leading to a softening of the bones. Surgery to remove the parathyroid glands abolishes the syndrome.

Symptoms of over activity include:
Excessive thirst
Excessive urination

## Adrenal Glands

The **adrenal glands** are two small glands that sit atop the kidneys and weigh about the same as a nickel. They produce hormone-like substances into the bloodstream. Among many other substances, the adrenal glands produce adrenaline (epinephrine). When the body is called to respond to stress, the adrenal gland is the primary gland that will react.

Under quiet conditions, there is very little adrenaline in the blood. However, under stress adrenaline is responsible for the "flight or fight" reaction. Adrenaline is responsible for the following:

Constricts smooth muscle
Causes gooseflesh and hair to "stand on end"
Dilates the pupils of the eyes
Constricts blood vessels often resulting in pallor
Dilates the coronary arteries
Dilates arteries to skeletal muscles
Increases heart rate and cardiac output
Relaxes bronchiole muscles allowing faster and easier breathing
Stimulates respiration
Inhibits movement of the digestive tract
Contracts gut sphincters
Inhibits the urinary bladder
Contracts ureters
Increases blood sugar
Stimulates metabolism

Increases blood coagulation

## Ovaries/Testes

In the female, the **ovaries** produce the female sex hormones estrogen and progesterone. They are also responsible for secondary sex characteristics. Those include: Development of breasts, axillary and pubic hair, and the female proportions of the body. In the male, the **testes** produce the male sex hormone testosterone. They are also responsible for secondary sex characteristics as the ovaries are in the female. Those secondary sex characteristics include: A deeper voice, pubic, axillary, and facial hair and the male shape of the body.

## Pineal Gland

The pineal gland, also known as the pineal body, is a pine cone shaped gland of the endocrine system. It produces several hormones including melatonin, a serotonin derived hormone that affects sleep patterns. It is located near the center of the brain between the two hemispheres. It has several functions. Besides secreting melatonin, it helps regulate endocrine functions, converts nervous system signals to endocrine signals, influences sexual development, and induces sleepiness.

## Thymus Gland

Located behind the sternum (breast bone) and in front of the heart, the thymus reaches its maximum size near puberty. It's composed of two identical lobes. Sometimes called the main organ of the lymphatic system, its primary function is to promote the development of T-lymphocytes. These T-lymphocytes, also called T-cells, are white blood cells that protect the body from organisms like bacteria and viruses. They also help control cancerous cells thus protecting the body from itself.

## Nervous System

The nervous system is the most complex system of the body. It detects stimuli (information), integrates that information with other inputs and makes appropriate reactions. Messages are sent through electrochemical impulses through nerves to muscles, glands and organs.

From the brain, the spinal cord extends approximately 16 to 18 inches through the spinal canal. The spinal cord is composed of 31 segments with nerves extending from either side to various parts of the body. Each nerve has a neuron – like a transfer station that receives and transmits nerve impulses from one part of the body to another. Each neuron has a cell body and thick cable-like extensions called dendrites that receive impulses from the body and long, thin processes called axons that carry impulses away from the cell body. Nerve impulses "jump" from one axon to another by way of an electrochemical reaction. That's why some chemical reactions, i.e. drugs, supplements, etc. can enhance or inhibit nerve flow.

The nervous system is divided into two divisions: The central nervous system (CNS), made up of the brain and the spinal cord; and the peripheral nervous system (PNS) connecting nerves to receptor sites.

The peripheral nervous system includes 12 cranial nerves. They are usually listed with Roman numerals. They are as follows:

I. Olfactory nerve – smell
II. Optic nerve – vision
III. Oculomotor – looking around
IV. Trochlear – eye movement
v. Trigeminal – facial feelings
VI. Abducens – eye muscles
VII. Facial – smile, wink, taste
VIII. Auditory – balance, equilibrium, hearing
IX. Glossopharengeal – swallowing, gag reflex

    X. Vagus – motor nerve for swallowing, talking,
       part of digestion
    XI. Spinal Accessory – shrugging shoulders
    XII. Hypoglossal – tongue movement

The peripheral nervous system is further divided into two parts:
    The Somatic nervous system
    The Autonomic nervous system

The somatic nervous system consists of afferent and efferent nerve fibers. The afferent nerve fibers carry information from the body to the central nervous system. The efferent nerve fibers carry information or messages for movement from the brain to skeletal muscles.

The autonomic nervous system, also called the involuntary nervous system, is further broken down into two branches called the sympathetic and parasympathetic nervous systems. The autonomic nervous system regulates functions that occur automatically in the body. Heart beat, breathing and digestion are a few of the normal functions regulated by the autonomic nervous system

The sympathetic nervous system, also known as the fight or flight system, responds to stress. Heart rate increases, blood pressure increases, circulation is restricted, eyes dilate, decreases digestion and the urinary process, increases breathing and generally it makes us more alert to react to a stressful situation. On the other hand, the parasympathetic nervous system does the opposite. It's also known as the rest and digest system. It reduces heart rate and blood pressure, increases circulation, contracts the bladder, increases digestion, slows breathing, and generally calms us down to a state of rest or relaxation. It helps us maintain a relaxed state.

# Chapter 4
## Meridians

Foreign to western medicine is a practice called meridian therapy. There are invisible channels in the body called meridians. The Chinese use the term "jing luo" which means channels, conduit, meridian. For centuries oriental medicine has maintained that "qi" or "chi" circulates through the body via these channels. Qi (Chi) is the flow of energy throughout the body via specific channels. In Japan it is called "ki," and in India, "prana" or "shakti." The ancient Egyptians referred to it as "ka," and the ancient Greeks as "pneuma." In Africa it's known as "ashe" and in Hawaii as "ha" or "mana." Although many critics and western medicine, with its close ties to the pharmaceutical industry, have argued their existence, obviously meridians have been involved in health care around the world for centuries. Research throughout the world has proven the existence and importance of meridians.

There are 12 major meridians involved in acupuncture and 8 extra meridians. These meridians, or energy pathways, have a beginning point and an ending point. Like a river, there are many tributaries and collaterals. The starting point of each meridian is usually an end point of a hand or foot. Each meridian is named after an organ or a function. The major meridians are: lung, kidney, gallbladder, stomach, spleen, heart, small intestine, large intestine, urinary bladder, pericardium, liver, and triple heater or triple warmer. There are many other minor meridians that are used to effect changes in the body. All meridians have specific routes and affect specific organs and body parts. By stimulating points along these meridians, positive changes can be made to the body.

The World Health Organization (WHO) has classified more than 400 acupuncture points along these meridians. In actual practice, there may be as many as 2,000 points used in different treatments. Each point is listed by name, number and meridian to which they belong.

When chi flows freely through the meridians, the body is balanced and healthy. When the energy becomes blocked, stagnated or weakened, it can result in dysfunction. This dysfunction can be in the form of physical, mental, or emotional ill health. Physically, an imbalance in an organ or organ system can lead to malfunction and eventually a dis-ease situation. Mentally and emotionally, an imbalance can lead to anger, depression, grief, self-pity, fear and more.

Acupuncturists stimulate specific acupuncture points with needles to counteract any imbalance that they may find. However, those acupuncture points react to various forms of stimulation. Laser stimulation, tapping, electrical impulse or simply rubbing specific points can cause a change. Obviously an acupuncturist has studied all related acupuncture points and can best stimulate all points necessary to affect a change. But some changes can be made by almost anyone. The acupuncturist stimulates certain points to restore balance to an imbalanced meridian.

Each meridian has a two hour period of the day and night where it is the primary, and strongest, meridian at the time. Each meridian is paired with an organ, system or another meridian. In this 24 hour cycle, each meridian is paired with another meridian. When one is strong the other is generally weak. By knowing this, one can determine which meridian is involved when symptoms reoccur as the same time each day. See appendix 6 for more details concerning the meridian clock.

## Lung

The lung meridian begins in the upper chest just anterior to the shoulder and travels along the inside of the arm to the tip of the thumb. This meridian is most active between 3 AM and 5 AM. Because the lungs are responsible for energy and respiration, an imbalance may lead to easily catching a cold, chronic fatigue, susceptibility to viral and bacterial infections, perspiration and inflammation problems, night sweats, dry cough, parched throat and mouth, low grade fever, red cheeks, altered sense of smell, and adverse skin conditions.

## Kidney

The kidney meridian starts at the tip of the little toe and goes along the sole of the foot, along the arch, around the medial malleolus (ankle bone), inside of the leg, to the top of the pelvic bone, along side of anterior mid line of the abdomen, jogs out two inches at the rib cage, then ends at the bottom of the clavicle. This meridian is active between 5 PM and 7 PM.

Typical symptoms of a kidney meridian that is out of balance are asthma, tinnitus, loss of hearing, dizziness, thirst, night sweats, low grade fevers, lassitude, fatigue, weak legs, tendency toward impotence in men and little or no menstruation in women, inability to metabolize water well, genital-urinary disorders, and low back pain. Emotionally an imbalance could affect willpower, determination, and a person's ability to cope.

## Gallbladder

The gallbladder meridian begins at the outer corner of the eye, circles behind the ear, down to below the skull, back up and over to the forehead, then back up and over the head and down the back of the head and lateral to the cervical spine, over the shoulders to the midpoint of the clavicle, down the side of the rib cage, to the gallbladder, to the waist, to the buttock, to the lateral side of the leg, in front of the lateral ankle bone and ending at the end of the fourth toe. The gallbladder meridian is active between 11 PM and 1 AM.

An imbalance in this meridian can cause liver pains, yellow discoloration on the tongue, skin and urine, bloating.

## Stomach

The stomach meridian begins below the eyes and just lateral to the nostrils. It travels to the medial corners of the eyes, to the bottom of the cheekbone, circles the mouth, to the jaw, to the mid clavicle, then descends through the nipples to just lateral of the umbilicus, to the pubic bone, to the outside of the legs and finally to the end of the second toe. The stomach meridian is active between 7 AM and 9 AM.

An imbalance emotionally can lead to feelings of worry, nervousness, pensiveness, and a lack of acceptance. Physically, an imbalance can lead to a burning sensation in the stomach, hunger, bleeding of the gums, constipation, and halitosis.

## Spleen

The spleen meridian begins at the tip of the big toe, ascends up the inside of the leg, to the groin, to the top of the pubic bone, to lateral of the umbilicus, to the outside of the rib cage. The spleen meridian is most active between 9 AM and 11 AM.

An imbalance in the energy of this meridian, can lead to diarrhea, constipation, bloating, loss of appetite, prolapsed internal organs, weak muscles, fatigue, lassitude, brain fog, absentmindedness, pasty complexion, diarrhea, cold limbs, and abdominal pain.

# Heart

The heart meridian goes through the chest to the axilla (armpit), along the inside of the arm, through the inner wrist and ends at the end of the little finger. It is most active between 11AM and 1 PM.

An imbalance in the heart meridian may result in chest pain, shortness of breath, panting, shallow breathing, dizziness, palpitations, frequent sweating, hot flashes/cold sweats, irritability, and insomnia. Emotionally it can cause anxiety and depression.

# Small Intestine

The small intestine meridian begins at the tip of the little finger, goes up the ulnar side of the arm to the posterior shoulder, up the side of the neck to just in front of the ear. This meridian is most active between 1 PM and 3 PM.

An imbalance of this meridian causes poor digestion, stomach distention, poor circulation, weakness in the legs, constant cold feeling, nerve pain, stiff/sore shoulders, swollen lymph glands, and acne.

# Large Intestine

The large intestine meridian begins at the base of the index finger and travels to the outside of the arm, to the top of the shoulder, above the scapulae to T1, over the shoulders to the mid clavicle up to the sides of the mouth to the lateral side of each nostril. The large intestine meridian is active between 5 AM and 7 AM.

Before expelling waste material, the large intestine extracts water it receives from the small intestine. If there is an imbalance in the large intestine meridian, the primary symptom would be abdominal pain. On an emotional level, an imbalance could manifest as difficulty holding on or letting go.

## Urinary Bladder

The bladder meridian begins at the inner corner of each eye; goes over the back of the head to the top of the neck; splits into four parts and descends (two on each side of the spine) to the buttocks and converge behind the knees. From there the meridian circles the lateral malleolus and ends at the end of the small toe. The bladder meridian is most active between 3 PM and 5 PM.

An imbalance in the bladder meridian may lead to neck and shoulder stiffness, back pain, urinary disease, and headaches. Emotionally, an imbalance can cause feelings of anger and an inability to express emotions.

## Triple Warmer

The triple warmer meridian controls the body as a whole. It controls metabolism, heat/moisture balance, and body temperature. Beginning at the end of the ring finger it travels through the posterior center of the wrist, through the elbow and back of the arm, up the neck lateral to the spine, it splits and part goes to the ear lobe and part to over the ears and to the medial point of the eyes to the cheeks. The triple warmer meridian is active between 9 PM and 11 PM.

Depending upon where the imbalance is most directed, symptoms may include any combination of the following: Fever, aversion to cold, headaches, sore throat, red/swollen tonsils, red tip of the tongue, profuse sweating, constipation, thirst, rapid pulse, cough, thirst, irritability, dry mouth, hot palms and soles, nausea, vomiting, and convulsions.

## Pericardium

The pericardium meridian begins just lateral to the nipple, ascends to the anterior shoulder, down the arm to the tip of the middle finger. The pericardium meridian is most active between 7 PM and 9 PM.

An imbalance of the pericardium meridian can cause heart disorder symptoms including chest pains and shortness of breath.

## Liver

The liver meridian begins at the end of the big toe, travels up the medial aspect of the leg to the groin, circulates through the external genitalia, and ascends to the free end of the eleventh rib. This meridian is most active between 1 AM and 3 AM.

An imbalance in the liver meridian causes headaches, stiff joints, vertigo, blurred vision, dry and painful eyes, headache, restlessness, jaundice, red face, dry skin, swollen and painful breasts, and menstrual disorders. Emotionally, an imbalance causes irritability, anger, depression, and a lack of control of emotions.

# Chapter 5
## Vitamins and Minerals

## Vitamins

Vitamins can be very confusing to most people. Too often we buy vitamins based on the latest TV commercial or advertisement in a magazine. It's easy to become confused when a salesperson in a store talks above your head and winds up selling you a bag full of vitamins, most of them you don't need.

Vitamins are "supplements." They supplement your diet. They provide vitamins that you may not get in your food. In the early 1950's, the Department of Agriculture announced that the ground that farmers use to produce our food was depleted in necessary minerals. Likewise, production farming and now the use of genetically modified food have left us deficient in vitamins necessary for optimum health. That's why it's necessary to supplement your diet with vitamins and minerals. For a healthy person who conscientiously works at eating healthy, a good, high quality multi-vitamin and mineral might be all that's needed to be healthy. Once a good foundation of vitamins and minerals is established, one can add specific vitamins and minerals to attack certain conditions.

Not all vitamins are created equal. Some are natural and some are synthetic. Natural vitamins occur naturally as ingredients in foods. Synthetic vitamins are produced in a laboratory. Although the synthetic vitamin's chemical components are similar to the natural vitamins, they are not as readily accepted by the body. Therefore, a portion of the vitamin itself is destroyed by the body before it is used. It's a good idea to occasionally refrain from taking your vitamins for a day or two to let the body rest and regenerate. One day each week or one week each month or two would be sufficient.

In order to quickly absorb information about vitamins, the following is a guide to reading the following chapter.

| | |
|---|---|
| RDA | Recommended Daily Allowance |
| SDA | Suggested Daily Allowance |
| Toxicity | An amount that may cause harm to the body. |
| Fat/Water Soluble | The way the supplement is dissolved in the body. Fat soluble vitamins are not readily dissolved in the body and can accumulate and become toxic. |
| Antagonists | Substances that work against the vitamin. |
| Synergists | Substances that assist, boost, or work in harmony with vitamins. |
| Sources | Substances from where the vitamin can be derived. |
| Mg | Milligrams |
| Mcg | Micrograms |
| IU | International Units |

## Vitamins

### Vitamin A  Retinol
RDA:  5,000 IU
SDA:  10,000 – 25,000 IU
Toxicity:   50,000 IU
Fat Soluble

### Antagonists:
Alcohol, coffee, cortisone, excessive iron, mineral oil, Vitamin D deficiency, estrogens, cortisol.

**Synergists:**

Vitamins B2, B12, C, E, Thyroxin, testosterone, Melanocyte Hormone, Growth Hormone, Zinc, Calcium.

**Sources:**

High – Liver (beef, pig, sheep, calf, chicken), fish oil (cod, halibut, salmon, shark, sperm whale), carrots, mint, kohlrabi, parsley, spinach, turnip greens, dandelion greens, palm oil.

Medium – Butter, cheese (except cottage, egg yolk, margarine, dried milk, cream, white fish, eel, kidneys (beef, pig, sheep), liver (pork), mangos, apricots, yellow melons, peaches, cherries (sour), nectarines, beet greens, broccoli, endive, collards, fennel, butterhead and romaine lettuce, squash (acorn, butternut, hubbard), chard.

Low – Milk, herring, salmon, oyster, carp, clams, sardines, grapes, bananas.

**Body Parts Affected:**

Bones, eyes, hair, skin, soft tissue, teeth.

**Deficiency Symptoms:**

Allergies, loss of appetite, blemishes, dry hair, fatigue, itching/burning eyes, loss of smell, night blindness, rough dry skin, sinus trouble, soft tooth enamel, susceptibility to infections.

**Signs and Symptoms of Toxicity:**

Allergic reactions, bone pain, blotchy, flaky, and itchy skin, blurred vision, diarrhea, edema, headaches, nausea, nervousness, sweating, tachycardia, tremors, and vomiting.

**Uses:**

Acne, alcoholism, allergies, arthritis, asthma, athlete's foot, bronchitis, colds, cystitis, diabetes, eczema, heart disease, hepatitis, migraine headaches, psoriasis, sinusitis, stress, tooth and gum disorders.

- Vitamin C will help protect against the toxic effects of Vitamin A, yet too much Vitamin C will deplete Vitamin A.
- Cold weather also depletes Vitamin A.
- When taking Vitamin D, use 1 part Vitamin D to 10 parts Vitamin A.
- When increasing the dosage of Vitamin F, increase the dosage of Vitamin A.
- Yet when increasing Vitamin A, increase the dosage of Calcium and Phosphorus

## Vitamin B1 Thiamine

RDA: 1 – 1.5 mg.
SDA: 2 – 10 mg.
Toxicity:    Unknown
Water Soluble

**Antagonists:**

Alcohol, coffee, fever, raw clams, sugar, stress, surgery, tobacco.

**Synergists:**

Vitamins B2, B6, B12, folic acid, niacin, Vitamin E, pantothenic acid, Growth Hormone, manganese, sulphur.

**Sources:**

High: Blackstrap molasses, brewer's yeast, brown rice, fish, meat, nuts, yeast, pork, outer grain kernels, bran, polishing, wheat germ, yeast, pork.

Medium: Gooseberries, plums, beans, green leafy vegetables, cauliflower, corn, peas. potatoes, all other grains, animals, mushrooms, all other grains.

Low: All other fruit and vegetables, coconut, some fish.

**Body Parts Affected:**

Brain, ears, eyes, hair, heart, liver, and peripheral nerves.

**Deficiency Symptoms:**

Beriberi, polyneuritis, numbness, slow heartbeat, edema, retarded growth, fatigue, weight loss, anorexia, G.I. complaints, anesthesia, hyperesthesia, loss of reflexes, depression, irritability, memory loss, muscular atrophy in the arms and legs.

**Uses:**

Growth, appetite, digestion, nerve activity, gastrointestinal tone, carbohydrate metabolism, energy production.

The need for B vitamins increases during times of stress, illness, or surgery.

Excessive use of alcohol or sugar destroys B vitamins. Since B vitamins are water soluble, they must be replaced every day. Alcoholics and diabetics often need more B vitamins. Thiamine assists in growth, digestion, appetite, nerve activity, energy production, and carbohydrate metabolism. It helps stabilize emotions and relieves irritability and depression. Thiamine also helps to produce hydrochloric acid in the stomach. B vitamin enzymes are poisoned by heavy metals.

**Vitamin B2 Riboflavin**

RDA:      Children: 0.6-1.2 mg
             Adults:1.5 (female), 1.7 (male)
SDA:      2-10 mg (adult)
Toxicity:  Unknown
Water soluble

**Antagonists:**

Alcohol, coffee, excessive sugar intake, tobacco.

**Synergists:**

Vitamins A, B complex, B6, B12, niacin, pantothenic acid, folic acid, biotin, insulin, growth hormone.

**Sources:**

High: Beef (kidneys, liver), chicken (liver), pork (heart, kidneys, liver), sheep (liver, kidneys), yeast.

Medium: Almonds (dry), asparagus, avocados, beans (kidney, lima, snap, wax), beet greens, broccoli, Brussels sprouts, cashews, cauliflower, cheeses, corn, cream, currants, dandelion greens, eggs, endive, kale, kohlrabi, lentils (dry), milk, oats, parsley, parsnips, peanuts, pecans, peas, rice bran, soybeans (dry), spinach, turnip greens, walnuts, watercress, wheat germ. Meats: bacon, beef, chicken, duck, fish, goose, lamb, pork, turkey, veal.

Low: Apples, apricots, artichokes, bananas, barley, beets, blackberries, blueberries, cabbage.

**Body Parts Affected:**

Eyes, hair, nails, skin, soft body tissues.

**Deficiency Symptoms:**

Cataracts, cracks and sores at the corners of the mouth, dizziness, itching burning eyes, poor digestion, retarded growth, red sore tongue.

**Uses:**

Acne, alcoholism, arthritis, athletes foot, baldness, cataracts, diabetes, diarrhea, indigestion, stress, antibody and red blood cell formation.

## Vitamin B3  Niacin, Niacinamide, Nicotinic acid

RDA:       13-18 mg
SDA:       50-5,000 mg
Toxicity:  Unknown
Water soluble

**Antagonists:**

Alcohol, antibiotics, coffee, corn sugar, excessive starches

**Synergists:**
B-complex, B1, B2, C, phosphorus

**Sources:**
Brewer's yeast, seafood, lean meats, milk products, poultry, desiccated liver, cooked rhubarb, peanuts.

**Body Parts Affected:**
Brain, liver, nerves, skin, soft tissues, tongue

**Deficiency Symptoms:**
Appetite loss, canker sores, depression, fatigue, halitosis, headaches, indigestion, insomnia, muscular weakness, nausea, nervous disorders, skin eruptions.

**Uses:**
Atherosclerosis, baldness, reduces LDL, increases HDL, reduces cholesterol (high), cystitis, facial oiliness, hypoglycemia, mental retardation, muscular disorders, nervous disorders, nausea in pregnancy, overweight, post operative nausea, stress, sun sensitivity, increases circulation, hydrochloric acid production, increases metabolism, helps sex hormone production. One California university is currently testing the effectiveness of 3,000 mg per day on dementia symptoms.

**Vitamin B5 Pantothenic Acid**
RDA:      0.15-10 mg
SDA:      20-100 mg
Toxicity:  Unknown
Water soluble

**Antagonists:**
Alcohol, coffee

**Synergists:**

B-complex, B6, B12, biotin, folic acid, vitamin C.

**Sources:**

Brewer's yeast, legumes, organ meats, salmon, wheat germ, whole grains, beef liver, mushrooms, elderberries, fresh orange juice.

**Body Parts Affected:**

Adrenal glands, digestive tract, nerves, skin

**Deficiency Symptoms:**

Diarrhea, duodenal ulcers, eczema, hypoglycemia, intestinal disorders, kidney trouble, loss of hair, muscle cramps, premature aging, respiratory infections, restlessness, nerve problems, sore feet, vomiting

**Uses:**

Allergies, arthritis, baldness, cystitis, digestive disorders, hypoglycemia, tooth decay, stress, antibody formation, vitamin utilization, conversion of proteins, fats, and carbohydrates to energy.

## Vitamin B6 Pyridoxine

RDA:        1.5-1.8 mg
SDA:        4 - 50 mg
Toxicity:   Unknown
Water soluble

**Antagonists:**

Alcohol, birth control pills, coffee, radiation (exposure), tobacco

**Synergists:**

B-complex, B1, B2, pantothenic acid, C, magnesium, potassium, linoleic acid, sodium

## Sources:

Blackstrap molasses, brewer's yeast, green leafy vegetables, meat, organ meats, wheat germ, whole grains, desiccated liver, prunes, brown rice, peas

## Body Parts Affected:

Blood, muscles, nerves, skin

## Deficiency Symptoms of Toxicity:

Acne, anemia, arthritis, convulsions in babies, depression, dizziness, hair loss, irritability, learning disabilities, weakness

## Uses:

Atherosclerosis, baldness, cholesterol (high), cystitis, facial oiliness, mental retardation, muscular disorders, nervous disorders, nausea in pregnancy, overweight, post operative nausea, stress, sun sensitivity, converts proteins, fats and carbohydrates to energy, antibody formation, growth stimulation, vitamin utilization.

## Vitamin B12  Cobalamin, Cyanocobalamin, Hydroxycobalamin

RDA:        3 mcg
SDA:        1,000 mcg, up to 15,000 mcg for short term
Toxicity:   None known
Water soluble

## Antagonists:

Alcohol, coffee, laxatives, tobacco

## Synergists:

B complex, B6, choline, inositol, C, potassium, sodium

## Sources:

Cheese, fish, milk, milk products, organ meats, cottage cheese, beef liver, tuna fish, eggs, shrimp, venison, lamb

**Body Parts Affected:**
Blood, nerves

**Deficiency Symptoms:**
General weakness, fatigue, apathy, nervousness, pernicious anemia, walking and speaking difficulties, mood swings, memory difficulties, mental fogginess, persistent sleep problems, weak immunity, irritability, digestive problems, hearing and vision loss, tingling extremities

**Uses:**
Alcoholism, allergies, anemia, arthritis, bronchial asthma, bursitis, epilepsy, fatigue, hypoglycemia, insomnia, over-weight, shingles, stress, metabolism, blood cell formation

### Vitamin B15 Pangamic Acid, Calcium Pangamate
RDA:      None stated
SDA:      Not known
Toxicity: Unknown
Water soluble

**Antagonists:**
Alcohol, coffee

**Synergists:**
B complex, C, E

**Body Parts Affected:**
Glands Heart, kidneys, nerves

**Deficiency Symptoms:**
Heart disease, nervous & glandular disorders

**Uses:**
Alcoholism, asthma, atherosclerosis, cholesterol (high), em-

physema, heart disease, headaches, insomnia, poor circulation, premature aging, rheumatism, shortness of breath, metabolism.

## Biotin Vitamin H, Coenzyme R

| | |
|---|---|
| RDA: | 150 - 300 mcg |
| SDA: | 300 - 500 mcg |
| Toxicity: | Unknown |

Water soluble

**Antagonists:**

Alcohol, coffee, raw egg white

**Synergists:**

B complex, B12, folic acid, pantothenic acid, C, sulphur

**Sources:**

Legumes, whole grains, organ meats, brewer's yeast, lentils, mung bean sprouts, egg yolk, beef liver, soybeans

**Body Parts Affected:**

Hair, muscles, skin

**Deficiency Symptoms:**

Depression, dry skin, fatigue, grayish skin color, insomnia, muscular pain, poor appetite

**Uses:**

Baldness, dermatitis, eczema, leg cramps, metabolism, B vitamin utilization.

## Choline

| | |
|---|---|
| RDA: | None Stated |
| SDA: | 100 - 1,000 mg |
| Toxicity: | Unknown |

Water soluble

**Antagonists:**
Alcohol, coffee, excessive sugar

**Synergists:**
Vitamin A, B complex, B12, folic acid, inositol, linoleic acid

**Sources:**
Brewer's yeast, fish, legumes, organ meats, soybeans, wheat germ, lecithin, beef liver, egg yolks, peanuts

**Body Parts Affected:**
Hair, kidneys, liver, thymus gland

**Deficiency Symptoms:**
Bleeding stomach ulcers, growth problems, heart trouble, high blood pressure, impaired liver and kidney function, intolerance to fats, decreased mental alertness (fog), lethargy, memory difficulties

**Uses:**
Alcoholism, atherosclerosis, baldness, cholesterol (high), constipation, dizziness, ear noises, hardening of the arteries, headaches, heart trouble, high blood pressure, hypoglycemia, insomnia, liver and gallbladder regulation, metabolism, lecithin formation.

## Folic Acid
RDA:      400 mcg
SDA:      1,000 - 10,000 mcg
Toxicity:   Unknown

**Antagonists:**
Alcohol, coffee, stress, tobacco

**Synergists:**
B complex, B12, biotin, pantothenic acid, vitamin C

**Sources:**
Green leafy vegetables, milk, milk products, organ meats, oysters, salmon, whole grains, brewer's yeast, dried dates, steamed spinach, canned tuna fish

**Body Parts Affected:**
Blood, glands, liver

**Deficiency Symptoms:**
Anemia, digestive disturbances, graying hair, growth problems

**Uses:**
Alcoholism, anemia, atherosclerosis, baldness, diarrhea, fatigue, menstrual problems, mental illness, stomach ulcers, stress, increase hydrochloric acid production, aids protein metabolism, aids red blood cell formation.

## Inositol

RDA:        None Stated
SDA:        100 - 1,000 mg
Toxicity:   Unknown

**Antagonists:**
Alcohol, coffee

**Synergists:**
B complex, B12, choline, linoleic acid

**Sources:**
Citrus fruits, brewer's yeast, meat, milk, nuts, vegetables, blackstrap molasses, whole grains, lecithin, fresh oranges, grapefruit, peanuts

**Body Parts Affected:**

Brain, hair, kidneys, liver, muscles

**Deficiency Symptoms:**

High cholesterol, constipation, eczema, eye abnormalities, hair loss

**Uses:**

Atherosclerosis, baldness, cholesterol (high), constipation, heart disease, over-weight, metabolism.

## Para Amino Benzoic Acid (PABA)

RDA: None stated
SDA: 10-100 mg
Toxicity: Excessive amounts may be toxic to some individuals.

**Antagonists:**

Alcohol, coffee, sulfa drugs

**Synergists:**

B-complex, folic acid, vitamin C

**Sources:**

Blackstrap molasses, brewer's yeast, liver, organ meats, wheat germ

**Body Parts Affected:**

Glands, hair, intestines, skin

**Deficiency Symptoms:**

Constipation, depression, digestive disorders, fatigue, gray hair, headaches, irritability.

**Uses:**

Baldness, graying hair, overactive thyroid, parasitic diseases, rheumatic fever, stress, infertility, enhances intestinal bacteria and blood cell formation, assists in protein metabolism.

External: burns, dark skin spots, dry skin, sunburn, wrinkles.

## Vitamin C (Ascorbic acid)

RDA:     45 mg

SDA:     250 - 5,000 mg

Toxicity: Excessive amounts can lead to diarrhea in some individuals. Vitamin C is water soluble and can be taken time released or 1,000 to 2,000 mg per hour until the stools become loose.

**Antagonists:**

Antibiotics, aspirin, cortisone, high fever, stress, tobacco

**Synergists:**

All vitamins and minerals, bioflavonoid, calcium, magnesium

**Sources:**

Cantaloupe, green peppers, cooked broccoli, citrus fruits, grapefruit, papaya, strawberries

**Body Parts Affected:**

Adrenal glands, blood, capillary walls, connective tissue, skin, ligaments, bones, gums, heart, teeth

**Deficiency Symptoms:**

Slow wound healing, teeth and gum defects, rough skin, achy joints, listlessness, weakness, scorbutic bone formation

In severe cases: Scurvy, megaloblastic anemia of infancy

**Uses:**

Alcoholism, allergies, atherosclerosis, arthritis, baldness, cancer, cholesterol (high), colds, cystitis, hypoglycemia, heart disease, hepatitis, insect bites, overweight, prickly heat, sinusitis, stress, tooth decay, bone and tooth formation, collagen production, synovial fluid production (joints), digestion, general healing

## Vitamin D (D2=Ergocalciferol, D3=Cholecalciferol)

Vitamin D3 demonstrates greater absorbability and efficacy

Best if taken with K2

RDA:     600 IU

SDA:     5000 – 10,000 IU

Toxicity:   Above 60,000 IU/day depending on age

**Antagonists:**

Mineral oil

**Synergists:**

Vitamin A, choline, C, F, K, calcium, phosphorus

**Sources:**

Egg yolks, organ meats, bone meal, sunlight, milk, salmon, tuna, sardines, shrimp

**Body Parts Affected:**

Bones, heart, nerves, skin, teeth, thyroid gland

**Deficiency Symptoms:**

Burning sensation in the mouth and throat, diarrhea, insomnia, myopia, nervousness, depressed feeling, poor metabolism, softening bones and teeth, achy bones, lowered immune system, darker skin, head sweating, obesity, gum disease, elevated blood pressure, sleepy feeling, fatigue, allergies, digestive issues (Crohn's, celiac, IBS)

**Signs and Symptoms of Toxicity:**

Nausea, thirst, diarrhea, excessive urination, muscular weakness, joint pain, increased serum calcium

**Uses:**

The gene Bax stimulates apoptosis, the process by which cells commit suicide when they go bad. In a study of 92 men and women, researchers found that the group given only Vitamin D increased their Bax 56% over the placebo group. Therefore, vitamin D helps the body eliminate unhealthy cell and replace them with healthy ones.

Studies have shown that 60,000 IU per day have been successfully used to eliminate MS symptoms. The optimum range for a blood test for vitamin D is 50-70 ng/ml.

Some of the many benefits of regularly taking vitamin D include: Acne, alcoholism, allergies, arthritis, cystitis, eczema, psoriasis, stress, calcium and phosphorus production, bone formation, metabolism, normal blood clotting, heart and other organ functioning.

## Vitamin E (d alpha tocopherol) (dl alpha tocopherol = synthetic)

RDA:       12 - 15 IU
SDA:       50 - 600 IU
Toxicity:   4,000 - 30,000 IU

**Antagonists:**

Birth control pills, chlorine, mineral oil, rancid fat and oil

**Synergists:**

Vitamin A, B complex, B1, inositol, C, F, calcium, phosphorus

**Sources:**

Dark green vegetables, spinach, broccoli, liver, wheat germ, vegetable oils, eggs, organ meats, desiccated liver, oatmeal, safflower oil, vegetable oil, peanuts, tomatoes, wheat germ oil, nuts including almonds, walnuts, hazelnuts and pecans, seeds

**Body Parts Affected:**

Blood vessels, heart, lungs, nerves pituitary gland, skin

**Deficiency Symptoms:**

Anemia, bleeding gums, bruise easily, capillary wall ruptures, dental cavities, low infection resistance, nose bleeds, poor digestion

**Signs and Symptoms of Toxicity:**

Although vitamin E is difficult to be toxic through food sources, yet an overdose with vitamin E supplements can cause bleeding (reduces the body's ability to form clots), hemorrhage and stroke. Hypervitaminosis E can lead to a vitamin K deficiency. Other signs and symptoms include: blotchy skin, increased blood level of triglycerides, decreased vitamin K activity and thyroid hormone production.

**Uses:**

Internal: Allergies, arthritis, atherosclerosis, baldness, cholesterol (high), crossed eyes, cystitis, diabetes, heart disease (coronary thrombosis, angina pectoris, rheumatic heart disease), menstrual problems, menopause, migraine headaches, myopia, overweight, phlebitis, sinusitis, stress, thrombosis, varicose veins, anti-oxidation, anti-clotting, male fertility, lung protection.

External: Heals burns, scars and wounds and reduces warts and wrinkles.

## Vitamin F Unsaturated Fatty Acids
**(Omega-3 = alpha-linolenic acid, Omega 6 = linoleic acid)**

RDA:        None Stated
SDA:        10% of total calories
Toxicity:   Not Known

**Antagonists:**

Radiation, x-rays

**Synergists:**

Vitamins: A, C, D, E, phosphorus

**Sources:**

Sunflower seeds, vegetable oils, wheat germ, nuts, leafy vegetables

**Body Parts Affected:**

Cells, glands (adrenal, thyroid), hair, mucous membranes, nerves, skin

**Deficiency Symptoms:**

Acne, allergies, diarrhea, dry skin, "alligator skin" or "chicken skin," dry, brittle hair, dandruff, eczema, gall stones, nail problems, underweight, varicose veins, fatigue, poor attention span, menstrual cramps

**Signs and Symptoms of Toxicity:**

Hypervitaminosis F is almost unheard of.

**Uses:**

Allergies, baldness, bronchial asthma, cholesterol (high), eczema, gallbladder problems or removal, heart disease, leg ulcers, psoriasis, rheumatoid arthritis, overweight, underweight, high blood pressure.

## Vitamin K (K1 = phylloquinone, K2 = menaquinone or MK7)

RDA:       None stated
SDA:       K1 = 200-500 mcg, K2 = 360-500 mcg
Toxicity:  None found

**Antagonists:**

Aspirin, antibiotics, mineral oil, radiation, rancid fats, x-rays

**Synergists:**

Unknown

**Sources:**

K1 - Green leafy vegetables, safflower oil, blackstrap molasses, yogurt, oatmeal, liver

K2 – hard and soft cheeses, kefir, raw butter, fermented vegetables, i.e. sauerkraut

**Body Parts Affected:**

Blood, liver, bones, arteries

**Deficiency Symptoms:**

Diarrhea, increased tendency to hemorrhage, miscarriages, nosebleeds, fatigue

**Uses:**

Bruising, eye hemorrhages, gall stones, hemorrhaging, menstruation problems, preparing women for childbirth, blood coagulation, helps prevent coronary heart disease, less calcification in the arteries, may help prevent wrinkles and varicose veins

## Vitamin P (Bioflavonoids)

RDA:      None stated
SDA:      500-3,000 mg
Toxicity:   Unknown

**Antagonists:**

Same as vitamin C

**Synergists:**

Vitamin C

**Sources:**

Fruits – apricots, cherries, grapes, grapefruit, lemons, plums.

**Body Parts Affected:**

Blood, capillary walls, connective tissue (skin, gums, ligaments, bones), teeth.

**Deficiency Symptoms:**
Same as vitamin C

**Uses:**
Asthma, bleeding gums, colds, eczema, dizziness (caused by inner ear), hemorrhoids, high blood pressure, miscarriages, rheumatic fever, rheumatism, ulcers, blood vessel wall maintenance.

# MINERALS

## Boron
RDA: None given
SR:   See below
Toxicity: None noted

**Antagonists:**
Any activity that consumes minerals, i.e. dehydration, exercise, alcohol

**Synergists:**
Other minerals

**Sources:**
Mined as 99% pure in Turkey and California

**Body Parts Affected:**
Joints, digestive tract

**Deficiency Symptoms:**
None noted

**Side effects:**
Herxheimer reactions (healing crisis) are sometimes experienced when resolving some conditions such as Candida. Muscle

cramping due to a loss of calcium have been experienced. This can be resolved by taking calcium and magnesium supplements.

## Signs and Symptoms of Toxicity:

Nausea, diarrhea, itchy skin, gas, bloated, hungry, frequent urination, increased libido

(Discontinue use for a few days and resume at a lower dosage.)

(Borax is rapidly and nearly completely excreted with the urine.)

## Uses:

Boron has been used to eliminate arthritis, reduce calcium loss from bones, increase testosterone levels, kill fungus as in Candida and toe fungus, vaginal thrush, vaginitis, skeletal fluorosis, and fibromyalgia.

## Dosage:

As a general rule, dissolve a lightly rounded teaspoonful (5-6 grams) of boron in 1 quart of a good quality water. This is the concentrated solution. Keep this from children.

Standard doses 1 tsp (5 ml) of concentrate mixed with water and taken with a meal. This contains 25-30 mg. Take one to two doses per day with a meal. For specific problems the dosage can be increased to three or more doses until the condition is resolved.

One doctor reported using 3 boron tablets (3 mg each) for 2-3 weeks to eliminate pain, swelling and stiffness of rheumatoid arthritis. He then placed his patients on 1 tablet per day as a maintenance dose.

A recent study showed that 100 mg of boron per day for one week showed a 50% increase in estrogen in women and a 50% increase in testosterone in men.

Boron has been successfully used as a fungicide to treat Candida. For low or medium weight people, 1/8 teaspoon of boron powder or for heavier people, ¼ teaspoon per quart of water. Drink the water throughout the day for 4-5 days a week until the condition is resolved. This same concoction is known as the Boron Detox due to its detoxification properties.

For vaginal thrush, one large gelatin capsule filled with boron or boric acid inserted at bedtime for several nights up to 2 weeks helps alleviate the condition. Alternatively the powder can be mixed with cool solidified coconut oil as a bolus or suppository.

## Calcium
    RDA:    800-1,400 mg
    SR:     1,000-2,000+ mg
    Toxicity: None Noted

**Anagonists:**
    Lack of exercise, stress.

**Synergists:**
    Vitamins A, C, D, F, iron, magnesium, manganese, phosphorus.

**Sources:**
    Whole milk, cheese, molasses, wheatgrass, green leafy vegetables, yogurt, bone meal, dolomite, almonds, liver, citrus fruits (pith), carob

**Body Parts Affected:**
    Blood, bones, heart, skin, soft tissue, teeth.

**Deficiency Symptoms:**
    Heart palpitations, insomnia, muscle cramps, nervousness, arm and leg numbness, tooth decay.

**Signs and Symptoms of Toxicity (hypercalcemia):**
    Nausea, diarrhea, weakness, dehydration, constipation, lethargy, possibly heart arrhythmia and mental imbalance.

**Uses:**

Arthritis, aging symptoms (backache, bone pain, finger tremors), foot/leg cramps, insomnia, menstrual cramps, menopause problems, nervousness, overweight, pre-menstrual tension, rheumatism, blood clotting, heart rhythm, nerve transmission, muscle growth.

Helps keep your body alkaline.

## Chromium

| | |
|---|---|
| RDA: | None stated |
| SDA: | 100-300 mcg |
| Toxicity: | None known |

**Antagonists:**

None

**Synergists:**

None

**Sources:**

Brewer's yeast, clams, corn oil, whole grain cereals.

**Body Parts Affected:**

Blood, circulatory system

**Deficiency Symptoms:**

Atherosclerosis, glucose intolerance in diabetics.

**Signs and Symptoms of Toxicity:**

Acute: Nausea, vomiting, diarrhea, muscle cramps, vertigo, fever, abdominal pain, kidney pain and possible failure, liver damage, organ failure, possible coma and death.

Chronic: Painful dermatitis, edema, painful eyes and mucous membranes, nasal and dental inflammation, bronchitis, rhinitis, sinusitis, liver failure, kidney failure, and possible lung cancer.

**Uses:**

Diabetes, hypoglycemia, glucose metabolism, helps keep blood sugar level normal.

## Copper

| | |
|---|---|
| RDA: | 2 mg |
| SDA: | 2-4 mg |
| Toxicity: | 40 mg |

**Antagonists:**

Zinc (high intake)

**Synergists:**

Cobalt, iron, zinc

**Sources:**

Legumes, nuts, organ meats, seafood, raisins, molasses, bone meal

**Body Parts Affected:**

Blood, bones, circulatory system, hair, skin.

**Deficiency Symptoms:**

General weakness, impaired respiration, skin sores.

**Signs and Symptoms of Toxicity:**

Acne, allergies, anemia, anorexia, anxiety, arthritis, asthma, attention deficit disorder, autism, candida, depression, dysmenorrhea, hypertension, hypothyroidism, manic depression, migraine headaches, muscle pain, nerve pain, PMS, sciatica, schizophrenia.

Eliminate by increasing zinc and magnesium levels in the blood.

**Uses:**

Anemia, baldness, promotes healing, hemoglobin & red blood

cell formation.

## Iodine
RDA:      100-130 mcg
SDA:      100-1,000 mcg
Toxicity:  Not known

**Antagonists:**
None

**Synergists:**
None

**Sources:**
Seafood, kelp tablets, iodized salt

**Body Parts Affected:**
Hair, nails, skin, teeth, thyroid gland

**Deficiency Symptoms:**
Cold hands and feet, dry hair, dry skin, dry mouth, irritability, nervousness, lowered IQ, reduced alertness, muscle pain, fibrosis, fibromyalgia, obesity

**Signs and Symptoms of Toxicity:**
Diarrhea, nausea, vomiting, weak pulse, burning sensation in the mouth, throat and stomach, hypothyroidism, elevated TSH levels.

**Uses:**
Atherosclerosis, hair problems, goiter, hypo/hyperthyroidism, increased energy, metabolism, promotes physical & mental development.

## Iron

RDA:      10-18 mg
SDA:      15-50 mg
Toxicity:  100 mg

### Antagonists:
Coffee, excess phosphorus, tea, zinc (excessive)

### Synergists:
Vitamin B 12, folic acid, vitamin C, calcium, cobalt, copper, phosphorus.

### Sources:
Blackstrap molasses, eggs, fish, organ meats, poultry, wheat germ, desiccated liver.

### Body Parts Affected:
Blood, bones, nails, skin, teeth.

### Deficiency Symptoms:
Breathing difficulties, brittle nails, iron deficiency anemia, pain skin, fatigue, constipation, decreased immunity

### Signs and Symptoms of Toxicity:
Anger, arthritis, birth defects, bleeding gums, cirrhosis of the liver, constipation, diabetes, diarrhea, dizziness, elevated blood pressure, fatigue, grayish color of the skin, headaches, heart damage or failure, hepatitis, hyperactivity, infections, insomnia, mental disturbances including mood swings, metallic taste in the mouth, nausea, premature aging, scurvy.

Eliminate by reducing protein intake and vitamin C intake, and increasing copper, manganese, vitamin B6 and zinc intake.

### Uses:
Alcoholism, anemia, colitis, menstrual problems, promotes

hemoglobin production, increases disease resistance.

## Magnesium

Magnesium citrate – inexpensive, mild laxative effect

Magnesium taurate – best for those with cardiovascular issues, easily absorbed

Magnesium malate – easily absorbed, good for those suffering with fatigue

Magnesium chloride – absorbed well, low in elemental magnesium, good for cell detox

Magnesium caronate – good for those with indigestion problems

Magnesium glycinate – best absorbable, safest for long term deficiency

Avoid Magnesium aspartate, glutamate, oxide or sulfate

| | |
|---|---|
| RDA: | 300-350 mg |
| SDA: | 300-500 mg (1,000 mg if active) |
| Toxicity: | 30,000 mg |

## Antagonists:

None, however, calcium supplements decrease the body's absorption of magnesium, as do soft drinks, fluoride, prescription drugs, alcohol, caffeine, excess sugar, diuretics and birth-control pills.

## Synergists:

Vitamins B6, C, D, calcium, phosphorus

## Sources:

Bran, honey, green vegetables, nuts, seafood, spinach, bone meal, kelp tablets.

## Body Parts Affected:

Arteries, bones, heart, muscles, nerves, teeth

## Deficiency Symptoms:

Depression, migraines, premenstrual irritability, confusion, disorientation, easily aroused anger, sensitivity to noise, seizures, coronary spasms, personality changes, muscle cramps, nervousness, rapid pulse, tremors, anxiety, fatigue, insomnia, hyperactivity, panic attacks, ADD, bladder problems, fibromyalgia, allergies, asthma and cardiac arrhythmias. Restless sleep with frequent nighttime awakenings have been noted in magnesium deficiency.

## Signs and Symptoms of Toxicity:

The first and most prominent sign of overdose is diarrhea.

## Uses:

Alcoholism, cholesterol (high), depression, heart conditions, kidney stones, nervousness, prostate troubles, sensitivity to noise, stomach acidity, tooth decay, overweight, promotes acid/alkaline balance, helps maintain blood sugar metabolism, relieves muscle contractions.

Magnesium should be taken before one retires for bed thus allowing it time to dispense throughout the body.

## Best forms:

Magnesium carbonate – has antacid properties, good for those with indigestion and acid reflux concerns

Magnesium chloride – good absorption, best for detoxing, boosts metabolism

Magnesium citrate – inexpensive, easily absorbed, mild laxative effect

Magnesium glycinate – one of the most bioavailable and absorbable forms, least likely to induce diarrhea, best option for correcting a long standing deficiency

Magnesium malate – highly soluble, vital component of enzymes, for people suffering from fatigue

Magnesium taurate – easily absorbed, no laxative properties, for people with cardiovascular issues

## Manganese

RDA:       None stated
SDA:       1-50 mg
Toxicity:  None stated

**Antagonists:**

Calcium, phosphorus – excessive intake of either

**Synergists:**

None specified

**Sources:**

Bananas, bran, celery, cereals, egg yolks, green leafy vegetables, legumes, liver, nuts, pineapples, whole grains

**Body Parts Affected:**

Brain, mammary glands, muscles, nerves

**Deficiency Symptoms:**

Ataxia(failure of muscle coordination), dizziness, ear noises, loss of hearing

**Signs and Symptoms of Toxicity:**

Neurologic symptoms similar to those of Parkinson's disease

**Uses:**

Allergies, asthma, diabetes, fatigue, Vitamin B 1 metabolism, Vitamin E utilization.

## Phosphorus

RDA:       800 mg
SDA:       800-1,000
Toxicity:  Not known

**Antagonists:**

Aluminum, iron, magnesium (excessive), sugar (excessive)

**Synergists:**

Vitamins: A, D, F, calcium, iron, manganese

**Sources:**

Eggs, fish, grains, glandular meats, meat, poultry, yellow cheese

**Body Parts Affected:**

Bones, brain, nerves, teeth

**Deficiency Symptoms:**

Fatigue, irregular breathing, loss of appetite, nervous disorders, overweight, weight loss

**Signs and Symptoms of Toxicity:**

Imbalance between phosphorus and calcium, kidney problems, possible psychiatric and motor disturbances, irritability, mood changes, compulsive behavior, reduced response speed.

**Uses:**

Arthritis, stress, stunted growth in children, tooth and gum disorders, helps regulate heart contractions, calcium and sugar metabolism.

## Potassium

|  |  |
|---|---|
| RDA: | None stated |
| SDA: | 100-300 mg |
| Toxicity: | Not known |

**Antagonists:**

Alcohol, coffee, cortisone, diuretics, laxatives, excessive salt, excessive sugar, stress

**Synergists:**

Vitamin B 6, sodium

**Sources:**

Dates, figs, peaches, tomato juice, blackstrap molasses, peanuts, raisins, seafood, apricots, bananas, flounder, potatoes, sunflower seeds, Swiss chard, spinach, broccoli, celery, avocado, Crimini mushrooms, Brussels sprouts, Romaine lettuce

**Body Parts Affected:**

Blood, heart, kidneys, muscles, nerves, skin

**Deficiency Symptoms:**

Acne, continuous thirst, dry skin, constipation, general weakness or fatigue, insomnia, muscle weakness or damage, nervousness, slow irregular heartbeat, weak reflexes, abdominal pain and cramps, and in severe cases, abnormal heart rhythms.

**Signs and Symptoms of Toxicity (hyperkalemia):**

Decreased blood pressure, diarrhea, fatigue, irritability, irregular heart beat, stomach cramps, vomiting, respitory failure, tingling sensation in the tongue, hands and feet.

Eliminated by taking calcium gluconate, sodium bicarbonate or a diuretic.

**Uses:**

Acne, alcoholism, allergies, burns, colic in infants, diabetes, high blood pressure, heart disease (angina pectoris, congestive heart failure, myocardial infarction), helps normalize heartbeat, relieves muscle contraction.

## Selenium

| | |
|---|---|
| RDA: | None stated |
| SDA: | 50 mcg. to 150 mcg. (20-30 mcg. in children) |
| Toxicity: | 400 mcg./day |

**Antagonists:**

Vitamin C and any processing has the tendency to destroy selenium.

**Synergists: Vitamin E.**

**Sources:**

Natural food sources include: Nuts (Brazil and walnuts), fish (tuna, cod, red snapper, and herring), beef and poultry, grains, onions, eggs, most vegetables, kelp, mushrooms, brewer's yeast, and milk.

**Body Parts Affected:**

Blood system, skin.

**Deficiency Symptoms:**

A few of the deficiency symptoms include: Muscle degeneration, muscular dystrophy, heart disease, premature aging, and liver damage. A prolonged severe deficiency can lead to cancer or even death.

**Signs and Symptoms of Toxicity:**

Symptoms of selenosis include: garlic breath, gastrointestinal disorders, hair loss, sloughing of nails and/or brittle nails, fatigue, irritability, and Amyotrophic Lateral Sclerosis (ALS) has been linked to selenosis.

**Uses:**

Selenium is a strong anti-oxidant. It prevents damage to red blood cells and slows the hardening of the tissues through oxidation. It protects against mercury toxicity and can help alleviate menopausal hot flashes.

**Sodium**
    RDA:      None stated

SDA:  100-300 mg
Toxicity: 14,000 mg

**Antagonists:**
Chlorine/potassium (lack of)

**Synergists:**
Vitamin D, potassium

**Sources:**
Salt, milk, cheese, seafood

**Body Parts Affected:**
Blood, lymph system, muscles, nerves

**Deficiency Symptoms:**
Loss of appetite, intestinal gas, muscle shrinkage, vomiting, weight loss

**Signs and Symptoms of Toxicity:**
Dehydration, fever, heat stroke

## Sulphur
RDA:  None stated
SDA:  Trace
Toxicity: Not known

**Antagonists:**
None specified

**Synergists:**
Vitamin B complex, B1, biotin, pantothenic acid

**Sources:**
Bran, cheese, clams, eggs, nuts, fish, wheat germ

**Body Parts Affected:**
Hair, nails, nerves, skin

**Deficiency Symptoms:**
Not known

**Uses:**
Collagen synthesis, body tissue formation, arthritis.
External: skin disorders (eczema, dermatitis, psoriasis)

## Zinc

| | |
|---|---|
| RDA: | 15 mg |
| SDA: | 20-100 mg (30 mg recommended) |

**Toxicity:**
Not known

**Antagonists:**
Alcohol, calcium and fiber (high intake), phosphorus (lack of), vegetarian diets

**Synergists:**
Vitamin A (high intake), calcium, copper, phosphorus

**Sources:**
Oysters, Brewer's yeast, liver, seafood, soybeans, spinach, sunflower seeds, mushrooms, pumpkin seeds, ginger root, whole grains

**Body Parts Affected:**
Blood, heart, prostate gland

**Deficiency Symptoms:**
Delayed sexual maturity, fatigue, loss of taste or smell, poor appetite, prolonged wound healing, retarded growth, sterility, increased susceptibility to infection, problems with acne, eczema, and psoriasis.

**Uses:**

Burn and wound healing (internal and external), carbohydrate digestion, prostate gland function, reproductive organ growth and development, vitamin B1, phosphorus and protein metabolism, alcoholism, atherosclerosis, baldness, cirrhosis, diabetes, high cholesterol, infertility.

Taking 45 mg daily has shown to lead to fewer infections and lower levels of oxidative stress.

Daily supplementation of zinc has been shown to reduce the risk of developing breast cancer by as much as 50%.

Research has noted that daily doses of 75 mg or more of zinc reduced the duration and severity of the common cold symptoms by an average of 42 percent.

# Chapter 6
## Amino Acids and Enzymes

## Amino Acids

Amino Acids are divided into two groups - essential and non-essential. Essential amino acids are those which cannot be produced in the body. They must be supplied to the body by one's diet. There are nine essential amino acids: Histidine, Isoleucine, Leucine, Lysine, Methionine, Phenylalanine, Threonine, Tryptophan, and Valine. The remaining 16 amino acids are non-essential and are created by transforming one amino acid to another. The transformation occurs primarily in the liver. Because of the transforming process, we must have an adequate supply of amino acids. Vegetarians, especially vegans, must be very observant of this in that a number of plant foods are deficient in amino acids. Most animal protein foods contain all of the essential amino acids, i.e., eggs, meat, milk, etc.

Amino acids are further classified as D or L. Dexyrotatory (D-), usually synthetic amino acids, means that they bend polarized light to the right. Levarotatory (L-), natural amino acids, bend polarized light to the left. These two classifications are mirror images of each other, yet the body more readily responds to the natural classification. Many manufacturers drop the L- and D- designations. The wise consumer will carefully read the labels to which is best for you. As with any supplement, a qualified wholistic healthcare professional should be contacted before adding a new supplement to your regime.

As with vitamins and minerals, taking too much of one amino acid will deplete the body of other amino acids. So, it is very important to take or consume a full range of amino acids to fully supply the body with its needs. However, unlike some vitamins and minerals, amino acids cannot be stored for later use. They must be supplied on a daily basis. Some common foods deficient in amino acids include:

| | | |
|---|---|---|
| Cereal grains | deficient in | Lysine |
| Gelatine | deficient in | Tryptophan |
| Legumes | deficient in | Methionine and Tryptophan |
| Rice and corn | deficient in | Threonine and Tryptophan |
| Soy beans | low in | Methionine |

## ESSENTIAL AMINO ACIDS

### L-HISTIDINE

**FOOD SOURCES:**
Most protein foods, including:
Cheese, eggs, milk, beef, pork, chicken, turkey, beans, peanut butter, tofu, and Greek yogurt

**COMPLEMENTARY MINERALS:**
Bromine
Chloride
Chromium
Potassium
Sodium
Zinc

**COMPLEMENTARY VITAMINS:**
Vitamin B3 (Niacin)
Vitamin B5 (Pantothenic Acid)

Vitamin C
Vitamin E

**GLANDS AFFECTED:**
Adrenal
Pineal

**TREATMENT APPLICATIONS:**
Histidine is used to form Histamine.

Histidine and Histamine are used to chelate trace minerals such as Copper and Zinc.

A deficiency can cause Tinnitus (ringing in the ear), most often in the right ear.

Other known conditions that have been treated include: hallucinations, paranoia, to improve sexual orgasm, impotence, and loss of sexual capability.

**SPECIAL NOTES:**
Histidine is obtainable from most protein foods. It is required by blood cells (red and white), bones, and the gastrointestinal tract for proper growth, repair, and functioning. Arginine is generally displaced by Histidine, so both should be taken together.

**L-ISOLEUCINE**

**FOOD SOURCES:**
Baked beans, Beef, Chicken, Cottage Cheese, Eggs, Fish, Legumes, Liver, Milk, and Soybeans.

**COMPLEMENTARY MINERALS:**
Calcium
Chromium
Magnesium
Selenium

Sulfur
Zinc

**COMPLEMENTARY VITAMINS:**
Vitamin A
Vitamin B Complex
Vitamin B-3
Vitamin B-12
Vitamin B-15
Vitamin C
Vitamin E

**GLANDS AND ORGANS AFFECTED:**
Eyes
Hypothalamus gland
Kidneys
Lymph glands
Pineal gland
Thymus gland

**TREATMENT APPLICATIONS:**
Maple Syrup Urine Disease

**SPECIAL NOTES:**
Maple Syrup Urine Disease is an accumulation of metabolites in the urine due to an imbalance of the amino acids Isoleucine, Leucine, and Valine. It is diagnosed by a sweet smelling odor in the urine.

L-Isoleucine deficiency can cause flu-like symptoms and gravel and hemoglobin in the blood.

## L-LEUCINE

**FOOD SOURCES:**
Baked beans, Beef, Chicken, Cottage cheese, Eggs, Fish, Liver,

Milk, Soybeans.

## COMPLEMENTARY MINERALS:
Calcium
Copper
Manganese
Selenium

## COMPLEMENTARY VITAMINS:
Vitamin A
Vitamin B Complex
Vitamin B-2
Vitamin B-12
Folic Acid

## GLANDS AND ORGANS AFFECTED:
Appendix
Lymph glands
Skin
Stomach
Thymus gland
Tonsils

## TREATMENT APPLICATIONS:
L-Leucine, along with L-Isoleucine, is used to treat Maple Syrup Urine Disease.

Other reported uses of L-Isoleucine include lowering blood sugar levels, relieving digestive problems, congested liver, damaged kidney, colon spasms, wound healing of skin and bones, and the inability to gain or lose weight.

## SPECIAL NOTES:
L-Leucine must be taken in a balanced proportion with Isoleucine and Valine to avoid nutritional conflict between these three.

## L-LYSINE

**FOOD SOURCES:**
Chicken, Eggs, Fish, Garbanzo beans, and Milk.
All Protein Foods.

**COMPLEMENTARY MINERALS:**
Calcium
Chromium
Iodine
Rubidium
Sodium
Zinc

**COMPLEMENTARY VITAMINS:**
Vitamin A
Vitamin B Complex
Vitamin B-2
Vitamin B-5
Vitamin B-6
Vitamin B-15
Vitamin C
Vitamin E
Niacin
PABA

**GLANDS AND ORGANS AFFECTED:**
Adrenal glands
Brain
Eyes
Hypothalamus
Pancreas
Pineal gland
Solar Plexus
Spine

Thyroid gland

**TREATMENT APPLICATIONS:**

L-Lysine has been used to alleviate anemia, depression, dizziness, fatigue, feeling of helplessness, and nausea. It has also been reported to be used in the treatment of Herpes Simplex and hypoglycemia.

**SPECIAL NOTES:**

Lysine helps with the absorption of calcium and the formation of collagen. Vitamin C aids in the process. Lysine should be taken with Methionine since one displaces the other.

## L-METHIONINE

**FOOD SOURCES:**

Egg yokes, Garlic, Onions, and Sarsaparilla.

**COMPLEMENTARY MINERALS:**

Chromium
Zinc

**COMPLEMENTARY VITAMINS:**

Vitamin A
Vitamin B-5
Vitamin B12
Vitamin C

**GLANDS AND ORGANS AFFECTED:**

Adrenal glands
Lymph glands
Thymus gland

**TREATMENT APPLICATIONS:**

Methionine helps prevent fat accumulation in the liver. It also helps prevent cholesterol build up by increasing the liver's pro-duction of lecithin. Methionine assists in protein synthesis and neutralizes free radicals (antioxidents). It stimulates hair growth and slows the aging process.

## SPECIAL NOTES:

Methionine has been shown to protect against cancer by car-rying the trace mineral Selenium to the body.

## L-PHENYLALANINE

Phenylalanine works best in the presence of vitamins B3, B6, C, copper and iron.

## FOOD SOURCES:

Egg whites, nuts, seeds such as cotton, sesame, and sunflower seeds.

Meats – Beef, chicken, turkey, pork, lamb, Alaskan native white fish, Pacific cod

Dairy – milk (especially whole milk), cheese, cottage cheese, Parmesan cheese

Soy

## COMPLEMENTARY MINERALS:

Calcium
Magnesium
Selenium
Sulfur

## COMPLEMENTARY VITAMINS:

Vitamin A
Vitamin B Complex
Vitamin B-3
Vitamin B15
Vitamin C
Vitamin E

## GLANDS AND ORGANS AFFECTED:
Eyes
Hypothalamus
Parathyroid gland
Pineal gland

## DEFICIENCY SYMPTOMS:
Swollen glands
Depression
Serous or mucous surface tumors
Rectal calculi

## TREATMENT APPLICATIONS:
Improves memory and alertness
Currently being used to treat depression, bipolar disorder, hyperactivity and Parkinson's disease
Pain killer for headaches, migraines, low back and neck pain, arthritis and menstrual cramps
Anxiety
Attention deficit-hyperactivity disorder (ADHD)

## SPECIAL NOTES:
Care should be taken when using Phenylalanine in that it has been known to elevate blood pressure. Taking too much Phenylalanine can cause headaches, insomnia, and irritability. DL-Phenylalanine is different than L-Phenylalanine in that it increases and prolongs the body's natural pain killing process. It decreases depression, including pre-menstrual depression. It increases the effects of acupuncture and electrical nerve stimulation. Phenylalanine reacts with Levodopa and MAOIs.

## L-THREONINE

## FOOD SOURCES:
Threonine is synthesized from aspartic acid.

Food sources high in threonine include: Cottage cheese, poultry, fish, meat, lentils, Black turtle bean, sesame seeds.

## COMPLEMENTARY MINERALS:
Calcium
Copper
Manganese
Selenium

## COMPLEMENTARY VITAMINS:
Vitamin A
Vitamin B complex
Vitamin B-2
Vitamin B-12
Folic Acid

## GLANDS AND ORGANS AFFECTED:
Appendix
Lymph glands
Peyer's patches
Skin
Stomach
Thymus gland
Tonsils

## DEFICIENCY SYMPTOMS:
Dysmenorrhea (painful menstruation)
Intermittent spotting
Inflamed uterus
Ovarian cysts
Indigestion
Intestinal malfunction
Sore throat

**TREATMENT APPLICATIONS:**

Threonine has been used for many female problems including painful or difficult menstruation, ovarian cysts, irritated uterus, gastrointestinal difficulties, and certain food allergies, especially fats.

**SPECIAL NOTES:**

Threonine prevents fatty build up in the liver. It is also an important element in collagen, elastin, and enamel protein.

## L-TRYPTOPHAN

**FOOD SOURCES:**

Beef, Chicken, Eggs, Fish, Milk, Soybeans

**COMPLEMENTARY MINERALS:**

Calcium
Magnesium
Selenium
Sulfur

**COMPLEMENTARY VITAMINS:**

Vitamin A
Vitamin B-3 (Niacin)
Vitamin E

**GLANDS AND ORGANS AFFECTED:**

Lung
Lymph glands
Parathyroid gland
Spleen
Thymus

**DEFICIENCY SYMPTOMS:**

Arthritis

Dermatitis (especially at the back of the hands and neck)
Insomnia
Schizophrenia

## TREATMENT APPLICATIONS:

Tryptophan is a precursor to Serotonin, an inhibitory neuro-transmitter in the brain. An increase supply of Tryptophan will decrease the activities of neurons and will help induce sleep and calmness. L-Tryptophan has been used to ease or alleviate migraine headaches. Some emotional disorders, including anxiety and depression, have been greatly helped by using Tryptophan. It helps produce Niacin which counteracts the effects of nicotine. Tryptophan helps reduce blood pressure, blood fats, and cholesterol.

## SPECIAL NOTES:

Tryptophan helps utilize the B complex vitamins. Note that Tryptophan elevates blood histamine levels.

## L-VALINE

## FOOD SOURCES:
Valine is biosynthesized from proteins, i.e., meats, dairy products, soy products, beans, and legumes.

## COMPLEMENTARY MINERALS:
Copper
Magnesium
Manganese
Sulfur

## COMPLEMENTARY VITAMINS:
Vitamin A
Vitamin B complex

Vitamin C
Vitamin E

**GLANDS AND ORGANS AFFECTED:**
Appendix
Duodenum
Heart
Liver
Lymph glands
Peyer's Patches
Posterior Pituitary gland
Skin
Spleen
Thymus
Thyroid
Tonsils

**DEFICIENCY SYMPTOMS:**
Erythema (abnormal reddening of the skin)
Insomnia
Mental and emotional disturbances
Nervousness
Spitting up blood
Throat and rectal inflamation

**TREATMENT APPLICATIONS:**
Valine has been used successfully in treating the above disorders as well as in combination with Leucine and Isoleucine to treat Maple Syrup Urine Disease.

**SPECIAL NOTES:**
Human insulin is made up of Alanine, Cystein, Serine, and Valine.

## NATTOKINASE

### FOOD SOURCES:

Nattokinase is an enzyme extracted and purified from a Japanese food called natto. Natto is made from fermented soy beans. During the fermentation process a bacteria (Bacillus natto) is added. Nattokinase is produced when the bacteria acts on the soy beans. Recently other processes have been found to produce Nattokinase. This enzyme exhibits a strong fibrinolytic activity.

### GLANDS AND ORGANS AFFECTED:

The entire cardiovascular system is benefitted by Nattokinase.

### DEFICIENCY SYMPTOMS:

There are no known deficiency symptoms associated with nattokinase.

### TREATMENT APPLICATIONS:

Nattokinase is a known blood thinner and clot buster. It helps to reduce blood clots, lower blood pressure, decreases the risk of stroke and reduces varicose veins. It has been shown to help prevent DVT (Deep Vein Thrombosis). Some studies have shown it helpful with Alzheimer's disease and diabetes. The recommended dosage is 2,000 to 4,000 FU (fibrolytic units)/day. Authorities recommend 1,000 - 2,000 in the morning and the same dosage in the evening.

### SPECIAL NOTES:

Nattokinase should not be taken if pregnant, have any blood disorders or if the body is losing too much blood. It should never be used while taking any other blood thinner including aspirin. Possible side effects include: inability of the blood to clot, bruising, bleeding, nausea, dizziness, and severely reduced blood pressure.

# NON-ESSENTIAL AMINO ACIDS

Non essential amino acids can be manufactured in the body whenever the essential amino acids are present. In other words, our bodies produce non-essential amino acids even when we don't get them from the food we eat.

## ALANINE

### SOURCES:
Dairy products, eggs, fish, gelatin, meat, seafood

Beans, bran, brewer's yeast, brown rice, corn, nuts, seeds, soy, yeast

Alanine is synthesized in the body from Acetaldehyde or Aspartic Acid.

### COMPLEMENTARY MINERALS:
Calcium
Chromium
Magnesium
Selenium
Sulfur
Zinc

### COMPLEMENTARY VITAMINS:
Vitamin A
Vitamin C
Vitamin B complex
Vitamins B - 2, 3, 12, 15
Vitamin E
PABA
Pantothenic Acid (B 5)

### GLANDS AND ORGANS AFFECTED:
Brain

Eyes
Hypothalamus
Pineal
Thyroid
Thymus

**DEFICIENCY SYMPTOMS:**
Depleted, burned out feeling
Fatigue
Convulsions
Mental degeneration
Spastic movements
Muscle contractions
Night sweats
Tics or twitches

**TREATMENT APPLICATIONS:**
Boosts the immune system via lymphocyte production
Helps regulate blood sugar
Boosts the adrenal glands
Reduces the symptoms of benign prostate hypertrophy when taken with glycine
Muscle building, repair and endurance

**SPECIAL NOTES:**
Alanine is used as a food seasoning.
Deficiency symptoms are often caused by poor diet and/or insufficient rest.

## L-ARGININE

**FOOD SOURCES:**
Beef, pork, dairy products, poultry, seafood, wild game, gelatin, buckwheat, flour, granola, lupins, cooked soybeans, nuts including peanuts, seeds, wheat germ, oatmeal

Arginine is synthesized in the body from ornithine, but too slowly to fulfill all the body's requirements.

**COMPLEMENTARY MINERALS:**
Calcium
Magnesium
Selenium
Sulfur

**COMPLEMENTARY VITAMINS:**
Vitamin A
Vitamin B complex
Vitamin B3 (Niacin)
Vitamin B15
Vitamin C
Vitamin E

**GLANDS AND ORGANS AFFECTED:**
Appendix
Eyes
Hypothalamus
Lymph
Parathyroid
Peyer's Patches
Pineal
Skin
Thymus
Tonsils

**DEFICIENCY SYMPTOMS:**
Inflamation, especially of the veins
Intestinal disorders
Sterility

**TREATMENT APPLICATIONS:**

Increases muscle mass and decreases body fat in body builders

Tinnitus

Antidote for some allergies

**SPECIAL NOTES:**

Arginine deficiency has been thought to be the cause of cellulite accumulation

When balanced with Lysine, it helps avoid cold sores (herpes eruptions) Inhibits the growth of several types of tumors, especially mammary tumors

Aids in wound healing

Stimulates the immune system, especially severely ill or injured patients

Stimulates the thymus gland

Assists in liver regeneration

Detoxifies ammonia

## L-ASPARAGINE

**FOOD SOURCES:**

Asparagus

**COMPLEMENTARY MINERALS:**

Chromium

Zinc

**COMPLEMENTARY VITAMINS:**

Vitamin A

Choline

Inositol

Niacin

**GLANDS AND ORGANS AFFECTED:**

Liver

Lymph
Thymus

**DEFICIENCY SYMPTOMS:**
Gallbladder dysfunction
Liver disorders

**TREATMENT APPLICATIONS:**
Asparagine is used in the treatment of brain and nervous system disorders.

**SPECIAL NOTES:**
Asparagine is synthesized in the body from Asparic acid.
Asparagine metabolizes toxic ammonia in the body.

## L-ASPARTIC ACID:

**FOOD SOURCES:**
Legumes such as garbanzo beans, lentils, and soybeans
Nuts such as almonds, flaxseeds, peanuts, and walnuts
Animal sources such as beef, eggs, salmon, and shrimp

**GLANDS AND ORGANS AFFECTED:**
Hormonal glands
Nervous system

**DEFICIENCY SYMPTOMS:**
Hypo hormonal conditions, i.e., hypothyroid, hypopituitary, etc.
Altered nervous system response and reaction

**TREATMENT APPLICATIONS:**
Aspartic acid is used to relieve fatigue and increase stamina.

**SPECIAL NOTES:**

Through enzymatic reaction, Aspartic acid is produced in the body from ammonia and Fumaric acid.

Aspartic acid is used by the body to manufacture the essential amino acid theonine.

This amino acid detoxifies ammonia and helps protect the liver.

Aspartic acid is a mineral transporter

It helps form Ribonucleotides, precursors of RNA and DNA.

Aspartic acid helps neutralize milk allergies.

## L-CARNITINE

**FOOD SOURCES:**

Muscle and organ meats

Chicken, Eggs, Fish, garlic, onions, and all protein foods to provide Lysine and methionine (for transformation)

**GLANDS AND ORGANS AFFECTED:**

Testes

Blood

**DEFICIENCY SYMPTOMS:**

Ketosis

Cardiomyopathy

Skeletal muscle weakness

Hypoglycemia

**TREATMENT APPLICATIONS:**

Reduce fatty acids and triglycerides

Possible male infertility

Treatment of Ketosis (a build up of Ketone bodies or fat waste) in the blood

Strengthens the heart

Anti-ischemic

Reduces the possibility of heart attack

**SPECIAL NOTES:**

In the presence of sufficient amounts of Vitamin C, B-6, and Niacin (B-3), Carnitine is obtained in the body by the transformation of Lysine and Methionine.

It has been noted that frequent use of Safflower oil (Vitamin F) in application to the skin causes a deficiency of Carnitine. Symptoms may include sore throat, chest pain, and a heavy feeling in the throat.

Men have a higher carnitine levels than women, the highest amounts are found in the testes and provides mobility and fertility to the sperm.

Carnitine regulates Ketones in the blood. If unchecked, the blood can become acidic and Calcium, Magnesium, and Potassium can be lost in the urine which can become fatal.

## CITROLINE

**FOOD SOURCES:**

Rind of a watermelon
Made from ornithine and arginine

**GLANDS AND ORGANS AFFECTED:**

Liver
Kidneys

**DEFICIENCY SYMPTOMS:**

Iron deficiency

**TREATMENT APPLICATIONS:**

Increased energy

**SPECIAL NOTES:**

Manufactured in the liver by Lysine.
Converted to Arginine then to Ornithine in the kidney.
Converts ammonia to urea and excreted in the form of urine.

## L-Cysteine &L-Cystine

### SOURCE:
The body forms Cysteine from Serine and Methionine.

### BODY PARTS AFFECTED:
Blood
Skin

### DEFICIENCY SYMPTOMS:
Age spots
Arteriosclerosis
Arthritis
Skin disorders

### TREATMENT APPLICATIONS:
Healing the skin from burns, cuts, and surgical operations

### SPECIAL NOTES:
Cysteine is required to properly structure certain enzymes, hormones, and neuropeptides that contain sulfur.

As an antioxidant and free radical scavenger, Cysteine can protect proteins, fats, and nucleic acids (RNA and DNA). Free radical damage to cells can lead to age spots, aged skin, arthritis, hardening of the arteries, and certain types of mutagenic disorders, i.e., cancer.

Cysteine can help protect from the adverse effects of smoking and drinking.

Cysteine may help protect against toxins from pollution.

## L-GLUTAMIC ACID

### FOOD SOURCES:
Wheat gluten
Wheat protein

**COMPLEMENTARY MINERALS:**
Chromium
Manganese
Potassium
Sodium
Zinc

**COMPLEMENTARY VITAMINS:**
B complex
Vitamin B-3 (Niacin)
Vitamin B-5 (Pantothenic Acid)
Vitamin B-6
Vitamin C

**GLANDS AND ORGANS AFFECTED:**
Adrenals
Pancreas
Spine

**DEFICIENCY SYMPTOMS:**
Fatigue
Irritability
Increased urination
Mood swings
Possible contributing cause of Epilepsy, Hepatic coma, Muscular Dystrophy, and
mental retardation.

**TREATMENT APPLICATIONS:**
Enhance brain activity
Chronic Fatigue Syndrome
Multiple Sclerosis

**SPECIAL NOTES:**
Glutamic acid accepts ammonia throughout the body and is

transformed to Glutamine. It is transformed in the liver to urea and excreted by the kidneys. By absorbing ammonia, it protects the brain from excessive ammonia. A prominent agent in brain metabolism, Glutamic acid and its derivatives make up about half of the amino acids in the brain. The brain is made up of approximately 90% protein. It is an important factor in the Krebs Cycle of energy.

## L-GLUTAMINE

**FOOD SOURCES:**
Beet juice
Wheat protein

**COMPLEMENTARY MINERALS:**
Calcium, Selenium
Chromium, Sulfur
Magnesium, Zinc

**COMPLEMENTARY VITAMINS:**
Vit. A
Vit. B-3 (Niacin)
Vit. E

**GLANDS AND ORGANS AFFECTED:**
Heart
Lymph
Thymus

**DEFICIENCY SYMPTOMS:**
Difficulty breathing (dyspnea)
Cardiac difficulties
Flu-like symptoms

**TREATMENT APPLICATIONS:**

Glutamine attaches to ammonia in the central nervous system and takes it to the kidneys for elimination.

It is known to improve IQ.

It has been used to help with petite mal epilepsy, schizophrenia, and senility.

It helps improve ulcers.

**SPECIAL NOTES:**

Glutamine is essential for the synthesis of niacin.

**L-GLYCINE**

**SOURCE:**

Glycine is biosynthesized in the body from the amino acid serine.

**COMPLEMENTARY MINERALS:**

Magnesium

Sulfur

**COMPLEMENTARY VITMINS:**

Vit. A

Vit. B-complex (especially B2, B3, PABA)

Vit. C

Vit. E

**GLANDS AND ORGANS AFFECTED:**

Bones

Heart

Liver

Spleen

Thyroid

**DEFICIENCY SYMPTOMS:**

A deficiency can lead to convulsions due to over-excitability of the brain.

**TREATMENT APPLICATIONS:**
Glycine has been used effectively to treat progressive muscular dystrophy.

It is an inhibitory neurotransmitter in the CNS.

## L-HYDROXYPROLINE

**FOOD SOURCES:**
Gelatin

**COMPLEMENTARY MINERALS:**
Calcium
Chlorine
Fluorine
Lithium
Magnesium
Sodium
Sulfur

**COMPLEMENTARY VITAMINS:**
Vit. A
Vit. B2
Vit. B3
Vit. C
PABA

**GLANDS AND ORGANS AFFECTED:**
Bones
Cartilage
Connective tissue
Ligaments
Skin

Tendons

## DEFCIENCY SYMPTOMS:
Bone decay
Dizziness
Hyper thyroid
Overtaxed nervous system
Rickets
Sciatic neuralgia
Tooth decay

## TREATMENT APPLICATIONS:
Helps increase calcium absorption
Prevents hardening and loss of function of some organs

## ORNITHINE

## SOURCES:
Ornithine is a product of the action of arginase on L-Arginine creating urea.

## GLANDS AND ORGANS AFFECTED:
Liver

## DEFICIENCY SYMPTOMS:
Visual field and visual sharpness reduction
Cataracts
Night blindness
Fatigue

## TREATMENT APPLICATIONS:
Converts into other amino acids
Releases growth hormones
Helps athletes in training, especially in weight training
Increases energy

Used to fight cirrhosis

Helps excrete ammonia

## L-PROLINE

**FOOD SOURCES:**

Casein (milk protein)

Beet sugar

Molasses

**COMPLEMENTARY MINERALS:**

Aluminum

Calcium

Chromium

Phosphorus

Selenium

Sulfur

Zinc

**COMPLEMENTARY VITAMINS:**

Vit. A

Vit. B complex

Vit. B2 & Vit. B12

Trypsin & Chymotrypsin

Folic acid

**GLANDS AND ORGANS AFFECTED:**

Bones

Duodenum

Heart

Liver

Spleen

Stomach

Thyroid

**DEFICIENCY SYMPTOMS:**

Ringing in left ear (tennitis)

If prolonged, can result in "gyrute atrophy" affecting vision and the eye

## TREATMENT APPLICATIONS:

Converts into other amino acids

Releases growth hormones

## L-SERINE

## SOURCES:

Synthesized from metabolism, primarily from protein

## COMPLEMENTARY MINERALS:

Calcium

Chromium

Magnesium

Selenium

Sulfur

Zinc

## COMPLEMENTARY VITAMINS:

Vit. A

All B vitamins

Vit. C

Vit. E

Folic acid

## GLANDS AND ORGANS AFFECTED:

Brain

Eyes

Hypothalamus

Stomach & Pancreas

Pineal gland

Spine

**DEFICIENCY SYMPTOMS:**
Cough
Increased sensitivity
Irritability
Nervousness
Seizures
Small head
Psychomotor retardation
Retarded growth

**TREATMENT APPLICATIONS:**
Assists enzymes in digestion
Helps in the construction of RNA and DNA
Natural skin moisturizing factor

## L-TAURINE

**SOURCES:**
From the biosynthesis of methionine and cysteine
Found only in animal products
Second most abundant amino acid in human milk
Metabolized in the liver

**COMPLEMENTARY MINERALS:**
Calcium
Chromium
Potassium
Sodium
Zinc

**COMPLEMENTARY VITAMINS:**
B complex
Vit. B6
Vit. C
Vit. E

## GLANDS AND ORGANS AFFECTED:
Bones
Duodenum
Heart
Liver
Parathyroid gland
Pineal gland
Pituitary gland
Thyroid gland

## DEFICIENCY SYMPTOMS:
Epileptic seizures
Visual impairment
Memory loss
Fat allergy
Heart problems due to retaining potassium
Excessive alcohol consumption depletes Taurine

## TREATMENT APPLICATIONS:
Promotes the regulation of blood sugar
Anticonvulsant
Helps maintain proper bile composition
Helps keep cholesterol soluble
Helps prevent gall stones
Prevents loss of potassium from the heart muscle
Prevents calcium and potassium waste during stress or weight
loss

## L-TYROSINE

## FOOD SOURCES:
Aged cheese
Avocados
Ripe bananas
Beer

Chicken livers
Pickled herring
Wine
Yeast

**COMPLEMENTARY MINERALS:**
Calcium
Magnesium
Selenium

**COMPLEMENTARY VITAMINS:**
Vit. A
Vit. B5 (Pantothenic Acid)
Vit. C
Vit. E

**GLANDS AND ORGANS AFFECTED:**
Adrenal gland
Anterior pituitary gland
Lymph
Peyer's patches
Skin
Thymus
Tonsils

**DEFICIENCY SYMPTOMS:**
Fatigue

**TREATMENT APPLICATIONS:**
Relieve stress
Improve cognitive and physical performance
Suppresses the appetite
Anti-depressant
Controls anxiety
Better sleep when taken with L-Tryptophan

Causes the release of growth hormones causing muscle growth and reduces fat

Precursor to epinephrine, nor epinephrine, and thyroxin

Anti-oxidant

## Enzymes

Enzymes are proteins necessary for every chemical reaction of the body. Without enzymes, vitamins, minerals and hormones cannot be utilized by the body. Enzymes digest food. They affect every cell, tissue, organ and fluid in the body. They are catalysts for every chemical reaction of the body.

There are three categories of enzymes – metabolic, pancreatic and plant (food) enzymes. **Metabolic enzymes** are produced in the body and are responsible for chemical reactions in the body including moving, breathing, talking, thinking and even immunity. They are necessary for all stages of digestion. **Pancreatic enzymes**, approximately 22 of them, are secreted mainly from the pancreas but also from the mouth to the small intestine. They are necessary for proper digestion of food. The third category is **plant (food) enzymes.** These are present in all raw plants. However, GMO's significantly alter their usefulness and effectiveness. These enzymes work in the mouth, stomach and small intestine. One thing to remember is that all enzymes are heat sensitive. Any process that involves temperatures above 118 degrees will destroy enzymes. That involves cooking, pasteurization, microwaving and canning. Digestive enzymes should be taken <u>with </u>food so that the digestive process can run smoothly and be more effective.

Some of the most common digestive enzymes are:

Protease – digests proteins

Amylase – digests carbohydrates

Lipase – digests fats

Disacchaaridases – digest sugar

Cellulase – digests soluable fiber

To properly nourish every cell in every part of our bodies, it takes over 1,000 nutrients each day. According to Dr. Dicqie Fuller in her book "The Healing Power of Enzymes," it takes (in their proper amounts):

    19 minerals
    13 vitamins
    9 amino acids
    1 protein
    1 fat
    1 water
    1 carbohydrate
    1,300 enzymes

So obviously, if all the above are not available in the diet, supplementation is necessary.

Here's a quick review of digestion with a close look at the role of enzymes. Digestion begins when food is adequately chewed. The salivary glands begin the process by secreting the digestive enzymes amylase, lipase and some protease. Raw fruits, vegetables and whole grains contain cellulase to break down soluable fiber to a digestable form. Cellulase is not produced in the human body and must be taken by supplementation or from plants.

In the upper part of the stomach, amylase digests up to 60% of carbohydrates, protease up to 30% of protein, and lipase up to 10% of fat. Hydrochloric acid and pepsin continue to break down food in the stomach. Hydrochloric acid from the blood, within the first hour of digestion, increases the acidity (pH 3.0 – 1.5) in the lower portion of the stomach to deactivate the plant enzymes. At that point chief cells secrete pepsin to further break down protein. This action maintains the stomach pH below 3.0 so that pepsin can continue working.

From the stomach, the contents flow through the pyloric valve into the duodenum (upper part of the small intestine). An alkaline substance called bicarbonate is combined at this point with bile from the gallbladder and pancreatic enzymes to reactivate food enzymes. In the next section of the small intestine (jejunum), di-saccharidases are secreted to further digest sugar. The majority of nutrients from digested food are absorbed into the blood in the small intestine. The digestion continues through the last section of the small intestine (ileum) until it reaches the ileo-cecal valve. At that point the liquefied nutrients are passed into the large intestine where the liquid and salts are absorbed into the blood stream and feces are formed.

**Serrapeptase** is a proteolytic enzyme that digests protein. However, recent studies have shown that it also helps eliminate internal organ scar tissue and reducing or eliminating arterial plaquing. It has been shown to be as effective, or more so, than non-steroidal anti-infammatory drugs (NSAIDs) in blocking pain or in curbing inflammatory reactions. Clinical trials have shown success in treating arthritis, carpal tunnel syndrome, fibrocystic breast disease, lung and sinus conditions. And there are no known side effects.

# Chapter 7
## More System Boosters

## HERBS FOR HEALING

Any plant that is used for food, flavoring, medicine, or perfume can be considered an herb. They are used throughout the world for culinary, medicinal, aromatic, and spiritual uses. Regardless of the many studies and successes over the years, in the United States, modern medicine will probably never accept the efficacy of medicinal herbs because of the influence of the pharmaceutical companies. It is virtually impossible to have a study published because many of these doctors sit on the editorial boards of journals and publications.

Nonetheless, herbs have been used for healing for many years. Chinese herbal medicine used herbs since before the first century. The Ayurveda medicinal system in India is based on herbs. Archaeological evidence has shown the use of medicinal plants as far back as the Paleolithic period, over 60,000 years ago. The Sumerians over 5,000 years ago created a list of plants and listed remedies. Several ancient cultures wrote about the medicinal use of plants. The Egyptians wrote about medicinal plants in their Egyptian medicinal papyri and in tombs. During the 3rd century B.C., the Greeks wrote about herbs in the Diocles of Carystus, and in the 1st century B.C. by Krateuas. Over the centuries, thousands of doctors and healers have used herbs for healing.

There are several terms associated with herbs that are helpful to know:

- Infusions – hot water extracts of herbs through steeping, i.e., chamomile or mint
- Decoctions – long-term boiled extracts, i.e., roots or bark
- Maceration – old infusion of plants with high mucilage content, i.e., sage or thyme
- Tinctures – alcoholic extracts of herbs
- Extracts – liquid, dry or nebulisates
- Liquid – lower ethanol percentage than tinctures, made by distilling tinctures
- Dry – plant material evaporated into a dry mass and produced as capsule or tablet
- Nebulisate – a dry extract created by freeze drying
- Essential oils – extracts that are generally applied to the skin
- Inhalation – in aromatherapy, used as a therapy to help change moods

**IMPORTANT:** Several of these herbs should not be used if pregnant, nursing, or have a medical condition that requires specific medication. Be sure to research thoroughly or discuss usage with a naturopath, holistic doctor or holistic pharmacist.

The following are a few herbs and some specifics about them:

## Alfalfa
**Parts used:** Herb
**Best time:** Before meals
**Contains:** Vitamins A, D, E, K, calcium, iron, magnesium, phosphorus, potassium, silicon, 8 digestive enzymes.
**Action:** Helps with rheumatoid arthritis, lupus, ALS
    Combats allergies
    Strengthens the heart
    Relieves muscle fatigue

## Aloe Vera
**Parts used:** Leaves
**Best time:** External – any time, Internal - evening
**Contains:** Calcium, iron, lecithin, manganese, potassium, sodium, zinc
**Action:** Externally – cuts, burns, wounds, skin irritations, insect bites
    Internally - stops internal scar tissue, helps with gastritis, constipation, hyperaciditiy, stomach ulcers
    Helps detoxify

## Ashwagandha
**Parts used:** Roots and berries
**Best time:** Any time
**Contains:** Alkaloids, steroidal lactones
**Action:** External – Helps with tumors, carbuncles, ulcers
Eases tension, anxiety and fatigue
Increases concentration
Boosts endurance
Increases DHEA, precursor hormone to testosterone, estrogen and progesterone
Aids in sleep
Decreases blood sugar levels

## Black Cohosh
**Parts used:** Root
**Best time:** Bedtime
**Contains:** Vitamins A, B5, inositol, calcium, iron, magnesium, phosphorus, potassium, silicon
**Action:** Acts as a sedative
    Contains estrogen – helps many female conditions
    Relieves childbirth and menstrual pain
    Helps dispel uric acid
    Neutralizes blood toxins
    Normalizes blood pressure

May prevent many palvic conditions
May stimulate vaginal lubrication

## Black Walnut
**Contains:** Vitamin B5, calcium, iodine, iron, magnesium, manganese, phosphorus, potassium, silica
**Action:** External – skin conditions such as poison oak and ring worm
Internal - helps oxygenate the blood to destroy parasites
Dries lactating mother's milk

## Blessed Thistle
**Parts used:** Herb
**Best time:** Anytime, best in afternoon
**Contains:** Vitamin B-complex, calcum, iron, manganese, phosphorus,potassium
**Action:** Improves digestion and circulation
Stimulates memory
Balances hormones – helps with cramps, headaches, menopause
Stimulates mother's milk
Strengthens the heart, liver, lungs, kidneys

## Burdock
**Parts used:** Root
**Best time:** Morning or afternoon
**Contains:** Vitamins A, B-complex, C, E, PABA, copper, iodine, potassium, zinc, sugar, lappin, resin, inulin, mucilage, some tannic acid
**Action:** Helps regulate hormone levels
Helps eliminate gout, eczema, skin conditions
Increases urine flow to clear the kidneys of uric acid and wastes
Helps break down calcium deposits and reduce joint swelling
Helps purify the blood

## Cayenne
**Parts used:** Fruit

**Best time:** Any time, best in the afternoon
**Contains:** Vitamins A, B-complex, C, calcium, iron, some magnesium, phosphorus, potassium, sulfur, capsaicin
**Action:** Acts as a catalyst to enhance the effectiveness of other herbs
Helps improve circulation and strengthen the heart
Topically helps stop bleeding and relieves pain

## Cascara Sagrada
**Parts used:** Bark
**Best time:** Bedtime
**Contains:** Vitamin B-complex, aluminum, calcium, lead, manganese, potassium, strontium, tin
**Action:** Helps discharge gallstones
Helps relieve constipation

## Celery
**Parts used:** Root and seed
**Best time:** Morning until noon
**Contains:** Vitamins A, B, C, calcium, iron, magnesium, phosphorus, potassium, silicon, sulfur

**Action:** Helps alkalinize the body
Helps with arthritis, low back pain, neuralgia, incontinence, gout

## Chamomile
**Parts used:** Flower
**Best time:** Anytime
**Contains:** Vitamin A, calcium, iron, magnesium, manganese, potassium, zinc, the amino acid tryptophan
**Action:** External – Relieves sore muscles and swelling
Wash for open sores and eczema
Internal – Helps alleviate pain from drug withdrawal, menstruation
Soothes the stomach and releases gas as in colic

Helps induce sleep

Helps reduce inflammation

## Chanca Piedra (Stone breaker)
**Parts used:** Entire plant – roots, stem, leaf
**Best time:** 2-3 times daily
**Contains:** Rutin, B-amyrin, geraniin, quercetin, dibencylbutirolactone, gallic acid, ethyl ester, stigmasterol, alkaloid phyllanthoside
**Action:** Antilithic (expelling stones), liver protective, pain-relieving, hypotensive, antispasmodic, antiviral, antibacterial, diuretic, antimutagenic, hypoglycemic.

Further actions: Expels stones, supports kidneys, increases urination, relieves pain, protects and detoxifies the liver, reduces inflammation, kills viruses, clears obstructions, lowers blood sugar, blood pressure and cholesterol, expels kidney and gallbladder stones.

## Chaparral
**Parts used:** Leaves
**Best time:** Afternoon
**Contains:** Aluminum, barium, chloride, molybdenum, potassium (high), silicon, sodium (high), sulfur, tin
**Action:** External – helps for herpes, eczema, hemorrhoids, skin diseases, arthritic pain

Internal – Helps to detoxify the body

Has been used to treat venereal disease and some forms of cancer

## Chickweed
**Parts used:** Tops
**Best time:** Early morning and/or late evening
**Contains:** Vitamins A, B-complex, C, D, calcium, copper, iron, manganese, molybdenum, phosphorus, zinc
**Action:** External – helps with burns, boils, skin conditions, swollen testes, sore eyes

Internal – helps with ulcers and inflamed bowels

Has antiseptic properties for the blood

## Comfrey
**Parts used:** Leaves and root
**Best time:** Anytime
**Contains:** Vitamins A, C, calcium, copper, iron, magnesium, phosphorus, potassium, zinc, 18 amino acids
**Action:** External – helps heal wounds, burns, open sores
    Internal – Helps with ulcerated GI system
    Helps expedite the repair of broken bones
    Aids digestion
    Destroys amoebic-like bacteria
**Caution:** Do not take if on MAO inhibitors.
    It's best not to take internally for an extended length of time.
    Best use: Make a poultice of
        4 cups chopped comfrey leaves and mix with
        ¼ cup of olive oil, coconut oil, or almond oil
        Wrap the paste with a cotton cloth
        Apply directly to the affected area for 30 minutes
        Once or twice per day for 10 days

## Culver's Root
**Parts used:** Flower
**Best time:** Any time
**Contains:** Cinnamic acid, glycoside, gum, mannitol, phytosterols, resin saponins, tannins
**Action:** Helps with liver congestion and constipation
    Used to treat liver, gallbladder, constipation, colitis, hepatitis
    Caution: Avoid using with bile duct obstruction, gall stones, internal hemorrhoids, menstruation, pregancy

## Dandelion
**Parts used:** Leaves and root
**Best time:** Any time
**Contains:** Vitamins A, B-complex, C, E, calcium, cobalt, copper, iron, nickel, phosphorus, potassium, sodium, tin, zinc
**Action:** External – juice is helpful in drying up warts

Has been used on acne, blisters, and corns

Has been used to strengthen the kidneys, liver, and pancreas

Internal – has been helpful with gallstones and jaundice

## Devil's Claw

**Parts used:** Leaves, secondary tubers

**Best time:** Any time

**Contains:** Aceteoside, harpagia, iridoid glycosides, luteolin, procumbine, phytosterols

**Action:** Internal – helps clean toxins from blood cells, muscles and joints

Helps to remove uric acid

Has been used to help arthritis, arteriosclerosis, gallstones, gout, and liver disease

## Echinacea

**Parts used:** Root

**Best time:** Evening

**Contains:** Vitamins A, C, E, copper, iodine, iron, potassium, sulfur

**Action:** Elevates the white blood cell count

Stimulates the lymphatic system

Purifies the blood

Acts as an antiseptic to remove viral formations

Removes toxins from the blood

Increases immunity

Lowers cholesterol

Strengthens the pancreas, liver, spleen and kidneys

## Evening Primrose

**Parts used:** Bark, oil from leaves, seeds, flowers

**Best time:** Any time

**Contains:** Vitamin F, magnesium, potassium, silicon, sulfur, zinc gammalinolenic acid

**Action:** Helps lower cholesterol

Inhibits formation of plaque and clots in arteries

Helps detox the liver
Helps relieve the itching, swelling, crusting and redness of eczema

## Eyebright
**Parts used:** Leaves, stem, flowers
**Best time:** Any time
**Contains:** Beta-carotene, vitamin C, choline, essential oil, euphrastanic acid, glucose, glycosides, mannose, phenolic acids
**Action:** External – as a poultice to treat the redness, swelling and visual disturbances caused by blepharitis and conjunctivitis
Internal - Strengthens eye tissues, soothes eye strain
Clears vision
Helps fight eye infections
Helps treat poor memory
Helps treat vertigo

## Fennel
**Parts used:** Seeds
**Best time:** Before a meal
**Contains:** Vitamin E, potassium, sodium, sulfur
**Action:** Settles stomach acid, good for colic, cramps, appetite suppressant
Helps increase the flow of mother's milk and menstrual flow
Intestinal stimulant and antiseptic
Sedative for small children
Used for pain relief, mild diuretic, anticonvulsive

## Fenugreek
**Parts used:** Fruit, stem, leaves
**Best time:** Any time
**Contains:** Vitamins A, B1, B2, B3, D, choline, iron, lecithin
**Action:** External – used as an insect repellant
Internal – Dissolves cholesterol and fat deposits in the blood stream
Destroys parasites

Anti-viral – fights lung infections

Expels mucus and phlegm from bronchial tubes

## Figs

**Parts used:** Fruit

**Best time:** Cool time of the day

**Contains:** Vitamins A, E, K, calcium, copper, iron, magnesium, potassium

**Action:** Relieves constipation and lung inflammation

## Garlic

**Parts used:** Bulb

**Best time:** Any time

**Contains:** Vitamins A, B1, C, calcium, copper, iron, manganese, potassium, selenium, sulfur, zinc, alliin (allicin when chopped – powerful antibiotic)

**Action:** External – Helps heal earaches, skin parasites, ringworm, warts

Internal – Helps resolve a cold

Dissolves cholesterol

Helps lower blood pressure

Helps reduce headaches, backaches, angina, dizziness

Kills parasites

As an enema – helps resolve bowel infections and kills parasites

As a douche – resolves yeast infections

May reduce the risk of some cancers, especially gastrointestinal

## Ginger

**Parts used:** Root

**Best time:** Any time

**Contains:** Vitamins A, B-complex, C, calcium, iron, magnesium, phosphorus, potassium

**Action:** A good transport herb by enhancing the effectiveness of other herbs

Relieves intestinal gas

Helps lower cholesterol
Stops nausea, morning sickness, motion sickness
Relieves stomach and colon spasms
Helps relieve constipation
Detoxifies the system
Helps decrease symptoms of colds and the flu
Helps sedate the central nervous system
Kills vaginal trichomonads

## Ginseng
**Parts used:** Root
**Best time:** Morning to mid day
**Contains:** Vitamins A, B1, B2, B3, B5, E, biotin, rutin, calcium, germanium, iron, magnesium, manganese, phosphorus, potassium, silicon, sulfur, tin
**Action:** Helps lower blood pressure and increase hormone levels
    Helps prevent arteriosclerosis
    Helps reduce cholesterol and blood sugar
    Helps detox chemicals, drugs and radiation
    Increases libido
    Helps boost the immune system

## Golden Seal
**Parts used:** Roots, rhizume
**Best time:** Any time
**Contains:** Vitamins A, B-complex, C, E, F, calcium, copper, iron, manganese, phosphorus, potassium, sodium, zinc
**Actions:** External – Helps reduce inflammation and clean sores
    Helps with eczema and ringworm
    Good for eyewash, mouthwash, gargle, vaginal infection
    Helps reduce pyorrhea and tonsilitis
    Internal – Helps lower blood sugar
    Helps stop infections and detoxify poisons
    Has antiviral and antibiotic properties
    Helps with gastrointestinal infections

## Gotu Kola
**Parts used:** Leaves, flower
**Best time:** Any time
**Contains:** Vitamins A, B-complex, E, C, K, magnesium
**Action:** Helps balance potassium and sodium
Lowers blood pressure and body temperature
Helps prevent depression, mental fatigue, and some mental disorders
Helps neutralize blood acids
Helps strengthen the hormonal system, especially the pituitary
Increases mental and physical power

## Hops
**Parts used:** Flower
**Best time:** Evenings
**Contains:** Vitamin B-complex, chlorine, copper, fluorine, iodine, iron, lead, magnesium, manganese, sodium, zinc, lupulin
**Action:** External – Helps with skin inflammation
Internal – Relaxes the liver and gallbladder, thereby increases bile flow
Helps increase digestion
Increases appetite
Helps calm a nervous stomach, eliminate gas and intestinal cramps
Induces urination
Reduces libido
Helps induce sleep

## Hawthorn
**Parts used:** Berries
**Best time:** Any time
**Contains:** Vitamins B-complex andC, beryllium, choline, iron, nickel, phosphorus, potassium, silicon, sodium, sulfur, tin, zinc
**Action:** Helps control cholesterol and break up fats
Helps strengthen a weak heart

Helps improve vascular sufficiency and irregular heart beat

Has antispasmotic properties and helps prevent hardening of the arteries

Helps neutralize acid conditions of the blood

Helps normalize blood pressure

Reduces heart inflammation and arteriosclerosis


## Hydrangea

**Parts used:** Leaves and roots

**Best time:** Any time

**Contains:** Calcium, iron, magnesium, phosphorus, potassium, sodium, sulfur

**Action:** Helps keep the kidneys free from deposits

Prevents pain when passing kidney stones or gallstones

Helps ease the pain of arthritis and gout


## Kelp

**Parts used:** Whole plant

**Best time:** Morning to noon

**Contains:** Vitamins A, B-complex, C, E, K, over 30 minerals

**Action:** Stimulates the thyroid gland

Boosts the endocrine system

Helps absorb and eliminate toxins

Protects against heavy metal and radiation toxicity


## Licorice

**Parts used:** Root

**Best time:** Evening

**Contains:** Vitamins B-complex, E, biotin, pantothenic acid, niacin, chromium, iodine, manganese, zinc

**Action:** Increases blood pressure when body is out of balance

Helps balance blood pressure, electrolytes and fluid levels when body is in balance

Stimulates the immune system

Helps the production of white blood cells

Used to treat hypoglycemia, addison's disease, and rheuma-
toid arthritis
Mild laxative
Inhibits viral growth
Consumes sodium and potassium at a high rate

## Lemon
(Although not considered an herb, lemon's healing properties de-
served inclusion here.)
**Parts used:** Peel and juice
**Best time:** Any time
**Contains:** Vitamins, B-complex, C, thiamin, riboflavin, pantothenic
acid, calcium, copper, folate, iron, magnesium, potassium, biofla-
vinoids
**Action:** Promotes healthy mucus membranes, skin, and vision
Aids in digestion
Helps dissolve kidney stones
Helps in cancer treatment
Protects cells
Regulates the immune system
Tranquilizing effect calms anxiety
Antiviral properties reduce healing time for oral and genital
herpes

## Lobelia
**Parts used:** Seeds
**Best time:** Any time
**Contains:** Cobalt, copper, lead, selenium, sodium, sulfur
**Action:** External – Used to wash infected areas of skin disease
Stimulant in small doses, sedative in large doses
Over dose can cause nausea, vomiting, convulsions

## Mandrake
**Parts used:** Root, leaves, fruit
**Best time:** Any time

**Contains:** Tropane alkaloids
   Use extreme caution – can effect the central nervous system
**Action:** Has anti-tumor properties
   Helps detox mercury poisoning
   Kills intestinal worms
   Helps clear venereal warts
   Rejuvenator for sterile women
   Over dose symptoms include: nausea, vomiting, diarrhea, fever
   Abortive, anodine, anti-inflammatory, anti-spasmotic, emetic,
   hallucinogenic, hypnotic, sedative


**Marigold**
**Parts used:** Flower
**Best time:** Any time
**Contains:** Vitamins A and C, phosphorus
**Action:** External – As a salve for burns and wounds
   As drops for earaches
   As douche or suppository to heal infections, ulcers, pruritus
   Helps sinus problems including nasal mucus discharge
   Internal - As a tea, helps heal hemorrhoids
   Cellular healing


**Marshmallow**
**Parts used:** Root, flower, leaves
**Best time:** Any time
**Contains:** Vitamins A, B-complex, pantothenic acid, calcium, io-
dine, iron, sodium, zinc
**Action:** External – Used as a poultice for bee stings
   Internal – Helps release phlegm
   Helps relax bronchial tubes
   Used for healing lung ailments
   Removes mucus from lungs
   Removes stones and gravel from kidneys
   Helps with emphysema, diabetes, burns, bruising, vaginal in-
fections, high blood pressure

blood pressure

Increases milk flow for lactating women

## Mullen

**Parts used:** Leaf

**Best time:** Any time

**Contains:** Vitamins A, B-complex, D, iron, magnesium, potassium, sulfur

**Action:** External – Heals wounds and sores

Helps with open wounds, shingles, hives, hemorrhoids

Internal –Stops chronic cough (smokers, whooping)

Induces sleep

Reduces pain

Loosens and expels mucus

Ear infections (best remedy) 2-3 warm drops, 2-3 times per day

Helps with sinusitis, inflamed kidneys, swollen joints

## Myrrh

**Parts used:** Resin

**Best time:** Early morning and late evening

**Contains:** Terpenoids(anti-inflammatory, antioxidant), sesquiter-penes (affects the brain), certain gums, resin, essential oils, ca-dinene, dipentene, limonene, eugenol, cuminaldehyde, cinnamaldehyde, acetic acid, formic acid and others.

**Action:** External – as a douche, treats uterus and vaginal infections

Helps relieve skin rash

For sore throats – combine with red raspberry for mouthwash and gargle

Internal – Anti-bacterial

Helps: With dental problems – gingivitis, plaque buildup, bleeding gums

With bronchitis and mucus accumulation in the lungs

Heal the stomach and colon

Purge stagnant blood from the uterus

With arthritic conditions

With amenorrhea, dysmenorrheal, menopause, and uterine tumors

Lower cholesterol (LDL) and increase HDL

Respitory problems, i.e., congestion, cough, sore throat

Digestive problems, i.e. diarrhea, dyspepsia, flatulence, hemorrhoids, upset stomach

Strengthen the immune system


## Nettle (Urtica dioica)

**Parts used:** Leaves or roots

**Best time:** Anytime

**Contains:** Vitamins A, C, calcium, iron, manganese and potassium

**Action:** It's an astringent, anodyne, anti-rheumatic, ant-allergenic, diuretic,tonic, styptic, expectorant, anti-spasmodic, anti-histamine, and more.

External –helps stop bleeding

Minimizes skin conditions, including dandruff

Stimulates the lymphatic system

Helps relieve symptoms of arthritis, asthma, menopause, BPH

Alleviates diarrhea

Reduces nausea

Stimulates the lymphatic system and boosts immunity

Helps remove uric acid from joints

Promotes milk production in lactating women

Strengthens the fetus in pregnant women

Helps reduce menstrual cramps and bloating

Reduces inflammation

Reduces incidents of prostate cancer

Eliminates allergic rhinitis

Helps with GI problems, i.e. IBS, constipation

As a mouth wash, prevents plaque and reduces gingivitis

Relieves neurological disorders like MS, ALS and sciatica

Helps destroy parasites and worms

Helps support the thyroid gland, spleen, and pancreas

**Caution:** May cause stomach upset in some people

This could interact with certain medications. See your pharmacist before taking.

## Olive Leaf

**Parts used:** Leaf

**Best time:** Any time

**Contains:** Antioxidants (double amount in green tea 400% higher than vitamin C), polyphenols, flavonoids

**Action:** May reduce infarct volume and brain edema

Helps improve blood-brain barrier permeability

May help in treating cancerous tumors of the liver, prostate, colon, skin and breast

Effective in reducing or eliminating a cold or the flu

## Oregano (Wild Marjoram)

**Parts used:** Leaf

**Best time:** Anytime

**Contains:** Vitamins A, B6, C, E, K, fiber, calcium, folate, iron, magnesium, and potassium, rosmarinic acid (antioxidant), beta-caryophyllin (anti-inflammatory), carvacol and thymol (antimicrobial phytochemicals)

**Action:** Antibacterial and antifungal

Helps stop a cold or flu within a day or so(See "Common Cold" or "Flu")

Kills MRSA as liquid or vapor (essential oil dilution of 1 to 1,000 with water)

Helps with upper respiratory infections

Helps eliminate phlegm from lungs

Helps with acne, bronchitis, dandruff, earache, fatigue, headaches, menstrual cramps, parasites, toothache

Anti-inflammatory

Useful for sinus infections, urinary tract infections (UTIs), yeast infections, and food-borne illness, athlete's foot

## Papaya
**Parts used:** Fruit, leaves
**Best time:** Any time after a meal
**Contains:** Vitamins A, B-complex, C, D, E, K, calcium, iron, magnesium, phosphorus, potassium, sodium, digestive enzyme papain
**Action:** External – Used to relieve ringworm
    Dissolves corns, warts, pimples, dead tissue
    Internal – Expels worms (seeds with honey)
    Stops constipation and/or diarrhea
    Helps with bleeding ulcers
    Induces abortion

## Parsley
**Parts used:** Leaves
**Best time:** Any time
**Contains:** Vitamins A, B1, B2, B3, C, folic acid, calcium, cobalt, copper, iron potassium, silicon, sodium, sulfur
**Action:** Lowers blood pressure
    Stimulates lymph glands
    Relaxes uterine tissue
    Helps with blepharitis, conjunctivitis, kidney and bladder infections
    prostatitis
    Caution: do not use during pregnancy – induces labor pains and dries up mother's milk

## Passion Flower
**Parts used:** Leaves and flowers
**Best time:** Late evening
**Contains:** Indoles, flavenoids
**Action:** Helps lower blood pressure
    Slows the pulse rate
    Stimulates respiration
    Acts as a sedative for insomnia
    Helps with headaches, neuralgia, epilepsy, convulsions, sciatica

## Pennyroyal

**Parts used:** Tops, flowers
**Best time:** Any time
**Contains:** Keytone pulegone
**Action:** External – Relief from insect bites – mosquito, tick, chigger, gnats

Relieves rashes and itching

Internal –Helps eliminate toxins through sweating

Helps eliminate gas

Stimulates menstruation

CAUTION: May cause spontaneous abortion. Do not use if pregnant.

## Peppermint

**Parts used:** Leaves
**Best time:** Anytime
**Contains:** Vitamins A, C, E, choline, copper, inositol, iodine, iron, magnesium, niacin, potassium, silicon, sulfur
**Action:** External – As an enema, helps with colon problems

Internal - Opens sinuses (inhale 5-10 drops in 2 quarts of water)

Soothes a stomachache

Helps with digestion, morning sickness

Helps alleviate colic, constipation, stomach cramps, gas, heartburn, morning sickness, motion sickness, vomiting

Suppresses type A influenza virus

## Raspberry

**Parts used:** Leaves, roots, berries
**Best time:** Anytime
**Contains:** Vitamins A, B, C, D, E, F, calcium, iron, magnesium, phosphorus
**Action:** External – As a douche – strengthen the uterine wall

Internal - Helps lower high blood pressure and high blood sugar

Decreases eye mucus
Relieves painful menstruation
Normalizes menstrual flow
Alleviates abdominal cramps
Stops morning sickness, false labor pains
Eases childbirth and decreases labor pains
Enriches the colostrums in breast milk
Caution: can cause loose stools

## Red Clover
**Parts used:** Flowers
**Best time:** Morning
**Contains:** Vitamins A, B-complex, C, F, P, calcium, cobalt, copper, magnesium, manganese, molybdenum, nickel, phosphorus, selenium, sodium, tin
**Action:** External – As a wash or salve for burns, psoriasis, shingles, acne
As a mouthwash – gargle for sore throat
Internal – Blood purifier for spasms, lung congestion, bronchitis, whooping
cough
Has been used to treat cancer
Help lactation for nursing mothers

## Rose Hips
**Parts used:** Fruit, petals, buds
**Best time:** Daytime
**Contains:** Vitamins A, B-complex, C, D, E, P, rutin, calcium, iron, potassium, silica, sodium, sulfur
**Action:** Helps alleviate diarrhea, headaches, cramps, dizziness

## Rosemary
**Parts used:** Leaves
**Best time:** Any time
**Contains:** Vitamins A, C, calcium, iron, magnesium, phosphorus,

potassium, sodium, zinc
**Action:** External – As a mouthwash for halitosis
    Internal – Helps alleviate depression
    Helps lower blood pressure
    Improves circulation
    Strengthens the liver and heart
    Alleviates gas, colic, indigestion, nausea, fever
    Soothes nerves
    Helps regulate menses

## Safflower
**Parts used:** Flower
**Best time:** Afternoon
**Contains:** Vitamins F, K
**Action:** Helps remove phlegm from the lungs
    Detoxify uric acid
    Alleviate flu and fever
    Produce perspiration
    Lower cholesterol
    Has been used as a remedy for jaundice

## Sage
**Parts used:** Leaves
**Best time:** Late morning to evening
**Contains:** Vitamins A, B-complex, calcium, phosphorus, potassium, silicon, sodium, sulfur
**Action:** External – Helps stop yeast infections when used as a douche
    As a rinse – stimulates hair growth and removes dandruff
    As a tea or enema – helps expel worms
    Internal –Decreases mucus in sinuses, lungs, throat
    Helps with memory, concentration, fatigue
    Helps with stomach pain, diarrhea, gas, colds and flu
    Helps dry up breast milk
    Helps stop night sweats and perspiration

## Sarsaparilla
**Parts used:** Root
**Best time:** Late morning to evening
**Contains:** Vitamins A, B-complex, C, D, iodine, iron, manganese, silicon, sodium, sulfur, zinc, progesterone, testosterone
**Action:** External – Helps heal sores, pustules, wounds, ringworm
    Helps remove mercury and heavy metals from the blood
    Helps strengthen nerve tissue
    Helps hair growth
    Helps increase urine flow, dispel gas, increase sweating
    Has anti-inflammatory and detoxing properties
    Acts as a catalyst to help absorb nutrients

## Saw Palmetto
**Parts used:** Fruit
**Best time:** Any time
**Contains:** Vitamin A, alkaloids, resin, dextrin, glucose, several oils
**Action:** For mucus membranes, acts as a sedative and anti-inflammatory
    Sedates muscles
    Helps reproductive organs
    Combats diabetes
    Reduces the prostrate
    Helps the reproductive organs

## Slippery Elm
**Parts used:** Inner bark
**Best time:** Any time
**Contains:** Vitamins C, E, F, K, P, calcium, copper, iodine, iron, manganese, phosphorus, potassium, selenium, sulfur, zinc
**Action:** External – as a poultice, heals sores, wounds, burns, poison oak/ivy, skin infections
    As a douche – reduces inflammation and burning
    Internal –Helps eliminate mucus inflammation of the mouth, throat, lungs

Helps with sore throat
Relieves constipation and diarrhea
Neutralizes stomach acids

## Ta Heebo (Pao D' Arco)

**Parts used:** Inner bark
**Best time:** Any time
**Contains:** Iron, zinc
**Action:** Has antibiotic properties
    Used in Brazil as a cancer remedy
    Used as a foot bath to kill toe fungus

## Thyme

**Parts used:** Leaves
**Best time:** Evening
**Contains:** Vitamins B-complex, C, D, iodine, silicon, sodium, sulfur
**Action:** External – Combine oil with vegetable oil to treat ring-worm, athlete's foot, scabies, crabs, lice
    Soak 45 minutes with thyme in bath to stop itchiness
    As a fomentation – heals wounds, warts, varicose veins
    As a douche – Helps alleviate leucorrhea
    Acts as a germicide, antiseptic, parasiticide due to thymol
    Helps treat hookworms
    Treats bronchitis, laryngitis, whooping cough, diarrhea, gastritis, gas, colic, lack of appetite

## Uva Ursi

**Parts used:** Leaves
**Best time:** Evenings
**Contains:** Allantoin, arbutin, tannins
**Action:** External – Add 1 cup to bath for skin infections, hemorrhoids, and after childbirth – helps restore womb to normal size
    As a douche – for vaginal infections
Internal - Used for nephritis, cystitis, urethitis, kidney and bladder stones

Reduces excessive sugar in the system

Helps reduce kidney inflammation

Antiseptic and pain reliever

Caution: is a vasoconstrictor to the uterus – do not use during pregnancy

## Valerian

**Parts used:** Root

**Best time:** Early morning and late evening

**Contains:** Copper, lead, magnesium, potassium, zinc, alkaloids, valeric acid, formic acid, malic acid, tannins, gums, resin

**Action:** A substitute for valium

A strong sedative

Relaxes muscles

Helps heal erysipelas, hives, shingles, eye inflammation, muscle pain

Caution: prolonged use can lead to depression

## White Oak Bark

**Parts used:** Bark

**Best time:** Any time

**Contains:** Vitamin B12, calcium, cobalt, iodine, iron, lead, phosphorus, potassium, strontium, sulfur, tin

**Action:** External – used for scabs, wounds, sores, poison oak, insect bites

As a douche for vaginal infections

As an enema for hemorrhoids

As a fomentation for swollen glands, goiter, lymphatic swelling

Internal – helps stop bleeding in the stomach, lungs, rectum

Stops diarrhea

Helps gallstones and kidney stones pass

## White Willow

**Parts used:** Bark

**Best time:** Any time

**Contains:** Salicin
**Action:** Alternative to aspirine
    External – For skin irritations
    As a gargle for sore throat
    Internal – Helps alleviate headaches, fever, joint and back pain, neuralgia and arthritis pain
    Helps alleviate kidney, bladder and urethra irritations

## Wild Yam
**Parts used:** Root
**Best time:** Any time
**Contains:** Two steroidal saponins
**Action:** Used to increase progesterone
    Used as an antiseptic for the liver, spleen, pancreas and gallbladder
    The American Indians used wild yam for birth control

## Witch Hazel
**Parts used:** Leaves and bark
**Best time:** Any time
**Contains:** Vitamins C, E, K, P, copper, iodine, manganese, selenium, zinc
**Action:** External – Used for bed sores, wounds, poison oak/ivy, insect bites
    psoriasis, as a soothing aftershave, ingrown nails, bruises, swelling cracked or blistered skin, insect bites, varicose veins, hemorrhoids
    Used as a mouthwash for inflamed mouth and throat
    As a douche – Stops vaginal discharges and infections
    Internal – Stops excessive menstruation and hemorrhages in the stomach, bowels, lungs, and uterus

## Yellow Dock (Rumex crispus)
**Parts used:** Leaves and root
**Best time:** Any time

**Contains:** Vitamins A, B-complex, C, calcium, iron, manganese, nickel, potassium, sulfur, oxalic acid

**Action:** External – helps with eczema, hives, psoriasis, cradle cap, sores,itching

    Internal – inhibits growth of staph and E. coli bacteria

    Acts as a laxative by stimulating bowel flow

    Can help stop or slow cancer growth

    Caution: Take in moderation to avoid irritating the urinary tract and risk of kidney stones

    During lactation – may have a laxative effect on infants

## Additional Herbs and their benefits:

Boswellia – relieves arthritis and joint pain

    Best results if taken with turmeric, ashwagandha and ginger

Chaste tree – reduces PMS symptoms, i.e. irritability, depression, headaches, breast tenderness – best if taken with St. John's Wort

Cranberry – urinary tract infections (UTIs)

Feverfew – helps reduce the frequency of migraine headaches

Ginko –helps with memory problems as in Alzheimer's, forgetfulness

Milk thistle – Silmarin in the seeds help protect the liver and helps treat

hepatitis and alcoholic cirrhosis

Psyllium – Mucilage in the seeds helps both diarrhea and constipation. Drink a lot of water when taking psyllium

St. John's Wort – 900 mg per day helps mild to moderate depression, may reduce the effectiveness of birth control pills

Valerian – Many studies have shown its effectiveness with insomnia

White willow bark –Contains salicin (relative of asprin) helps relieve pain. Can cause stomach distress, avoid giving it to children.

## CELL SALTS

Toward the end of the 19th century Dr. Wilhelm Heinrich Schussler created a system of medicine called the Theory of Biochemic Therapeutics. He concluded that if the body became deficient in essential minerals, this imbalance would cause health problems. He based his theory on the physiological fact that both the structure and vitality of the organs of the body are dependent upon certain necessary quantities and proper apportionment of its organic constituents.

After a great deal of research, Dr. Schuessler identified 12 mineral salts, or tissue salts, that were essential for normal body function at a cellular level. He determined that any imbalance in any one or more of these salts led to specific health problems and diseases. But that balance could be restored by taking the necessary mineral salt.

Mineral salts are taken in small doses, melted under the tongue and quickly absorbed into the bloodstream. Cell salts are used to directly replace deficiencies in the cells, thereby relieving symptoms or affecting a cure.

Generally, cell salt dosage is four tablets for adults and two tablets for children taken three times a day until the condition is cured. In acute cases, the remedy can be taken every half hour until relief is obtained.

Cell salts can be taken individually or in combination with other cell salts. They can be taken at the same time or spread throughout the day. Often the most indicated cell salt is taken first and then others added as the symptoms are relieved. However, a "shotgun" approach of taking different ones at the same time seems to work as well as alternating the different salts throughout the day.

There are usually no side effects, but occasionally a healing crisis (Jarisch Herxheimer, or Herx Reaction) may occur. In this reaction the symptoms get worse before they get better due to the detoxification of the body. Positive improvement usually occurs within the first few weeks of treatment. If the symptoms persist, a qualified holistic practitioner or naturopath should be consulted.

Cell salts are generally numbered for ease of identification. The following is a description of the 12 cell salts. Uses will also appear under "Symptoms." An asterisk (*) indicates primary therapy.

### #1  Cal. flour (Elasticity Salt)
**Names:** Calcium Fluoride, Calcarea Fluorica
**Chemical Formula:** $CaF_2$
**Body Parts Affected:** Bones, elastic tissue, teeth, joints
**Function:** Aids in the elasticity of tissues of skin, muscles and blood vessels
   Preserves elastic power of tissues
   Heals spinal disc problems, skin fissures/cracks and anal fissures
   Helps heal hemorrhoids
   Improves some vision impairment
   Helps prevent dental decay
**Symptoms:**   Cracks in the skin
   Loss of elasticity
   Sluggish circulation
   Loose or decaying teeth
   Enamel problems
   Prolapsed uterus
   Varicose leg veins
   Rough, chapped or cracked skin
   Testicular swelling or hardening
   Conjunctivitis
   Constipation
   Dizzy spells
   Hyperkeratosis (thickening of the skin)
   Myositis
   Osteomyelitis
   Joint pain

Periostitis
General swelling
Ulcers
Excessive menses
Fevers (alternate 4, 5, and 7 in that order)
Red, brown, black coloring around eyes
Wrinkles under the lower lid of the eye, crow's feet
Shiny skin
Small white scales on the upper eye lid
Yellow offensive nasal discharge
Translucent tips of the teeth
Teeth sensitive to cold or touch
Loose teeth
Rough hard cracked tongue
Cracked lips
Helps prevent and reduce stretchmarks
Bleeding gums
Chronic sinusitis

**Dosage:**      Adults – 4 tablets, three times per day
Under 6 – 2-3 tablets per day


## #2 Calc. phos (Nutrition Tonic)

**Names:** Calcium Phosphate, Calcarea Phosphorica
**Chemical Formula:** $Ca_3PO_4$
**Body Parts Affected:** Bones, muscles, nerves, connective tissues, teeth
**Function:** Aids normal growth and development, restores tone and strength, aids digestion, aids bone and teeth formation
**Symptoms:** Poor circulation
Bone weakness
Rickets
Anemia
Arthritis
Backache
Bone inflammation

Brittle of soft bones
Broken bones
Craving for smoked meats
Dental cavities
Diabetes
Eczema
Swollen glands
Gout
Headaches
Hemorrhoids
Hernia
Incontinence
Infections
Swollen knees
Indigestion
Nerve pain (sharp)
Osteoporosis
Smoking
Teething problems
Tonsilitis
Toothache
Parasites
Nasal polyps
Fatigue
Can be used with Ferr. Phos to treat anemia

**Dosage:** Adults – 4 tablets, 3 times per day
Children 1-6 – 2 tablets, 3 times per day

## #3 Calc. sulph (Blood Purifier)

**Names:** Calcium Sulphate, Calcarea Sulphrica
**Chemical Formula:** $CaSO_4$
**Body Parts Affected:** Blood, Skin
**Function:** Blood purifier and healer, removes waste products from the blood, assists the liver in the removal of waste products, skin and tissue support. Assists Kali Mur.

**Symptoms:** Acne
   Abscesses
   Mouth ulcers
   Gum boils
   Slow-healing wounds
   Frontal headaches
   Neuralgia
   Catarrh
   Colds
   Boils
   Burns
   Conjunctivitis
   Cradle Cap
   Diarrhea
   Enlarged glands
   Hang nails
   Prone to infection
   Itching feet
   Mastitis
   Sore throat
   Yellow mucus discharge

**Dosage:** Adults – 4 tablets, 3 times per day
      Children 1-6 – 2 tablets, 3 times per day

Works well in combination with Kali. Mur and Nat. sulph.

## #4 Ferr. phos (First Aid Salt)

**Names:** Ferrum Phosphoricum, Iron Phosphate
**Chemical Formula:** $Fe_3PO_4$
**Body Parts Affected:** Muscles, Nerves, Hair, Blood Vessels
**Function:** First aid, oxygen carrier, supplementary remedy, anti-inflammatory, strengthens blood vessel walls

**Symptoms:**

| | |
|---|---|
| Congestion | Inflammation – joint, muscle |
| Inflammatory pain | Incontinence |

Fever
Rapid pulse
Anemia
Arthritis
Bedwetting
Bronchitis
Cuts
Cough
Cystitis
Diarrhea
Earache
Eye inflammation
Head cold
Headache
Heart palpitations
Hemorrhoids
Hernia
Hoarseness

Indigestion
Injuries
Morning sickness
Stiff neck
Nose bleeds
Painful periods
Heavy periods
Pneumonia
Prolapse
Tinnitis
Respitory problems
Muscle strain

A little powered Ferr. Phos applied directly to a cut or wound can stem bleeding

**Dosage:** Adults – 4 tablets, 3 times per day
Children 1-6 – 2 tablets, 3 times per day


## #5 Kali. mur (Glandular Tonic & Blood Conditioner)

**Names:** Kalium muriaticum, Potassium Chloride
**Chemical Formula:** $KCl$
**Body Parts Affected:** Blood, muscles, saliva
**Function:** Blood conditioner (cleans and purifies), treats burns, aids digestion
**Symptoms:**

Bronchitis
Feverish colds
Tonsillitis
Catarrh
Whitish discharges

Asthma
Varicose veins
Chronic feet and leg swelling
Testicular swelling
Morning sickness in pregnancy

Swollen glands
Childhood eczema
Ear aches
Eustachian tube blockage*
Burns
Chronic cystitis
Cracking noises in ear
Pale-yellow stools
Diarrhea
Hemorrhoids
Lymph node swellings
Throat infections
Head colds with mucus congestion

Heart palpitations
"Chicken skin" on arms/legs
Scurvy
Sore throat
Small pox
Toothache with gum swelling
Milky white to grey tongue
Sweet taste
Colitis
Cysts

**Dosage:** Adults – 4 tablets, 3 times per day
Children 1-6 – 2 tablets, 3 times per day

## #6 Kali. phos (Nerve Nutrient)

**Names:** Kalium phosphate, potassium phosphate
**Chemical Formula:** K3PO4
**Body Parts Affected:** Nerves, brain cells
**Function:** Nerve nutrient and antiseptic
**Symptoms:**

Nervous tension
Nervous indigestion
Nervous headaches
Stress
Anxiety and worry
Depression
Insomnia
Bad breath
Shingles
Restless Leg Syndrome
Nervous asthma
Night terrors
Back ache

Mental and physical exhaustion
Poor memory and concentration
Hoarseness
Swollen lymph nodes
Smoke sensitivity
Body odor
Weakened heart due to stress
Slimy, corrosive discharges
Offensive vaginal discharges
Stomach aches
Lack of lecithin in tissues
Loss of energy
Hunger feeling after eating

| | |
|---|---|
| Painful menstruation | Poor circulation |
| Agoraphobia | Vertigo |
| Facial gray/ash color | Sciatic nerve pain |
| Hair loss | Bedwetting |
| Panic attacks | Foul taste in the mouth |

**Dosage:** Adults – 4 tablets, 3 times per day
 Children 1-6 – 2 tablets, 3 times per day

## #7 Kali. sulph(Skin Salt)

**Names:** Kalium sulphate, Potassium sulphate
**Chemical Formula:** $K_2SO_4$
**Body Parts Affected:** Lungs, skin, mucus membranes, uterus, eyes, pancreas
**Function:** Oxygenates the cells and tissues of the body
**Symptoms:**

| | |
|---|---|
| Whooping cough | Cough with mucus rale |
| Jaundice | Inflammed mucosa |
| Predisposition to sinusitis | Conjunctivitis |
| Predisposition to otitis media | Painful joint movement |
| Dandruff | Facial neuralgia |
| Wandering limb pain | Alternating hot/cold feelings |
| Eustachian tube infections | Scanty/late menstruation |
| Nausea while pregnant | Yellow/greenish vaginal discharge |
| Extreme thirst | Sulfur smelling gas |
| Anal itching | Brittle nails |
| Diseases of the nail beds | Bladder infections |
| Chronic asthma | Eczema |
| High fever | Eye infections |
| Chronic gastritis | Overeating |
| Pharyngitis | Foul smelling nasal discharge (Ozeona) |
| Full feeling in stomach | Abdominal pain (lower right) |
| Abdominal bloating | Scalloped edges of tongue |
| Hyperpigmentation on face | Vitiligo |

White spots in beards          Dull taste in mouth
Pancreatic pain eased with fasting
Headaches due to warm rooms, stuffy atmospheres and in evening
Sticky, slimy yellow skin exudate

**Dosage:** Adults – 4 tablets, 3 times per day
Children 1-6 – 2 tablets, 3 times per day

## #8 Mag. phos (Nerve Relaxant)

**Names:** Magnesium phosphate
**Chemical Formula:** Mg3PO4
**Body Parts Affected:** Muscles, nerves
**Function:** Anti-spasmotic, ensures smooth movement of muscles
**Symptoms:**

| | |
|---|---|
| Muscle cramps/spasms | Nervousness |
| Restlessness | Exhaustion |
| Spasmotic intestines with gas | Headaches with sharp pains |
| Whooping cough | Spasmodic coughs |
| Sharp/piercing nerve pains | Peritonsillar abscess |
| Sciatica (usually right side) | Flatulence |
| Hiccups | Neuralgia |
| Writers cramp | Prostatitis |
| Eye twitches | Double vision |
| Stomach cramps | Heartburn |
| Perpetual yawning | Bronchial asthma |
| Chorea | Phantom limb pain |
| Colic | Bedwetting (enuresis) |
| Menstrual cramps | Sleeplessness |
| Nightmares | Remedy for addictions |
| Involuntary movement of hand | Constipation |
| Involuntary shaking of the head | Muscle weakness |
| Painful urination | Red spots on face, neck, chest |
| Tooth ache aggravated by cold or touch | |

**Dosage:** Adults – 4 tablets, 3 times per day
Children 1-6 – 2 tablets, 3 times per day

For quick results, can be dissolved in hot (but not boiling) water and sipped.

## #9 Nat. mur (Water Distributor)

**Names:** Naturium muriaticum, Sodium chloride
**Chemical Formula:** NaCl
**Body Parts Affected:** Digestive tract, glands
**Function:** Aids in digestion and water metabolism, assists in glandular function
**Symptoms:**

| | |
|---|---|
| MS symptoms | Toenail fungus |
| Craving for salty foods | Clear, thin, watery discharges |
| Clear, thin nasal discharges | Dry skin |
| Dry lips | Itchy skin |
| Hay fever | Loss of taste or smell |
| Headaches with constipation | Diarrhea |
| Vaginal dryness | Cracked nipples during/after pregnancy |
| Dandruff | Excessive sweating |
| Insufficient sweating | Sun allergies |
| Cold sores | Chronic cystitis |
| Gingivitis | Excessive or insufficient saliva |
| Heartburn | Excessive thirst |
| Hemorrhoids | Poor-quality sleep |
| Weak eye sight | Drowsiness, fatigue |
| Muscular weakness | Skin blisters |
| Hang nails | Hives (urticaria) |
| Insect bites | Addison's Disease |
| Bright's Disease | Chronic knee swelling |
| Parasites | Herpes |
| Diaper rash | Fungal skin diseases |
| Difficulty gathering thoughts | Restless and fidgety |
| Arthritis | Bloated feeling after eating |
| Cold sensation in extremities | Excessive tearing or dry eyes |
| Bulimia | Loss of hair |

Dry tongue                  Blisters on edge of tongue

Taste of metal

Large pores on nose, cheeks, chin or forehead

Polyurea (frequent urination)

Hydrocele (testicular watery swelling)

Orchitis (inflammation of testicles)

Leucorrhea (white vaginal discharge)

Morning sickness with vomiting of water, frothy phlegm

Toothache or facial neuralgia with flow of tears and saliva

Whooping cough, dry cough, cough with phlegm, persistant tickling cough

Can be immediately applied to stings and bites.

**Dosage:** Adults – 4 tablets, 3 times per day

            Children 1-6 – 2 tablets, 3 times per day


## #10 Nat. phos (Acid Neutraliser)

**Names:** Naturium phosphate, Sodium phosphate

**Chemical Formula:** $NaPO_4$

**Body Parts Affected:** Stomach, liver, Gallbladder

**Function:** Helps maintain acid-alkaline balance, helps regulate the liver and Gallbladder, aids in the assimilation of fatty acids.

**Symptoms:**

| | |
|---|---|
| Colic | Gout |
| Upset stomach | Heartburn |
| Indigestion | Joint pain and stiffness |
| Joint swelling | Body odor |
| Smelly feet | Jaundice |
| Nausea | Greenish-yellowish sour diarrhea |
| Kidney/gallstones | Gouty arthritic joints |
| Red buttocks/diaper rash | Morning sickness in pregnancy |
| Vertigo | Acid reflux |
| Dyspepsia | Acne |
| Boils | Cystitis |

Fatigue

Chronic gastroenteritis

Skin pustules

Wounds difficult to heal

Candida*

Grinding teeth

Sore or scabby outer ears

Sore throat

Frequent urination

Irregularity of sexual desires

Cradle cap

Pimples all over the body

Hives

Yellow, creamy discharge from eyes

Red, greasy nose

Blackheads around nose

Stinging blisters at tip of tongue  Sour and bitter taste

Skin chafing with soreness and redness

Eczema of the skin when accompanied with acrid, creamy, yellow secretions.

Severe headaches on top of head

Heart palpitations and irregularities

Irregular menstrual periods when accompanied with acid leucorrhea

Increased vaginal discharge – yellowish to brownish

**Dosage:** Adults – 4 tablets, 3 times per day

Children 1-6 – 2 tablets, 3 times per day

## #11 Nat. sulph (Water Eliminator)

**Names:** Natrium sulphate, Sodium sulphate

**Chemical Formula:** $Na_2SO_4$

**Body Parts Affected:** Kidneys, liver, gallbladder

**Function:** Eliminates excess water

**Symptoms:**

Edema (tissue fluid)

Water retention

Bloated appearance

Constant shivering attacks

Exhaustion

Daytime fatigue

Jaundice (bilious type)

Flu

Hepatitis

Nausea

Bitter taste in the mouth

Greenish appearance before vomiting

Bluish-red coloring on nose

Swollen eye sacks

Coppery taste in mouth
Predisposition to liver/gallbladder disease
Sharp, tearing cutting pains in left chest/left hip – can only lay on right side
Liver area feeling of pain and pressure
Frequent flatulence with foul smelling gas
Diarrhea in the morning and vomiting of bile
Top remedy for head injuries/epilepsy after a head injury
"Alcohol nose" – dark red in a chronic condition – toxic overload
Greenish-brown or gray coating on back of tongue or
Slimy thick white mucus coating

**Dosage:** Adults – 4 tablets, 3 times per day
Children 1-6 – 2 tablets, 3 times per day

## #12 Silica (Toxic Eliminator)

**Names:** Silicon dioxide, Silicic oxide
**Chemical Formula:** $SiO_2$
**Body Parts Affected:** Blood, skin, nails, hair, bones, connective tissue, mucus membranes.
**Function:** Cleanser and detoxifier
**Symptoms:**

| | |
|---|---|
| Pimples | Boils |
| Styes | Sensitivity to light and noise |
| Shivering | Skin abscesses with suppuration |
| Cracked, brittle or split nails | Tendency to catch colds |
| Gland disorders | Dull hair |
| Irritating cough | Night sweats |
| Poor memory | Ulcerated nose |
| Hemorrhoids | Leucorrhea |
| Abscesses | Absent mindedness |
| Allergies | Arteriosclerosis |
| Bruises | Renauld's Syndrome |
| Fistulas | Lung infections |
| Lymphoma | Otitis media/externa |

Overexertion

Strong thirst

Swallowing difficulties

Tonsilitis with pus

Wrinkles

Keloids (raised scars)

Stretch marks

Cold but warm inside

Hang nails

Rushes of blood to head

Swollen glands

Tissue infections

Ulcers on the tongue

Foul smelling feet

Vaccination reactions

Scleroderma (hardening of tissues)

Hip joint disease/pain

Carbuncles (boils) especially in Spring

Loss of taste

Chronic dyspepsia (poor digestion) with belching

Offensive discharge (Ozeana with fetid)

Trigeminal neuralgia (face ache) with small lumps/nodules on face and scalp.

Lupus with discharge of thick matter

Translucent skin quality in temple area

Crow's feet wrinkles at corners of eyes

Upper eyelids shrunken and the lid looks deeply indented

Sensation of hair on tongue

Taste of fat in the mouth

Taste of blood in the mouth, especially in the morning

Involuntary twitching of eyes or face muscles

Headaches from the occiput moving towards the eyes

Sweaty, sore feet with raw flesh between the toes

Irritable and nervous exhaustion

Twitching movements when falling asleep (not restless leg syndrome)

Distinct aversion to hot or warm cooked meals, especially meat

Thin, pus forming, caustic, putrid secretions

**Dosage:** Adults – 4 tablets, 3 times per day

Children 1-6 – 2 tablets, 3 times per day

The cell salt known as "BioPlasma" is a combination of all 12 tissue salts. This is good to use if unsure of which cell salt to use. Cell salts in homeopathic form bypasses the digestive system, which may have been the cause of the deficiency to begin with.

## Essential Oils

An essential oil is simply the oil of a plant from which it is extracted. The aromatic compounds are extracted from the seeds, bark, roots, stems, and flowers. Essential oils are concentrated hydrophobic liquids containing highly volatile aromatic compounds. Therefore they are used quite extensively in aroma therapy. They are also used in cosmetics, perfumes, incense, flavoring for some foods and aroma for some household cleaning products.

Essential oils have been used throughout history for many different applications. The Egyptians used essential oils in their medical practices, for beauty treatments, religious ceremonies, and food preparation. The Greeks used essential oils for their practices of therapeutic massage and aromatherapy. The Romans used the oils to promote health and personal hygiene. History records that the Chinese, Persians and Indian Ayurvedic practitioners quite extensively used essential oils extracted from aromatic plants.

In 1937 a French chemist, Rene-Maurice Gattefosse, healed a badly burned hand using pure lavender oil. Later Dr. Jean Valnet used therapeutic grade essential oils to treat injured soldiers during World War II. His treatments were very successful. Dr. Valnet became a world leader in developing aroma therapy practices. The research and practice of aromatherapy and the use of essential oils has continued to this day.

When reading the history of healing, one will generally find some reference to oils of plants used liberally for healing. Many "primitive" countries or regions still rely on plant oils as their medication. However, as we became more sophisticated and pharmaceutical companies became more powerful, the use of essential oils, along with other natural substances, ran out of favor with the medical world. Aroma therapists and others interested in natural healing held onto the use of plant oils to heal certain conditions.

Today very extensive distillation processes are used to extract essential oils. The appropriate plant harvested at the right time and specific plant parts along with a meticulously controlled extraction process are required for successful extraction. Most often the oils are extracted by a process of distillation.

There are three common methods of administering essential oils: aromatic diffusion (inhalation), topical (transdermal) and internal as a dietary supplement. Using a diffuser or rubbing two drops in the palm of the hand and inhaling can affect moods, opens airways, and kills bacteria and viruses in the air. Topically, a few drops rubbed into the skin can give comfort and support the immune system. They can be applied to the suboccipital area (posterior base of the skull), bottoms of the feet (large pores = qick absorption), over the heart (calming), localized (directly to the area of concern). Taking essential oils internally supports the immune system and helps the mouth, throat and digestive system. There are several ways of taking essential oils internally. Holding one or two drops under the tongue for twenty seconds then swallowing, or place into a glass of water and drink or drop into an empty capsule and swallow as any other supplement. Be aware that not all essential oils can be taken internally. Thouroughly research and check with a holistic healthcare provider before taking any essential oil internally.

Essential oils can be used individually or in combination with other essential oils. As with many modalities, some work better with some than others. A bit of experimentation helps to find the best combination for that particular condition and that particular person. For most adults, 2 to 4 drops at a time is sufficient. Remember, frequency equals effectiveness. For best results, use a small amount frequently. For children, 1 to 2 drops at a time is enough. For small children and people with very sensitive skin, dilute one drop of essential oil with one teaspoon of fractionated, or organic, coconut oil. For most essential oils it's best not to apply undiluted oil directly on the skin. Diluting in an oil for massage or water for other uses is recommended.

For most conditions, especially if the condition is a minor one, one or two treatments per day is enough. If the condition is more persistent, some have used 2-4 drops every 2-3 hours. Chronic or severe conditions sometimes require a combination of essential oils at a time, 2-4 times per day.

As a reference, the following chart might be useful:
1% dilution – 1 drop of EO per 1 tsp. carrier oil or 6 drops of EO per 1 oz. carrier oil
3% dilution – 3 drops of EO per 1 tsp. carrier oil or 18 drops of EO per 1 oz. carrier oil
5% dilution – 30 drops of EO per 1 oz. carrier oil

There are many essential oils from all over the world used for a myriad of conditions. A complete guide for using essential oils is too extensive to present here. However, please note that there are more indications and uses for each essential oil than is listed here. The following is a list of some of the most popular and commonly used essential oils:

### Basil *(Ocimum bisilicum)*
**Indications:** Mental fatigue, migraine headaches, scanty menstrual periods
**Actions:** Anti-inflammatory, antibacterial, antiviral, antispasmodic, decongestant
**Uses:** Abdominal cramps, amenorrhea, bee sting, bursitis, chronic fatigue, chest infections, Crohn's disease, diabetes, earache, Epstein-Barr, fatigue, insect bites, migraine headaches, restless leg syndrome, tendinitis, vertigo

### Bergamot *(Citrus bergamia)*
**Indications:** Depression, stress, agitation, intestinal parasites, in-

flammation, insomnia, vaginal candida
**Actions:** Antiseptic, antibacterial, anti-inflammatory, calming
**Uses:** Depression, stress, irritability, respiratory infection, bronchitis, Sore throat, thrush, tonsillitis, urinary tract infection

## Cedarwood *(Cedrus atlantica)*
**Indications:** Anger, arteriosclerosis, bronchitis, hair loss, nervous tension, skin disorders (acne, psoriasis), urinary tract infections
**Actions:** Anti-inflammatory, antiseborrhoeic, antiseptic, antispasmodic, astringent, diuretic, emmenagogue, expectorant, insecticide, tonic
**Uses:** Arthritis, reduces skin peeling and redness, prevents wound Infection, relieves spasms of the heart, nerves, intestines, muscles, respiratory system, conditions like asthma and restless leg syndrome, relieves toothaches, protects the gums, stops diarrhea, helps relieve hypertension, arthritis, gout, UTI's, stimulates menstruation, normalizes menstrual cycle, removes phlegm from respitory tracts, mosquito and insect repellant

## Chamomile *(Matricaria recutiita)*
**Indications:** Restlessness, tension, stress, insomnia, headaches, Inflammation (bursitis, tendonitis), carpal tunnel syndrome
**Actions:** Anti-inflammatory, antispasmodic, anti-infectious, antibacterial, antispasmodic, decongestant
**Uses:** Calming, helps regenerate skin, blood cleanser, depression, muscle tension, insomnia, skin conditions, eczema, restless legs (for skin conditions, consult a holistic doctor to determine possible allergy)

## Cinnamon *(Cinnamomum verum)*
**Indications:** Bacterial infections, vaginitis, vaginal yeast infection
**Actions:** Antibacterial, anti-viral, antimicrobial, anti-infectious, anti-fungal
**Uses:** Helps increase circulation, helps with diabetes, halitosis, diverticulitis, mold exposure, hypoglycemia, MRSA, and above indications

## Clary Sage
**Indications:** Weak gums and skin, skin rashes, gassy stomach, hormone imbalance, irregular or painful menses, anxiety, nervousness, hysteria, impotence, loss of libido, wounds, high blood pressure, muscle pains, respitory ailments, stress
**Actions:** Anticonvulsive, antiseptic, antidepressant, antispasmodic, aphrodisiac, astringent, blood pressure regulator, painkiller
**Uses:** Stress – inhale or diffuse (2-3 drops is sufficient) Abdominal pain, muscle pain – equal amounts (5-6 drops) of CS and a carrier oil (coconut , almond or olive) and apply to the affected area
Skin conditions: Mix equal amounts of CS and coconut oil and apply directly to the skin

Can be mixed with other essential oils to enhance or complement the desired effects.

Caution: Clary sage should not be used when taking alcohol or any Narcotic products. Pregnant or nursing ladies should avoid CS. Avoid giving to small children or infants

## Clove (*Syzygium aroomaticum*)
**Indications:** Infections (wounds and respiratory), infectious deseases, toothache, pain, indigestion, gas, nausea
**Actions:** Antimicrobial, antioxidant, anti-inflammatory, antiseptic, Analgesic, bactericidal, thins the blood
**Uses:** Stops bad breath, numbs the gums, blood thinner, helps eliminate thrush, viruses, candida, chicken pox, fungal infections, gingivitis, herpes simplex, mold infection
(Do not use if on a blood thinning medication)

## Coriander (*Coriandrum sativum*)
**Indications:** Diabetes, blood sugar imbalance
**Actions:** Anti-inflammatory, sedative
**Uses:** Stabilize blood sugar, diabetes, supports pancreatic function

## Eucalyptus (*Eucalyptus globules/polybractea/radiata*)
**Indications:** Skin conditions, intestinal/digestion problems, in-

flammation (bronchitis, conjunctivitis, sinusitis, vaginitis), cold, congestion, hay fever, candida, herpes, hypoglycemia
**Actions:** Antibacterial, anti-infectious, anti-inflammatory, antiviral, expectorant
**Uses:** Sinus congestion, sinusitis, ear and eye inflammation, respiratory infections, acne, skin infection, vaginitis, shingles, ulcers, wounds, insomnia, stress (calming effect), depression

### Frankincense *(Boswellia carteri)*
**Indications:** Asthma, depression, inflammation, mental fatigue
**Actions:** Antidepressant, antitumoral, astringent, digestive, expectorant, diuretic, emmenagogue, immunostimulant, sedative, tonic, uterine and vulnerary.
**Uses:** Insect bites, arthritis, depression, bronchitis, inflammation, seizures, headaches, herpes, stress, high blood pressure, stimulates neurotransmitters, improves memory and mental clarity.
Oil of choice for brain disorders.

### Frankincense has a frequency of 147 MHz, well within the healing range.
(A healthy body will generally have a frequency between 62 and 78 MHz. Disease patterns usually develop at 58 MHz and below.) Frankincense has been shown to be very effective against cancer cells especially when used along with thyme.

### Geranium *(Pelargonium graveolens)*
**Indications:** Bleeding, blisters, skin conditions (dermatitis, eczema, psoriasis, vitiligo), impetigo, dry skin, gall stones, tumor growth
**Actions:** Antibacterial, antifungal, anti-inflammatory, anti-infectious, astringent, hemostatic (stops bleeding), dilates bile ducts, helps cleanse oily skin
**Uses:** Helps clear skin conditions, shingles, bleeding, hormonal imbalances, blisters, detoxification, flushes gall stones, liver disorders, vertigo

## Grapefruit *(Citrus x paradisi)*
**Indications:** Appetite, cellulite, digestion, obesity, stress, toxic condition
**Actions:** Antidepressantt, antiseptic, disinfecting, detoxifying, diuretic, fat dissolving
**Uses:** Helps suppress addictions and appetite, eating disorders, stress, pre-menstrual tension, metal toxicity, obesity (fat dissolving characterists), fatigue

## Helichrysum *(Helichrysum italicum)*
**Indications:** Blood clots, inflammation, excess phlegm, fever, cuts, wounds, acne, coughs, indigestion, infection, hard or excess mucus, acne, gallbladder disorders, bloating, stomach aches, liver disorders
**Actions:** Anticoagulant, anti-inflammatory, antimicrobial, antiseptic, antispasmodic, emollient, expectorant,febrifuge, fungicidal, mucolytic
**Uses:** Helps reduce fever, gives relief from colds, softens the skin, helps dissolve blood clots, reduces inflammation, diuretic, protects against infection, loosens phlegm and protects against accumulation, inhibits fungal infections, detoxifies the liver, helps reduce arthritis, sinusitis, colitis, neuritis, fights fungal infections including candida

## Lavender *(Lavandula angustifolia)*
**Indications:** Skin conditions (acne, dermatitis, eczema, burns, sunburns, Dandruff, rashes, poison oak/ivy, itching), anxiety
**Actions:** Analgesic, anticonvulsant, anti-inflammatory, antiseptic, antitumoral, sedative
**Uses:** Promotes tissue regeneration, speeds wound healing, heals burns, promotes calming, used for dandruff, headaches, insomnia, muscle spasms, hives, nervous tension, skin conditions, high blood pressure, headaches, insomnia, stress, depression

## Lemon *(Citrus limon)*
**Indications:** Respiratory, bladder and ureter infection, anxiety, digestive problems, sore throat, anemia
**Actions:** Antibacterial, anti-infectious, antiseptic, antiviral, disinfectant
**Uses:** Improves the immune system, improves circulation and digestion, strengthens nails, helps with herpes, shingles, sore throats, high blood pressure, helps minimize or eliminate depression

## Lemongrass *(Cymbopogon flexuosus)*
**Indications:** Bladder and urinary tract infections, edema, fluid retention, digestive disturbances, torn tendons and ligaments, metal toxicity, high cholesterol, gastritis
**Actions:** Anti-inflammatory, sedative, helps regenerate connective tissues, strengthens vascular walls, stimulates the thyroid, promotes blood flow and lymph flow, detoxifies, antifungal
**Uses:** Helps improve digestion, circulation, eyesight, sore throat, headache, respiratory difficulties, helps heal connective tissue, decreases cholesterol, helps stabilize the thyroid, helps soothmuscle spasms

## Melaleuca *(alternifolia, ericifolia, quinquenervia)*
**Indications:** Elevated mucous in respiratory and urinary tracts, high blood pressure, bronchitis, fungal infections, respiratory infections, sore throat, tonsillitis, vaginal thrush, acne, athlete's foot, eczema
**Actions:** Antibacterial, antiviral, anti-inflammatory, anti-infectious, antiparasitic
**Uses:** Acne, athlete's foot, Candida, cuts, ear infection, eczema, fungal infections, herpes simplex, hives, rashes, shingles, Thrush, hemorrhoids, vaginal douch to treat yeast

## Myrrh *(Commiphora myrrha)*
**Indications:** Bronchitis, diarrhea, gingivitis, hyperthyroidism,

thrush, vaginal thrush, ulcers, viral hepatitis
**Actions:** Anti-inflammatory, antiviral, anti-infectious, antiparasitic, supports hormones and the immune system, antidepressant
**Uses:** Helps balance the thyroid, stops bleeding gums, soothes and heals cracked skin, helps curb negative emotions, helps with asthma, candida, eczema, fungal infections, digestion, sore throats, wrinkles

## Orange *(Citrus aurantium)*
**Indications:** Chest pain (angina), insomnia, menopause
**Actions:** Anticoagulant, anti-inflammatory, antitumoral, sedative, improves circulation
**Uses:** Diarrhea, jaundice, heartburn, respiratory infections, digestive disturbances, lowers cholesterol levels, mouth sores, fluid retention, skin inflammation

## Peppermint (*Mentha piperita*)
**Indications:** Upset stomach, indigestion, bronchitis, diarrhea, heartburn, hot flashes, headaches, nausea, motion sickness, throat infections
**Actions:** Antibacterial, antifungal, antiparasitic, anti-infectious, decongestant, expectorant, anti-inflammatory for the intestinal and urinary tracts
**Uses:** Soothes digestion, improves concentration, improves mental accuracy, tension headaches, may help with Bell's palsy, morning morning sickness, fever, diarrhea, food poisoning, eases toothaches, arthritis, skin conditions (eczema, dermatitis, psoriasis)

## Pine (*Pinus sylvestris*)
**Indications:** Arthritis (rheumat*oid*), bronchitis, diabetes, sinusitis, severe infections.
**Action:** Antidiabetic, anti-infectious, antifungal, antiseptic, antihypertensive, sexual stimulant
**Uses:** Relaxes muscles (topically), stimulates the respiratory system,

helps with cuts, coughs, fatigue, gout, lice, stress, urinary infection, helps stimulate the adrenal glands and increase blood pressure

## Rosemary (*Rosmarinus officinalis*)
**Indications:** Respiratory and lung infections, hypertension/hypotension, arthritis, menstrual disturbances, hair loss, cardiac arrhythmia, indigestion
**Action:** Antibacterial, antifungal, antiseptic, antiparasitic, antispasmodic, stimulates mental clarity, analgesic, antioxidant, expectorant, anti-inflammatory
**Uses:** Helps lower cholesterol, helps combat hair loss by stimulating the scalp (massage 5-6 drops on scalp after shower), vaginal infection (1-2 drops around or in the vagina), improve memory by diffusing or an inhaler, inhale via nasal inhaler or diffuse for headaches, (use similar methods for: stress relief, respiratory problems, improved gallbladder function)
(CAUTION: do not injest. Not to be used by ladies who are pregnant or breastfeeding)

## Sandalwood (*Santalum album*)
**Indications:** Bronchitis, cystitis, herpes, skin tumors, low testosterone
**Action:** Stimulates the pineal gland (center for emotions)
**Uses:** Helps normalize skin hydration, helps with cystitis, skin infection, nervous tension, depression, menstrual problems, skin infection, helps balance testosterone levels

## Thyme (*Thymus vulgaris*)
**Indications:** Congestion from a cold, infections, parasites, acne, cuts, sores, eczema, oral conditions, high blood pressure, hormonal imbalance
**Action:** Antiseptic, antibacterial, antispasmodic, hypertensive
**Uses:** Helps reduce high blood pressure, reduces cholesterol, triglyceride and LDL levels, increases HDL levels, fights bronchitis, fights oral conditions including sore throat, balances hormon lev-

els, fights fungal and bacterial infections, helps alleviate skin condtions including rashes and acne, helps eliminate eczema, helps improve progesterone production

### Ylang Ylang (*Cananga odorata*)
**Indications:** Heart conditions (arrhythmias, tachycardia, brady-cardia, palpitations), Anxiety, depression, high blood pressure, impotence, hair loss, insomnia
**Action:** Antispasmodic, helps regulate blood pressure and heart-beat
**Uses:** Ylang Ylang may help lower high blood pressure, stimulate the adrenal glands, calm the spirit, calm rapid breathing, impotence, spark hair growth

## Homeopathic Remedies

Homeopaths dilute a substance in distilled water or alcohol in a vial (called dynamisation or potentisation), and then vigorously shake the vial and strike a soft object with the combination for one minute. Some use 10 hard strikes against a soft object. The process is called succession and it is believed to activate the "vital energy" of the diluted substance to make it stronger.

On a bottle of homeopathic solution, a number will follow the name. That number refers to the diluting of the substance. Hahne-mann created a system of numbering called the centesimal or C scale. This refers to diluting a substance by a factor of 100 at each stage. A 2C dilution requires one part of a substance to be diluted in-to 100 parts of water or alcohol, then one part of that solution to be diluted into another 100 parts of water or alcohol. A 10 C solution requires that the process is repeated 10 times. In homeopathy, the more dilute the solution the higher the potency. Homeopaths con-sider the more dilute the substance the stronger and deeper-acting the remedy. There are other similar scales, such as the X scale and the decimal or D scale. They are relatively the same. Hahnemann used the 30 C solutions for most conditions that he encountered.

Although this procedure makes it seem like a very weak solution, the effectiveness is great. *Jenna came in the office with her arms and legs covered with poison oak. Her job required that she walk through thick woods marking out trails to be converted into logging roads. Her dog followed her everywhere she went. She would change clothes when she finished surveying an area, however, her dog would rub against her legs to show affection. That affection transferred the poison oak from his fur to her skin. She was treated with a homeopathic poison oak remedy and NAET. After the homeopathic and two NAET treatments, Jenna's skin was clear and she was able to walk through the woods without contracting poison oak.*

The following is a list of some homeopathic remedies and conditions they are reported to help. This list is by no means conclusive. As with so many other remedies, some work for some people. Some remedy may work for a specific condition while sometimes a combination of remedies may work. A Traditional homeopath will generally use only one remedy for a specific condition while a Functional homeopath may use several remedies for one condition. Again, this list is simply to help you become aware of what's available to help with your health. Contact a Homeopath or natural health care doctor who is familiar with homeopathy to get more information and specific insight into homeopathy. Disclaimer: This list is for information only. It is not designed to diagnose or present a cure.

| | |
|---|---|
| Aconitum napellus | Sudden high fever with dry skin |
| Aesculus hippocastanum | Hemorrhoids |
| Apis melifica | Swelling from insect bites or allergies |
| Arnica Montana | Traumatic pain, muscle soreness |
| Arsenicum album | Food poisoning symptoms |
| Belladonna | Sudden onset of high fever with perspiration |
| Borax | Arthritis pain, canker sores |

| | |
|---|---|
| Bryonia | Muscle & joint pain relieved with rest |
| Calcarea phosphoric | Growing bone pains |
| Cantharis | Blisters, bladder pain |
| Carbo vegetabailis | Abdominal bloating with gas |
| Caulophyllum thalictroides | Menstrual cramps |
| Causticum | Bed-wetting, incontinence |
| Chamomilla | Teething pain |
| Chelidonium majus | Indigestion, nausea |
| Cimicifuga racemosa | Painful menstruation with upper back pain |
| Cina | Nervousness, irritability, insomnia in children |
| Cinchona officinalis | Diarrhea with gas and bloating |
| Cocculus indicus | Motion sickness |
| Coffea cruda | Insomnia with mental activity |
| Cuprum metallicum | Leg cramps, muscle cramps |
| Dulcamara | Joint pain worsened by damp weather |
| Euphrasia officinalis | Eye discharged |
| Ferrum phosphoricum | Low fever |
| Gelsemium sempervirens | Apprehension, fever |
| Hamamelis virginiana | Hemorrhoids |
| Hydrastis canadensis | Postnasal drip |
| Hypericum perforatum | Nerve pain |
| Ignatia amara | Nervousness, hypersensitivity from daily stress |
| Kali carbonicum | Pain and weakness in lower back |
| Kali iodatum | Colds with frontal sinus pain |
| Kali muriaticum | Nasal congestion with white discharge |
| Kali phosphoricum | Tension headache from mental stress |
| Kali sulphuricum | Colds with yellow discharge |
| Lachesis mutus | Menopausal hot flashes |

| | |
|---|---|
| Ledum palustre | Insect bites |
| Lycopodium clavatum | Bloated abdomen due to gas |
| Mezereum | Sinus pain |
| Natrum muriaticum | Runny nose from allergies |
| Phosphoricum acidum | Poor concentration due to over-work |
| Pulsatilla | Colds with thick yellow nasal discharge |
| Rhus tox | Joint pain improved with motion |
| Rumex crispus | Dry cough aggravated by breathing cold air |
| Ruta graveolens | Eye strain from artificial light or computer use |
| Sabina | Heavy menstruation |
| Sepia | Mood swings |
| Silicea | Fatigue and irritability from overworking |
| Spongia tosta | Croupy cough |
| Sulphur | Skin rash aggravated by heat and water |
| Sulphur iodatum | Nasal discharge from colds or the flu |
| Symphytum officianale | Promotes bone healing |
| Tabacum | Motion sickness with cold sweat improved with fresh air |
| Urtica urens | Skin rash due to allergies |
| Zincum metallicum | Leg cramps |

# Chapter 8
## NAET and EAV

### Nambudripad's Allergy Elimination Technique (NAET)

One might ask how and why did a chiropractor get involved with treating allergies. I hear that a lot but there is no quick and easy answer to give. For 20 years I had treated back and joint pain using standard chiropractic procedures. Our patients ranged from 3 months old to 101 years old, grade school, high school, college, Olympic and professional teams and individuals. However, many times patients would tell me that they had been treating with this doctor or that doctor or this specialist or that specialist with no success at all in getting to the root of their concerns. Even as a chiropractor, I knew that "popping the back" wasn't always the answer.

After hearing about a system that eliminated allergies and thereby helping other conditions, a trip was planned to meet the doctor who researched and developed the system known as NAET. Dr. Devi Nambudripad, D.C., L.Ac, R.N., Ph.D., M.D. and her team spent years developing a process that is now taught all over the world. Thousands of healing practitioners from all backgrounds are successfully employing her protocols. The procedure is called NAET (Nambudripad's Allergy Elimination Technique).

When we think of allergies we think of coughing, sneezing, wheezing, and blowing. Granted those are reactions to some allergens that some enjoy. However it is much more involved than that. During consultation, most patients will admit to one or two allergies and sometimes none at all. However, after testing they may demonstrate 20, 30 or even more allergies or sensitivities. Those sensitivities may be from exposure to industrial or household pollutants, herbicides, pesticides, pollens, animals, foods and much more. They can occur at any age and to anyone. A distinction is made here between an allergy (immediate reaction) and a sensitivity (delayed reaction). Allergies or sensitivities and their reactions may vary greatly between individuals.

Allergies can be classified as:
    Ingestants – food, water, chemical
    Inhalants – dust, chemicals
    Contactants – latex, fabrics, chemicals
    Injectants – drugs (recreational or prescription)
    Infectants – viruses, bacteria, parasites
    Physical agents – radiation, UV, cold, hot

Some of the most common food allergies include:
    Eggs
    Milk
    Soy
    Cheese
    Nuts and seeds
    Fish
    Shellfish
    Corn
    Oats
    Wheat, Rye, Barley
    Spices
    Vitamins
    Minerals
    Vegetables
    Cooking ingredients

Milk and dairy
Sugars
Viruses
Bacteria

Some of the contact allergens tested include:
Animal epithelia and dander
Fabric
Plastics
Insects
Grass
Pollen
Weeds
Trees
Flowers
Dust
Chemicals

A partial list of symptoms may include (they may vary a bit):
Headaches
Swelling of the nasal mucosa
Respiratory problems
Eye irritation, including redness and swelling
Sneezing
Coughing
Sore throat
Wheezing
Fatigue
Dizziness
Full or bloated feeling
Impaired hearing
Memory lapses
Mental fogginess
Anxiety
Depression

Muscle aches and pains
Joint pain, including arthritis
Itchy skin, including eczema and hives
Learning disabilities
Aggressive behavior
Hyperactivity
Weight gain/loss
Abdominal pain
Colon disorders
Digestive and elimination problems
And there are many more

When the body is viewed holistically, it's viewed somewhat differently than the standard "mainstream" way of looking at it. Everyone agrees that there's a nervous system, a cardiovascular system, an endocrine system, etc. However a holistic doctor will understand the energy system, in keeping with the oriental view of healing. Although disputed by some middle-of-the-road doctors, university studies have proven the existence of an unseen energy system that flows throughout the body. Modern high tech procedures have mapped out the rivers of energy that flow through the body. Surprisingly, they resemble almost exactly the pathways described by oriental doctors hundreds, if not thousands, of years in the past. This energy system has everything to do with how the body maintains health.

One of the most plausible views concerning allergies is that the allergies occur when the flow of energy in the body becomes interrupted. That interruption can come in many forms, such as food, drink, polluted air, and contact. According to ancient oriental healers, a healthy body is one in which its energy is in balance. When some force causes the body to become imbalanced, disease occurs.

Looking at the big picture, everything is comprised of energy. Every molecule has energy. And thusly, every cell of the body has energy. There are rhythms, frequencies, wavelengths, and electrical charges of the vibrating energy waves that make up everything we see. Those charges or frequencies can be measured and can be intensified or diminished. When those frequencies are interrupted, changes occur. When they occur in the human body, an imbalance is set up and the body will react to the imbalance. In some cases the immune system becomes compromised and the person becomes vulnerable to attacks from outside the body. Outside influences sometimes become overwhelming and the body reacts by creating antibodies. Under normal circumstances the body would simply take care of the attack and life would resume as normal. But occasionally the attack manifests as an allergic reaction.

Dr. Nambudripad, in her 1999 book "Say Goodbye to Illness," explains it this way:

"When the allergen's incompatible electromagnetic energy comes close to a person's energy field, repulsion takes place.This causes energy blockages in the meridians. These blockages cause imbalances in the body. The imbalances cause stagnation and illness which creates disorganization in the body function. The disorganization of the body and its function involve the vital organs, their associated muscle groups and nerve roots."

To prevent the allergen from causing further disarray after producing the initial blockage, the brain sends messages to every cell of the body to reject the presence of the allergen. This rejection will appear as repulsion, and the repulsion will produce different symptoms in the person like weak limbs, tiredness, aches, pains, insomnia, constipation, anger and many other such unpleasant symptoms."

According to oriental medicine the energy transportation system of the body is referred to as the meridian system. Simply put, these are unseen lines of energy that flow near the surface of the body. There are many acupuncture points (tiny reservoirs of energy) but only 12 acupuncture control points. They are located on either side of the spine from T1 (upper back) to L5 (lower back). By stimulating these control points, all the meridians can be affected. Stimulation can be by electrical shock, tapping, rubbing or laser. Dr. Nambudripad found that by tapping the control points in the presence of allergens and while breathing in certain ways, the body "resets" itself and will not react negatively to the allergens. The person is advised to stay away from the allergen(s) for 25 hours while the meridians reset. After that, there should be little or no reaction to the allergens.

Several years ago several of my colleagues felt it was difficult to avoid some things for 25 hours, i.e., plastic, fabric, etc. Therefore, a computer wizard was hired to develop a program that would assist the body in "resetting" its meridians. It was a natural transition for those of us who routinely use a computer system to do EAV work. Just three minutes connected to the computer system seemed to have the same effect as the 25 hours of avoidance. The patient simply connects to the computer system following the 20 minutes of rest. The computer system "finalizes" the treatment and the patient is advised to avoid the items that were treated. However, if they accidentally touch or eat a treated item within the 25 hours, all is not lost. The treatment will work anyway.

Because the nature of the treatment doesn't fit with a patient's preconceived paradigm, skepticism runs high when we begin a treatment. However, most skeptics become believers after we've done some muscle testing. The section on Muscle Reflex Technique explains how and why this works. For now, we'll just assume it does. The patient is tested with MRT before the treatment begins. Then he/she is given a glass filled with vials of allergens to be treated. Almost without fail, the patient will suddenly go weak. They may try with all their might but to no avail. The muscles can't withstand the pressure as before the vials were held. Then the vials are taken away. The patient becomes strong again.

As treatment begins, the patient lies down and raises one arm.

Again the muscles are tested without the vials. The patient is usually strong. When the vials are held and the muscles tested again, not surprisingly he/she gets weak. The patient holds onto the glass of vials throughout the treatment. After the treatment the same "weak" muscles are tested again. The patient is usually surprised at how strong they've become after only breathing and tapping the back. When they realize that the only difference was the treatment, they often become ardent believers in NAET.

*Bud had been a B-17 bomber pilot during WWII. He came to the office pale, body slumped forward, white headed with a grey/yellow tint to his skin. His daughter, a patient in our clinic, requested that we treat him to help him feel better and have more energy. During our consultation we discussed the fact that his kidneys and liver weren't fully functioning and he had diabetes. We tested him for allergies and organ weakness. After weekly treatmemts for four weeks his daughter informed us that when he began treatment, his oncologist had told him he had less than two months to live. He had stage 4 pancreatic cancer. He lived past his "death date." In fact, his treatments were reduced to semi-monthy.After 6 months his hair turned dark brown.His skin was back to its normal color. His liver and kidneys were now fully functioning. We would catch him sitting in the waiting room flirting with the little old ladies. His oncologist told him that the tumor on his pancreas had decreased in size to almost non-existant. He said, "I don't know what they are doing over there, but it's working. Keep it up." Bud lived another five and a half years and died from a completely unrelated infection.*

*Tami was a college student when she first contacted our office. She told us that, on two occasions while living at home, she was taken to the hospital with severe breathing problems caused by touching a peanut. Both times she had been pronounced dead and revived in the emergency room. She was told that she had had severe reactions to peanuts. She stated that she had tried shots, medications, avoidance and homeopathic medicine but none of it helped. She thought she would give NAET a try. After six NAET treatments she tested free from an allergy to peanuts. She went home and, with the car running, her mother let her touch a peanut – no reaction. She touched the peanut to her tongue – no reaction. She ate the peanut – no reaction. She said that in the years since then she eats peanut butter and jelly sandwiches like they were going out of style. She said, "I don't know how, but it works."*

## Electro Acupuncture by Voll (EAV)

Most patients suffer from functional disturbances. A functional disturbance occurs when no specific tissue or organ damage can be identified by conventional lab work or other pathological diagnostics. However, the patient continues to experience a myriad of symptoms.

Functional medicine, like functional blood chemistry and functional urinalysis, helps detect and identify disturbances. With functional energy medicine, energetic and regulatory disturbances can be detected prior to symptoms. For example, a person carries, and can pass along, the influenza virus up to a week before symptoms appear. A functional test performed during that week will provide clues that the virus is present and that symptoms will appear soon. However, a functional EAV test does NOT diagnose. Diagnoses can only be given from conventional testing.

Functional medicine, or bio-energetic medicine, combines computer and electronic technology with the ancient wisdom of traditional oriental medicine. As described earlier, energetic meridians or channels that form electrical pathways throughout the body was described centuries ago by ancient Chinese healers. They called the flow of energy along these pathways "Chi," others called it "prana." To stay healthy, these channels rely on the balanced and unblocked flow of life energy. The ability to stay healthy and fight off disease depends on the unrestricted flow of Chi.

In 1951 a researcher named Nivoyet discovered that acupuncture points have lower skin resistance, and therefore, higher conductivity than surrounding tissue. Then in 1952, Dr. Walter

Schmidt discovered that electrical resistance increased at a specific acupuncture point when the corresponding organ was malfunctioning. In 1953, German physician Dr. Reinhold Voll, consolidated these findings and developed a systematic approach for evaluating the body through skin resistance measurements. He developed a practice that became known as "Bio-electronic Functions Diagnosis & Therapy" (BFD). But it wasn't until 1978 that Dr. Helmut Schimmel, a West German physician and researcher, developed the Vega System. He called his system the "Vegatest Method" or VRT (Vegetative Reflex Test). He had spent 30 years researching and developing his method.

In 1979, James Hoyt Clarke introduced his Dermatron. This was the first Computerised Electro Dermal Screening (CEDS) system. After years of working to perfect a computer system that would be capable of taking electro-dermal measurements quickly, simply and accurately, he introduced the LISTEN (Life Information System Ten) System in 1991. With his new system, Clarke was able to test 18,000 substances.

In 1998, BioMeridian Industries introduced the BEST System. Working in a Windows format, it was capable of testing 29,000 substances. This system proved to be more accurate and convenient than previous systems. Because of these new advances, electro-dermal testing and bio-energetic technology gained popularity among practitioners around the world. Even though these systems are FDA approved, the FDA is very heavy-handed when it comes to the production and use of electro-dermal systems. Because of this, acceptance and popularity abounds in Europe and other countries and yet is suppressed in the U.S. With widespread clinical acceptance, scientific research has grown. Many scientific papers have been written and published extolling the accuracy and benefits of this new technology.

In 2003, G-Tech Systems introduced the Asyra system. Joe Galloway had been researching and working with electro-dermal systems for over 20 years. Besides vastly improving the software, the system allowed for single site testing rather than probing many sites.

Two hand-masses were employed rather than a probe that often caused pain when testing. In other words, the patient holds two cylinders during the test rather than having one hand poked many times. This proved to be faster and more accurate than previous systems. A detailed report is generated and printed to help the doctor determine the major concern and a possible course of action. The newest system has proven to be faster, more accurate and completely objective. What would have previously taken over an hour to complete, a thorough test can now be run in less than ten minutes.

The Asyra is loaded with a number of commonly used tests and some specialty tests to help determine the root causes of imbalance. Sometimes the comprehensive test alone is enough to give a direction to pursue. However, there are more extensive tests to help obtain a deeper picture as to what's happening in the body. Once the information is gathered, it can be sorted in different ways to give an accurate, personalized picture of that patient. After a thorough consultation and review of symptoms, the comprehensive analysis is generally run. Most often specialty tests are added to the comprehensive test to give a deeper view of what's happening in the body.

Some of the most common tests include:

| | |
|---|---|
| Acupuncture Evaluation | Homotoxicology Evaluation |
| Allergy/Sensitivity Profile | Hormonal Profile |
| Autism Panel | Metabolic-Digestive Profile |
| Constitutional Influence | Miasm Influence |
| Cranial Therapy | Neurotransmitter Profile |
| Degenerative Disturbance | Nosode Susceptibility |
| Dental resonance Profile | Nutritional Evaluation |
| Emotional Freedom Technique (EFT) | Symptom-Emotion Correlation |
| Emotional Stressors | Toxic Stressors |
| Environmental Sensitivity | Vertebral Profile |
| Food Sensitivity | |
| Gastrointestinal Panel | |

There are thousands of specific energetic tests available. A small sampling of those tests include:

Advanced Allergy Profile
Alzheimers Panel
Antibodies
Auric Field
Auricular Points
Bach Flowers
Bacteria
Brain Waves
Cellular Permeability
Cell Salts
Chemical Toxins
Chromosomes
Color Therapy
Crystal Signatures
Dairy Panel
Drainage
Enzymes
Fungus
Harmful Energies
Heavy Metals
Hormones
Inflammatory Panel
Inhalant Profile
Lyme Disease
And much more......

Meridians
Miasms
Mycoplasma
Mycotoxins
NAET
Neurotransmitters
Nutrient Deficiencies
Nutritional Maintenance
Organs
Oxidative Stress
Parasites
PH
Phenolics
Polarity
Protozoas
Reflexology Evaluation
Rife Frequencies
Sarcodes
Systems
Thyroid Evaluation
TMJ Stressors
Vaccines
Viruses

There are over 40,000 homeopathic, nutritional, herbal, and pharmaceutical items loaded in the Asyra system. The system also allows for additional substances to be loaded to give an unlimited range of tests.

# Chapter 9
## OTHER THERAPIES

A holistic practice will employ standard diagnostic and treatment procedures and protocols. Laboratory tests, x-ray studies, MRI's, CT scans, etc., are all commonly used when necessary. However, the holistic practice will often use procedures that are "non-standard" according to the medical world. Many of these "non-standard" tests, procedures, and treatments are more accurate and cost effective than the standard tests. But because most "non-standard" procedures are not covered by insurance companies and, therefore, not profitable most medical practices avoid "non-standard" procedures, tests and protocols.

Peer pressure is another restriction for some doctors to avoid holistic practice. Recently in our area, a very prominent medical physician lost his license. For many years he practiced without a single complaint or lawsuit. He had a good reputation for helping his patients with all kinds of disorders. His practice was considered holistic because he used some "non-standard" procedures along with his "standard" medical procedures. His big "sin" was that he often prescribed vitamins and minerals along with or instead of standard medicines. The state medical board, along with the police with guns drawn, raided his office. Files, medications and supplements were confiscated and his practice closed. His medical license was suspended on grounds of "practicing non-standard medicine." The word got out to all MD's in the state to refrain from deviating from the "standard" medical procedures of drugs and surgery.

Besides standard lab tests and urinalysis testing, several "non-standard" tests have been designed to give more specific information. See Appendixes 2 and 3 for more lab tests and urinalysis testing and how to read the reports.

## Muscle Response Testing

Many practitioners use a form of testing muscles to assist them in analyzing a problem or condition and often in the treatment of that condition. Muscle testing is also known as Bio-kenesiology, Applied Kenesiology (AK), Muscle Response Testing (MRT), Muscle Reflex Technique, Muscle Response Technique, Total Body Modification (TBM), Neuro Emotional Technique (NET), and Touch For Health. It was first introduced in 1964 by Dr. George Goodheart, a Detroit chiropractic physician. By using isolation techniques, a chiropractic procedure isolating one muscle from those around it, Dr. Goodheart could test the strength of one muscle alone. Through many experiments, trials and studies, he found that structural imbalance leads to disorganization of the entire body. This disorganization can lead to disorders of the glands, organs and central nervous system. In bioenergetic healing, as well as in acupuncture, this condition is termed an imbalance. When an organ or system is out of balance, eventually the body will suffer.

Dr. Goodheart penned the title of Applied Kenesiology to his form of muscle testing. It didn't take long for others to modify the technique and give it their own special name. Dr. John Thie developed a form of muscle testing and called it Touch For Health (TFH). He wrote a highly successful illustrated book by the same name and has taught his technique all over the world. Dr. Donald Lepore developed his own variation and called it Muscle Response Testing. In his book, The Ultimate Healing System, Dr. Lepore demonstrates how to test for toxicities, deficiencies and imbalances. He also demonstrates self testing.

When muscle testing, the patient can lie down, sit up or stand. A muscle is selected to be used for testing. Very often the deltoid muscle (shoulder muscle) is used because of its availability and strength. If there is a condition or anatomical reason for not using the deltoid, any other muscle that can be isolated can be used. The person to be tested extends an arm at a ninety-degree angle to the body – either in front or to the side. The hand is turned to where the thumb is pointing toward the floor. The person doing the test, the facilitator, then pushes with two fingers against the arm just above the wrist ( 5-10 pounds of pressure) to establish the strength of the testing muscle (indicator muscle) while the patient or subject resists. When testing in this way for allergies, the indicator muscle will immediately weaken when the person tested holds something they are allergic to. When the allergen or offending item is removed the muscle immediately returns to its original strength. It is commonly difficult for a person new to this form of testing to determine minute differences in muscle strength. However, with time and practice, it becomes easier to feel subtle changes. The mechanism of muscle testing is intricate, however, a simple version is this: A muscle can be strong when it's not challenged by something harmful to the body. If an allergen or a poison is brought close to the body in the non-testing hand, the God-given, innate intelligence of the body will attempt to protect the body by moving energy from the testing arm to the hand holding the offending item. The result is a weakness in the testing arm. Remove the offending item and the body no longer needs extra energy for protection and moves back to the testing arm. The result is re-established strength.

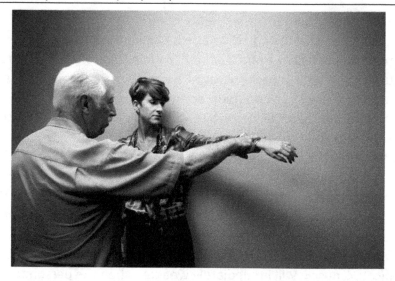

An alternative muscle to test could be the biceps muscle.

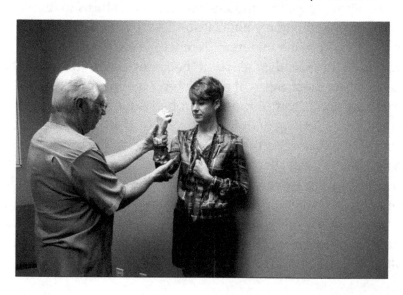

Muscle testing is arguably subjective. However, with practice, one can detect the most subtle changes in resistance with surprising accuracy. The same amount of pressure must be exerted each time a test is performed to get an accurate reading. Several of our patients rely on muscle testing to determine if certain vitamins, minerals, or even some foods would be beneficial for them to consume.

One form of muscle testing is called surrogate testing. If a person is too young or physically hampered in some way, a facilitator can muscle test a third person while that person is making contact with the patient. This utilizes energy conductivity to diagnose allergies and perform other tests with a person who otherwise could not be muscle tested.

## Ultrasound Therapy

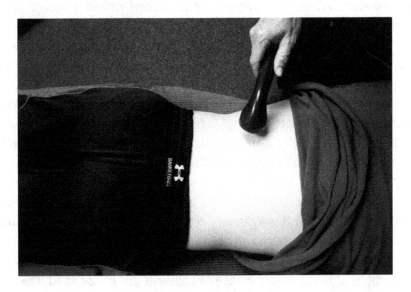

Two modalities that we rely on as adjunctive therapy are ultrasound and laser. Ultrasound therapy is an underutilized adjunct to help eliminate inflammation and expedite healing. Any "itis" in a diagnosis refers to an inflammation, i.e., arthritis – inflammation of a joint, tendonitis – inflammation of a tendon, bursitis – inflammation of a bursa, etc. Ultrasound uses ultra high frequencies (between 1 and 3 MHz), imperceptible to the human ear, to penetrate into the deeper layers of tissue. The sound range for a normal human ear is between 15Hz and 20 Hz.  As the sound waves penetrate, the tissue molecules are set into vibration. This vibration results in localized heat generation and increased blood flow to the target area. With the increased blood flow, fresh oxygen and nutrients are brought to the area thereby reducing inflammation and increasing elasticity. Some of the mechanothermochemical (physical, thermal, chemical, colloid chemical and biologic) effects include: Heat, micromassage, softens scar tissue, increases oxidation, reduces edema, disrupts tissue deposits such as spurs and calcium deposits and is mildly sedative. All this for the patient means reduced pain and greater range of motion.

The 1-2 inch diameter head of the ultrasound unit is called the transducer. When the transducer is placed on an affected area (skin) with a conductive or "coupling" agent (gel), the sound waves will penetrate into the tissue. Ultrasound therapy can also be performed with the transducer under water and the water acting as the coupling agent. Without the coupling agent or away from the skin, the therapy is almost 100% ineffective. At 1 MHz, ultrasound penetrates muscle tissue 9.0mm (approximately 3 inches) and at 3 MHz it penetrates approximately 3.0mm (slightly over 1 inch). For fat tissue the values are similar (50mm at 1 MHz and 16.5mm at 3 MHz). When a substance is added to the coupling get and ultrasound therapy is performed, it's called phonophoresis. The sound waves will drive the added ingredients into the tissues to contribute to the healing process.

Ultrasound plays an important role in the three phases of healing – inflammation phase, proliferation phase and the remodeling phase. Ultrasound stimulates the mast cells, white blood cells, platelets and macrophages during the intitial inflammatory phase. During ultrasound therapy the mast cells degrade releasing arachidonic acid which mediates the inflammation. This acid causes an increase in the inflammatory response essentially promoting the overall repair events.

During the next phase, the proliferative phase, the emphesis is more on restructuring the tissues. Fibroblasts and endothelial cells are targeted to produce scar tissue and to begin the rebuilding.

The final remodeling phase refines the temporary scar that was produced in the proliferative phase. The affected tissue takes on the characteristics of the surrounding unaffected tissue. The functional capacity of the scar tissue is enhanced and unless there was major damage, the area will be as good as it was before.

Our office has found that ultrasound therapy is the first line of defense for:

| | |
|---|---|
| Tendonitis | Arthritis |
| Sprains/strains | Bursitis |
| Muscle pain | Tennis elbow |
| Frozen shoulder | Scar softening |
| Plantar Fasciitis | Heel spur |
| Back/Neck pain | Carpal Tunnel Syndrome |
| Fracture repair | |

Ultrasound is not used:
Over a malignant or cancerous tumor
Over the sex organs
Over a pregnant uterus
If an infection, fracture or blood clot is suspected
If there is a risk of hemorrhage

## Low Level Laser Therapy (Cold Laser, Soft Laser)

Cold laser therapy is also known as low level laser therapy (LLLT), photobiomodulation (PBM), biostimulation laser, phototherapy and therapeutic laser therapy. In 2003 the North American Association of Laser Therapy (NAALT) defined phototherapy as "a therapeutic physical modality using photons of light from the visible red to the infrared spectrum for tissue healing and pain reduction." There have been over 2500 published articles and over 120 double blind studies showing the effectiveness of cold laser therapy.

Low level laser therapy is safe, effective, non-invasive, requires no drugs or medicines and has no adverse side effects when used properly. They were approved in 2001 by the FDA for the relief of pain. There are four classes of cold lasers as described by the U.S. government. They are based on their ability to do damage to the eye.

- Class 1 & 1m are the safest, have the lowest power and are the most popular for healing practitioners.
- Class 2 are the weakest lasers on the market and are being phased out.
- Class 3 & 3b lasers are very powerful and very sensitive to the surroundings.
- Class 4 continuous lasers are the most powerful and can cause damage to tissues if not strictly used properly.

A common safety factor is to treat all lasers as if they were the sun – don't look into the beam of a laser.

The lasers that are used in our office produce a coherent light that penetrates the skin 4-5 inches. The wave length of the lasers affects more than the superficial structures but also penetrates to the cellular level. No more than 5 to 7 minutes are required to attain the desired results. Some of the conditions commonly treated with phototherapy include: Carpal Tunnel Syndrome, soft tissue injuries, arthritis, muscle strains, tendonitis, swelling/edema, tennis/golfer's elbow, nerve regeneration, neck and low back pain, fibromyalgia, repetitive stress injuries, bone healing, joint sprains, wound healing, burns, thrush, mucositis, shingles, postoperative vomiting, and more. Cold lasers have been used for smoking cessation, many skin conditions, weight loss and scar and wrinkle removal. The disadvantages are: it takes several treatments to attain the desired goal and not all insurance companies cover the expense.

*Gina came to our office complaining that she had smoked for most of her life. She said she smoked about a pack of cigarettes each day. She hated it. She knew that smoking was not healthy,* smelled awful and cost her a lot of money each month. The stress of work and a divorce drove her to smoking as a release. She wanted to quit in the worst way. After one laser treatment and a session of TFT for smoking cessation, she turned her back on smoking and hasn't returned nor had the desire to smoke. Robin had a similar story except that she had a husband and three young children. She detoxed from drugs but continued to smoke two packs a day. After one TFT session and one laser treatment she stopped smoking completely.

Bob had suffered a traumatic accident that left him weak and in continous pain. The pain medications stopped working after a while. With manipulation and laser therapy to the general area and to specific trigger points, he was able to return to work with minimal discomfort.

## Thought Field Therapy

Another tool at the disposal of a holistic practice is Thought Field Therapy. Originally introduced by Frank Callahan, Ph.D., TFT has been used for emotional conditions such as: pain, trauma, anger, anxiety, additive urges, phobias, depression, rage, obsessions, guilt, shame, embarrassment and more. Since Dr. Callahan's book, Tapping the Healer Within, others have modified his procedures and renamed the technique EFT, NFT, etc. Properly done, the success rate is incredibly high.

I walked into my treatment room to find Susie in a ball in the corner crying. She told me that after 30 years of marriage, her husband announced to her, in front of their friends, that he was divorcing her. She was devastated. She asked to have a TFT to help her cope with the situation. It took five minutes to do the procedure and afterward she felt like a huge weight had been taken off her shoulders. Later her co-workers called to ask what we had done to Susie. They said that she was a completely different person.

Jennifer was a vibrant young lady of 24 years. She told me that she had been married for one year and now finds her marriage falling apart. She explained that she had been raped at the age of 14 and is now flashing back to that time. After 7 minutes of TFT, Jennifer said that the event now meant no more to her than if she had seen it on TV.

Sydney was at her wit's end. Following a very heart wrencthing divorce, her son began to lash out at her and his sister. Bradley was 12 years old and was large enough to cause pain in his outbursts if he wasn't careful. Sydney had taken him to various doctors and councellors but his attitude had not changed, his grades were very poor in school and he seemed to hate everyone. As a last resort she brought him to our office. He was was tested with the Asyra and treated with homeopathic drops designed especially for him and with TFT for his emotions.

Sydney informed us that the next day she noticed a change in Bradley. He was no longer angry, and in fact, was affectionate. His periods of exploding in anger were gone. After seven weeks he was continuing to improve. Only rarely did he get angry. He was running, laughing and being silly. His teacher, without knowing about the Asyra, drops or TFT, commented to Sydney that Bradley seemed happier, his grades had improved remarkably and his writing skills had even improved. She was so thankful to have the old Bradley back again.

TFT is a very valuable tool considering that many of the conditions we deal with daily stem, in one form or another, from stress. Most patients are truly amazed at the results and often return for treatment for other conditions. The procedure is quite simple. Both the doctor and patient concentrate on the problem to be solved. The patient is asked to rate how bad the condition makes them feel from 1 to 10 with 10 being the worst. The doctor taps on a specific acupuncture point while the patient performs some simple neurologic tasks. The doctor then taps on specific acupuncture points on the head, face and upper chest areas. The patient is asked again to rate how bad they feel with the first number that "pops" into their mind. The number will usually be less than the previous number. The procedure is repeated until the patient responds with a number as low as 1. Often the patient will notice an immediate change while at other times the change will not be noticed until a specific situation is encountered. Invariably the patient will notice a change. This procedure works almost 100% of the time if the patient truly "wants" it to work.

# Chapter 10
## Conditions

Volumes can and have been written regarding each of the conditions listed below. Many of these conditions are seen on a regular basis in a holistic office. In presenting recommendations for each, a great amount of emphasis was placed on presenting remedies that have been proven to work – either by direct observation or observations made by highly trusted doctors. As with so many other things having to do with health care, what works for one person might not work the same for the next person. Therefore, in some instances several remedies have been provided. Extra verbiage was kept to a minimum so that the focal point could be addressed quickly.

This is not an extensive list of conditions nor an exhaustive description of each. This is not meant to take the place of a qualified, holistic, natural healthcare provider. It is simply a tool to give the reader some insight into what can be done naturally to provide some assistance.

## Abscess (Tooth)

A dental abscess, or tooth abscess, is a collection of pus generally associated with a tooth. It's usually a bacterial infection that has accumulated in the soft pulp of a tooth (most commonly a dead area). A broken tooth, tooth decay or a failed root canal treatment can be the ultimate cause of the abscess. The following is a list of alternative treatments that have worked. These remedies may be taken individually or in combination.

**Drain the abscess** – If you want to quickly decrease the size of the sore, carefully sterilize a needle and gently, cautiously, prick the boil with one or two holes. Using a Q-tip, gently release the toxic pus by pushing on the abscess. Don't swallow any of the pus due to its toxicity. Rinse the mouth with hydrogen peroxide. Spit it out and repeat the rinsing step three times. On the third time, hold the hydrogen peroxide in the mouth for about 5 minutes then release. Again, don't swallow any of the H2O2 or the pus.

**The Cell Salt Silica** – Five small tablets dissolved under the tongue three times per day will help decrease the swelling and pain.

**Clove Essential Oil** – Helps kill the infection and relieve the pain. Brush teeth with clove oil and, using a Q-tip, rub it on the gums and on or into the affected tooth.

**Peppermint Essential Oil** – Helps kill the pain.

**Bragg's Apple Cider Vinegar** – Swishing around in the mouth for a few minutes helps disinfect and reduce the swelling.

**Oil Pulling** – To remove toxins from the abscess (and the rest of the body), coconut oil has been used for many years. It is not only anti-bacterial but also boosts the immune system. Swish 1 tablespoon of coconut oil in your mouth for 10-30 minutes. Do not swallow! Spit it out into a tissue or paper towel (not in the sink) and immediately rinse your mouth out.

**Oil of Oregano** – Oregano is an anti-viral, anti-bacterial, anti-fungal and anti-oxidant immune system booster. It helps kill the infection quickly.

**Raw Garlic** – There are many reasons for using garlic. In this instance, rubbing the juice from a clove of garlic directly on the abscess and surrounding area helps kill the infection and ease the pain.

## Abdominal bloating

It can be alarming when your abdomen feels full or distended. Pain and shortness of breath are rare symptoms of this condition. It can be frightening to have a bloated feeling and appearance for no apparent reason. I often hear: "I'm careful with what I eat and I don't eat very much. So why am I bloated?" It can be very frustrating.

Abdominal bloating can be caused by allergies, diet, constipation or even irritable bowel syndrome. Anytime food is not being digested properly gas and bloating can result. Sometimes simply changing the diet can relieve the symptoms. However, that doesn't address the cause of the condition.

We've found that the most common underlying cause of abdominal bloating is allergies. Avoiding dairy, gluten, red meat, artificial sweeteners, alcohol, carbonated beverages, fatty foods or greasy foods will help temporarily but that won't resolve the problem. A NAET evaluation for food allergies is a good starting point. While eliminating the allergies, a thorough evaluation of the gastrointestinal tract should be done.

Upper GI gas (belching or burping) often occurs when one ingests food, water or air too quickly. On the other hand, if there's insufficient hydrochloric acid in the stomach to properly break down food, it can produce a buildup of gas in the stomach. Likewise, if there's insufficient enzymes, amino acids and/or bacteria in the intestinal tract, "stomach growling," or flatulence (passing gas) will occur.

By eliminating allergies using NAETprocedures and restoring normal digestive flow, abdominal bloating can be eliminated.

Another form of abdominal swelling is a gastroenterological

condition known as ascites (or dropsy or hydroperitoneum), which refers to an accumulation of fluid in the peritoneal cavity (abdomen). The abdomen becomes distended and often uncomfortable. The causes vary from cancer, liver disease, alcoholism, tumors and chronic liver infection to drug abuse.

There are several remedies that have been proven beneficial in alleviating the symptoms. However, the cause of the condition should be determined and addressed so that this condition will be completely eliminated. The following may help:

**Garlic:** one-half teaspoon of fresh garlic juice to one-half cup of water taken two times per day for 2-3 weeks.

**Bitter melon (bitter gourd) root juice:** 25 ml of juice diluted in water and taken regularly three times per day can provide prompt relief.

**Punarnava** has been very effective against ascites. Pound out the dried roots to make a power. Add one teaspoon to lukewarm water and drink twice daily for effective relief.

**Polytrichum Juniperum** as a diuretic infusion is one of the better remedies for ascites. As an infusion, take one to two teaspoons of dried herb (or two to four teaspoons of fresh herb), place in a cup of hot water for approximately ten minutes and then strain.

## Acid Reflux (Heart burn, GERD, Peptic ulcer disease)

A burning sensation in the chest that sometimes travels up the throat is often referred to as heartburn. The cause of this sensation is generally due to the lower esophageal sphincter relaxes and allows some of the stomach contents to reflux (flow back up into the throat). The misconception, perpetuated by TV commercials, is that the stomach has too much acid. Therefore, acid-blocking drugs are often requested and prescribed. However, the stomach, like other organs of our body, produces less as we get older and not more. Acid reflux is very often the result of having too little acid in our stomach.

Sometimes, as the esophageal sphincter relaxes, part of the stomach itself can slip into the esophagus and thus create a hiatal hernia and that can lead to heartburn. Helicobacter pylori bacterial infection can also lead to acid reflux.

Several things can adversely affect the esophageal sphincter and cause it to relax. Some medications including beta blockers, aspirine and NSAID's can be causative factors. Smoking, drinking fluoridated water, alcohol, carbonated soft drinks or coffee, and eating foods such as chocolate, peppermint, high-fat foods can lead to acid reflux.

Some effective ways to eliminate acid reflux include:

Drink one tablespoon of Bragg's Apple Cider Vinegar in water or juice. Drink just before eating.

Take one or two capsules of betaine hydrochloric acid before eating.

Make ginger root tea by adding two or three slices of fresh ginger root to two cups of hot water. Let it steep for 20 minutes and drink the tea 10 to 20 minutes before the meal.

## Acne

Acne is an outward manifestation of an internal problem. Topical creams help mask the appearance but do nothing to resolve the problem. There are many causes for this condition but the most prevalent is allergies. The patient is first tested to determine what allergies the patient has and the severity. The patient is then treated for the allergies using NAET procedures. At the same time, the patient is given instructions on how to properly accomplish the Barnes Temperature Test for thyroid function. When thyroid function is low, blood circulation to the skin is diminished. Bacteria can accumulate and cause an inflammatory reaction on the skin. Pores become plugged and the visual signs of acne appear. Eliminating the allergies, elevating the thyroid function (if low), eating a good, balanced diet, taking the proper combination of vitamins, minerals, enzymes and amino acids, avoiding sugar and keeping the surface of the skin clean will help eliminate acne.

To help with the present eruptions, we suggest using Vitamin E and Vitamin F (unsaturated fatty acids). Both vitamins can be found in Safflower oil and Olive oil. If a fat allergy exists, that's usually a sign of a sulfur deficiency. By eliminating the allergy and the deficiency the skin should return to normal.

Constipation can also be a cause of acne. Without proper elimination, toxins will pass through the colon wall and into the blood. One route of escape is via the skin. If constipation is a concern, we suggest enemas, colonics, ionic foot baths and baking soda baths. See Appendix 4: Detoxification.

Cell Salt #12, Silica has been shown to help eliminate acne.

## Adrenal Exhaustion
## (Adrenal Fatigue Syndrome, Hypoadrenia)

The adrenal glands, one atop each kidney, are primary hormonal glands. They are the primary stress control systems of the body. Emotional, physical, mental, or environmental stress over a period of time can cause the body to exceed its ability to adjust to the demands placed on it. Over time, it can lead to adrenal fatigue or exhaustion. Depression, anger, infections, surgery, excessive exercise, excessive sugar intake, fear, and chronic illness are just a few of the stressors that can lead to adrenal fatigue.

Adrenal fatigue or insufficiency can occur when the adrenal glands do not produce adequate amounts of steroid hormones, especially cortisol and aldosterone. When this happens, many regulatory balances begin to malfunction. Studies are showing that some chemicals such as Roundup are disrupting hormonal systems.

Some of the signs and symptoms of adrenal fatigue are: chronic fatigue, brain fog, depression, chronic pain, fibromyalgia, hypoglycemia, craving for salty or fatty foods, inability to lose weight or a tendency to gain weight, reduced sex drive, a weak, jittery feeling, lightheadedness upon arising from a resting position, and many more. If left unattended, adrenal fatigue can lead to a complete adrenal exhaustion. This condition is often missed or misdiagnosed.

In a healthy body, the adrenal glands react to a stimulus with the flight or fight mechanism. Adrenaline is produced to help the individual to either fight the situation or run from it. When adrenaline is released into the blood stream it:

Constricts the smooth muscle of the skin (gooseflesh, hairs stand on end)
Dilates the eyes for more light
Constricts cutaneous blood vessels (white with freight)
Dilates blood vessels of the heart and skeletal muscles
Increases heart rate and cardiac output
Relaxes muscles of the lungs for better oxygen supply
Stimulates respiration
Inhibits digestion
Inhibits the urinary bladder
Contracts the sphincters of the gut
Increases blood sugar
Skeletal muscle fatigues less easily

Once the situation is resolved, the need for adrenalin is reduced and the body can return to its normal state. Very often in that return to normal, the person will become jittery and the body will uncontrollably shake.

Some symptoms of adrenal fatigue are:
Waking up tired even with a full night's sleep
Fatigue during the day for no known reason

Muscle weakness
Depression
Irritability
Muscle weakness or tension
Inability to concentrate
Bone loss
Increased allergies
Difficulty sleeping
Cravings for sugar and/or salt
Hair loss
Weight gain
Loss of balance or a dizzy feeling

Treatment for adrenal fatigue or exhaustion is not as difficult as it may seem. One of the first things to realize if the exhaustion has progressed is that the sodium-potassium balance is interrupted. In this case, sodium is too low to affect a normal balance. By adding a little sea salt to water and drinking a few sips, the balance can be restored and many symptoms fade away.

Diet is a major factor in adrenal recovery. The first step is to remove any toxic, chemical filled, or hard to digest foods from the diet. Avoid sugary foods such as candy, cereals and sweets. Most foods with gluten, I.e. breads pastas, etc. not only convert to sugar but most gluten foods are also laced with GMO's, pesticides and herbicides. Avoid high fructose corn syrup and artificial sweeteners.

Avoid processed foods. Most are full of fillers, preservatives and who knows what else. If the food has a shelf life of months, it's probably not good for the digestive system. The more organic the food is, the better it is for the human system. The food industry has abused the term "natural" to the point that it means nothing on the label.

Coffee can be beneficial if no more than 2-3 cups are consumed per day and taken in the morning.

Some good, easily digested foods are: Wild caught salmon, chicken, turkey, cruciferous vegetables (cauliflower, broccoli, brussel sprouts, etc.), nuts (esp. walnuts and almonds), seeds (pumpkin, chia, flax), coconut, olives, avocado, kelp, celtic or Himalayan sea salt.

Some nutrients help boost the adrenal system. Some of these are:
Vitamin B5
Vitamin B12
Vitamin C
Vitamin D3
Magnesium
Zinc
Fish oil
Ashwagandha
Holy basil

In our office we use a combination of EAV (Asyra) testing to give direction for treatment and to balance the body and give it a head start in the healing process. If a number of allergies are involved (and they usually are), we use some NAET treatments eliminate toxins and allergies. If the patient has had a urine or saliva test performed, those results are correlated with the Asyra results to help determine a course of treatment.

Some suggestions we make are:
Get plenty of sleep. Avoid staying up late and avoid watching TV or using the computer just before bedtime.
Minimize, as much as possible, work and relational stress.
Rest when tired. Take time during the day to relax.
Laugh a lot and avoid negative people and negative self talk.
Exercise regularly to keep the system balanced.
Use TFT for support for any traumatic experiences.
Use cell salts – 4,6,7,9 – 5 pellets each in water bottle. Sip all day.
Be patient. It may take 6-24 months to recover depending on severity.

## Allergies

A condition that causes an adverse or abnormal reaction to one or more substances is generally known as an allergy. An allergy is a reaction to something known as an allergen. These can be categorized into eight types:

- Inhalants: Dust, pollen, perfume, something inhaled through the nose
- Ingestants: Food, drink, vitamins, drugs, anything ingested
- Contactants: Poison Oak, fabric, chemicals, anything touched
- Injectants: Stings, drug injections, insect bites, anything injected through skin
- Infectants: Viruses, bacteria
- Physical agents: cold, heat, sun
- Molds, fungi, parasites, candida, yeast
- Emotional and genetic factors

When a person who is allergic is exposed to an allergen that they have trouble with, the body develops an excess of an antibody called immunoglobulin E (IgE). The reaction of these antibodies with the allergens causes a release of histamines and other substances which in turn causes allergic symptoms. It's a defense mechanism by the body's own immune system by sending antibodies to defend against allergens. Usually it's a slow development but once the activation process has begun, successive exposures have similar reactions.

The symptoms vary remarkably between individuals. Some have no symptoms at all while others can develop anaphylactic shock due to exposure.

Simply put, an allergy is a hypersensitivity of the immune system. A person's immune system may react to the environment, foods, chemicals (including medications) or a host of other factors. Any of these items may cause an excessive activation of particular type of white blood cells called mast cells and basophils. These "factors" are antibodies called Immunoglobulin E (IgE). The response to these antibodies is inflammatory and can be mild or severe, even deadly.

Symptoms of allergies may range from runny nose, itchy skin, eczema, hives, difficulty breathing, red and swollen eyes, to a full blown asthma attack. If the reaction is life-threatening, it's called anaphylaxis.

The medical treatment generally involves avoidance or steroid medications such as antihistamines and decongestants. As with most medications, they involve minimizing the symptoms. They are not meant to cure.

Alternatively, taking 2,000 mg of vitamin C daily has been shown to reduce the body's histamine level by 40%. In other words, that alone should reduce the body's reaction to allergens by 40%. 5-HTP has been used to reduce inflammation in the lungs. And too there are several herbs, cell salts, and essential oils that help reduce the symptoms of an allergy attack. However, the most successful treatment that we have found is with NAET (Nambudripad's Allergy Elimination Technique). We have found that, when performed properly, not only do the symptoms diminish but in most cases, any reaction to an allergen is eliminated. For more on this technique, see the section on NAET.

## Alzheimer's Disease

Alzheimer's disease (AD) is the most common form of dementia. First described by Alois Alzheimer, a German psychiatrist and neuropathologist, in 1906, it has become one of the most feared diseases of the older age group. It has been predicted that AD will affect 1 in every 85 people globally by 2050. When AD is suspected, the diagnosis can be confirmed with behavioral assessments and cognitive tests. These are usually followed by a brain scan. Some early symptoms of AD may include unexplained mood swings, language difficulties, confusion, short-term memory disturbances, changes in personality, and problems with attention and spatial orientation. On average people live 8 to 10 years after the diagnosis, but some can live with this for 20 years.

Alzheimer's disease has been categorized into three stages depending on each person's symptoms. Listed below are the three stages and symptoms associated with each.

**Stage 1 (Mild):**This stage can last 2 to 4 years.
- Less energetic and spontaneous
- Minor memory loss and mood swings
- May become withdrawn and avoid people and new places
- Become confused
- Difficulty organizing and planning
- Easily lost
- Exercise poor judgment
- Difficulty performing routine tasks
- Difficulty communicating and understanding written material
- Losing or misplacing things

**Stage 2 (Moderate):** Stage 2 can last 2 to 10 years. In this stage of AD the person becomes more clearly disabled. They may:
- Need assistance with more complicated tasks
- Forget recent events
- Become more disoriented and disconnected from reality
- Confuse past history with recent events
- Have difficulty comprehending a current situation, date or time
- Have trouble recognizing familiar people
- Have difficulty with reading, writing or understanding
- Have difficulty with speech
- No longer be safe to leave alone and may wander
- Become depressed, irritable, restless, apathetic or withdrawn

- Experience sleep disturbances
- Have more trouble eating, grooming and dressing

**Stage 3 (Severe):** Stage 3 may last 1 to 3 years. In this stage, people may:
- Lose the ability to speak, recognize people, feed themselves
- Lose control of bodily functions
- Lose almost all memory
- Sleep often
- Grunt or moan more commonly
- Become more vulnerable to illnesses, infections and respiratory problems

Early detection is important. The quicker a problem is detected, the easier it is to slow the progression or possibly stave off the process. It is important to classify the symptoms properly. Alzheimer's, dementia and mild cognitive impairment (MCI) can easily be confused. Infections, drug interactions, metabolic or nutritional disorders, brain tumors, depression and toxic states can all give dementia-like symptoms.

Medically, several drugs are used in the treatment of AD. Cholinesterase inhibitors such as Aricept, Cognex, Exelon, and Reminyl work by raising the level of acetylcholine in the brain (deficient in AD). In stages 2 and 3, Memantine is used to protect the brain neurons against the toxic effects of high levels of glutamate (released by damaged cells.

**Alternative/complementary treatment:**
Because toxic poisoning, especially aluminum and mercury, have been implicated in the cause of AD, a complete body detoxification is the first step in the preventive or healing process. The liver and colon would be logical places to start. See Appendix 4.

By doing resistive and endurance exercise for 30 minutes or more a day for 3-5 days each week you can reduce your chances of getting AD by up to 50%. Exercise can cause new synapses and blood vessels to form in the brain. It improves mood and helps with memory and problem solving skills.

Mental exercise can increase the number of neurons in the brain. Reading, learning poetry, playing card games, playing strategy games, doing crossword puzzles or jigsaw puzzles are examples of activities that require the use of the brain. Remember, whether it be mental or physical exercise, use it or lose it.

Research has shown that people with healthy diets are less likely to get dementia. Eating a well balanced diet of fruits, vegetables, grains and meats free from herbicides, insecticides, hormones and GMO's will help the body heal itself.

Researchers and scientists have not determined the actual causes of Alzheimer's disease. However, a number of treatment options have been tried over the years. Pharmaceuticals have not been able to "cure" the disease, only slow its progress. On the other hand, detoxing, exercise, good nutrition and supplementation have shown great promise, especially when taken in conjunction with proper AD medication. Be sure to consult with a pharmacist before mixing prescription medication and herbs or botanicals. The following is a list of what we recommend:

- Antioxidants, such as vitamin E (400-600 iu/day), alpha lipoic acid (10-50 mg three to five times per week), mangosteen, curcumin, and goji can be helpful in reducing the severity of Alzheimer's. Fresh vegetable and fruit juices have tons of beneficial antioxidants.
- B vitamins such as B6, folic acid (400-800 mcg/day), and B12 (800-1200 mcg/day) have been shown to lower homocysteine levels. High homocysteine levels in the brain are thought to cause neuronal damage leading to the progression of AD.
- High levels of niacin (1400-1500 mg/day spread throughout the day), especially from food sources (kale, spinach, legumes), may reduce the risk of age-related cognitive decline.

- Vitamin K2 (45-500 mcg daily) has shown helps increase vascular flow to the brain and might help prevent plaque deposition.
- Ginkgo biloba has been shown to improve cognition.
- Huperzine (huperzine Alpha) blocks the breakdown of acetylcholine. It has shown to be safe and clinically effective in mild to moderate cases. One study showed a 59% improvement when using huperzine A 400 mcg/day for 12 weeks.
- DHA (docosahexaenoic acid) protects the cognitive function in patients with mild, early stage AD. DHA is an omega-3 long chain polyunsaturated fatty acid. Omega-3 is essential for the brain. Taking 180 mg or more per day of DHA has shown to reduce the beta-amyloid build-up in the brain. Beta-amyloid is a protein that forms the characteristic brain plaques seen in patients with AD.
- Acetyl L-carnitine protects against beta-amyloid neurotoxicity. The dose should not be more than 100-300 mg/day a few times a week.
- Choline (100-500 mg 4-5 times/week) provides acetylcholine precursors. Acetylcholine is a neurotransmitter that affects learning and memory. Lecithin is a source of free choline.
- Other items such as curcumin, green tea and Blue green algae have shown beneficial uses in AD.
- Foods that contain some of the above nutrients include: Lentils (contains glucose for the brain), Chia seeds (omega-3 fatty acids (for brain cell communication and clearing the arteries), Brazil nuts (good source of monounsaturated fats and magnesium – along with almonds, walnuts and cashews), coffee (protects the blood-brain barrier and the brain from damaging elements and is high in antioxidants).

## Anemia

Anemia is the most common disorder of the blood. By definition it is a decrease in the number of red blood cells (RBCs) or the amount of hemoglobin in the blood that is less than the considered normal state. Hemoglobin, found in RBCs, carries oxygen from the lungs to the capillaries. If the proper amount of oxygen is decreased, a lack of oxygen to the tissues (hypoxia) leads to anemia. There are three main classes of anemia: excessive blood loss (hemorrhage or chronic low volume loss), blood cell destruction (hemolysis), or deficient RBC production (ineffective hematopoiesis).

Some common signs and symptoms include: Fatigue, dizziness, yellowing eyes, skin paleness, coldness and yellowing, low blood pressure, rapid heartbeat, palpitations, shortness of breath, muscular weakness, change in stool color, enlarged spleen. In severe cases: fainting, chest pain, angina, heart attack.

An EAV evaluation will reveal the most prevalent toxicities and deficiencies that may affect the blood. By taking the drops, most systems should balance. In addition, we recommend some nutritional therapy. Increasing the intake of iron, zinc, folate and vitamin B12 will help. B12 should be taken along with a vitamin B complex. Taking B12 alone will deplete levels of B3 and B6. If the body is low in zinc it will reject iron so it is important to balance zinc and iron. We also recommend a high potency multi vitamin and mineral.

Increasing the intake of vitamin B12, folate or folic acid and iron is best accomplished with supplements. However, increasing the consumption of certain organic, non-GMO foods will help. Some people are allergic to some of these foods, so care should be taken. Tuna, beef, eggs, liver and dairy products are good sources of vitamin B12. Dark leafy vegetables, dried beans, asparagus and oranges are good sources of folate or folic acid. Prunes, raisins, dried beans and apricots, liver and the herbs yellowdock and blackstrap molasses are good sources of iron.

# Arteriosclerosis

See Atherosclerosis.

# Arthritis

The term "arthritis" comes from the Greek *arthro* – joint plus *itis* – inflammation. Generally in an arthritic condition, the joint is inflamed, calcium is drawn from the surrounding bone (localized osteoporosis), calcium is laid down along the joint surfaces (causing decreased joint spacing), which causes stiffness and pain.

There are several forms of arthritis:
Osteoarthritis (degenerative joint disease) – from trauma or infection of a joint.
It can also be caused by chronic overuse.
Septic arthritis caused by a joint infection.
Rheumatoid arthritis is from an unknown cause.
Psoriatic arthritis is caused by severe psoriasis.
And there are many other forms.

Some common symptoms include: joint pain, swelling, stiffness (especially in the morning), inability to use the hand or foot due to difficulty in moving the joint, tenderness, fatigue and malaise, poor sleep, and unanticipated weight loss or weight gain.

We have found that ultrasound and chiropractic manipulation helps relieve the pain of arthritis. Ultrasound helps eliminate the inflammation in a joint and manipulation helps relieve the muscle spasm that often occurs.

Studies have shown that losing 10-20 pounds will eliminate most, if not all, of the symptoms in most cases. Walking and swimming laps is essential for those with osteoarthritis, even just walking 30 minutes per day helps. A program called Better Bones and Balance has demonstrated a reversal of osteoporosis that often accompanies osteoarthritis. Acupuncture has been beneficial in relieving symptoms in many cases.

Glucosamine sulfate is the only combination known to date to restore cartilage along joint surfaces. I underlined sulfate since there are two forms of glucosamine on the market today. Glucosamine sulfate (1500 mg once per day) has been shown to be beneficial in relieving the pain of arthritis. However, there are no studies that show that glucosamine hydrochloride has any beneficial effect on osteoarthritis. Taking more than 1500 mg per day has not shown to be any more beneficial than just 1500. Taking less than 1500 mg per day has shown to be a waste of time and money. It's best to take the 1500 at one time rather than splitting it up. When combined with 800 − 1200 mg of chondroitin and MSM, it was found that the pain and progression of osteoarthritis were both reduced. Care should be exercised if there is a sugar metabolism condition.

Capsaicin cream and transcutaneous electrostimulation (TENS) units are helpful in some cases by reducing substance P, a nerve ending impulse transmitting chemical, and by desensitizing nerve endings.

For years Boron was known as a "cure" for arthritis (all forms). However, big pharma and the FDA together suppressed the notion that anything non-chemical could help. Boron was discredited and put on the back shelf. Studies have shown that 1/8 to ¼ teaspoon of Boron in one liter of water and sipped throughout the day can eliminate arthritis. One to two liters of this combination per day is recommended.

Essential oils can be very helpful in reducing the swelling and pain caused by arthritis. When using essential oils, do a sensitivity test on your skin to determine if you have a reaction to a particular oil. It's always wise to consult your alternative holistic healthcare doctor before venturing off into unknown territory. That said, the following oils have worked for many people either individually or in combination. It's suggested that 3-6 drops of each oil (individually or in combination) combined with 1 ounce of coconut oil or another carrier oil, mixed and then applied to the affective area. Those oils are: Basil, Cayenne pepper, Chamomile, Eucalyptus, Frankincense, Lavender, Marjoram, Menthol, Peppermint and Rosemary. Rheumatoid arthritis sufferers have noted relief by using a combination of Frankincense, Ginger, Myrrh, Orange and Peppermint. Turmeric is an effective anti-inflammatory.

## Atherosclerosis

Atherosclerosis refers to the clogging of the arteries. Since this is not isolated to just one area it is referred to as a systemic problem. The problem can go unnoticed for years and only discovered by some debilitating event such as angina or heart attack.

There are 60,000 miles of capillaries (small blood vessels) in the body. When blocked, the body will form small vessels to compensate for the blockage. This process is called angiogenesis. Unfortunately, angiogenesis stops around the age of puberty. As we age, the larger blood vessels become stiffer and less elastic. This condition is called arteriosclerosis. Atherosclerosis, on the other hand, is caused by the buildup of fatty plaques in the artery. There has been a great deal of controversy as to why the arteries accumulate plaque. At the time of this writing, the most accepted cause is an inflammatory process within the arteries.

There are several natural substances that help combat arterial blockages. In many cases the blockages can be cleared completely, thus reducing blood pressure and the risk of stroke and heart attack.

**Natto**, a fermented product form the combination of boiled soybeans and the beneficial bacteria *Bacillus natto*. It's often called "vegetable cheese" because many people note that it tastes like cheese. The Japanese have used Natto for over 1,000 years to treat heart and vascular diseases, beriberi, and fatigue.

**Nattokinase**, often called "the poor man's clot buster," is an enzyme that is often used to clear arterial blockages. Nattokinase can effectively remove fibrous tissue and other clotting components by removing the fibrin deposit or clot rather than thinning the blood as most anticoagulant drugs do.

The drugs urokinase, streptokinase, and activase have been used with some degree of success but each has its own set of problems associated with it. Besides being very expensive and not readily available, the fibrinolytic activity (ability to dissolve clots and fibrous tissue) lasts for only about 4 to 20 minutes. However, the natural solution of natto and nattokinase, according to Japanese researchers, maintains its activity for four to eight hours. They noted that 100 grams of natto exhibits the same fibrinolytic activity as a therapeutic dose of urokinase.

Two precautions are noted for natto and nattokinase:
1. If taking warfarin (rat poison) to prevent blood clots, do not take natto or nattokinase. The high content of vitamin K in natto will impede the effectiveness of warfarin.
2. Natto or nattokinase should be taken with the evening meal or at bedtime, especially if at risk of stroke or heart attack. In this case it would be wise to keep some on hand in case of a heart attack or stroke.

As we age, the ability of our vascular system to dilate decreases. By taking **L-arginine** we can increase our blood flow. L-arginine is converted to nitric acid which helps the blood vessels to relax and dilate. Even a small increase in diameter can result in a large increase in blood flow, i.e. doubling the radius of a vessel results in a four fold increase in blood flow. Taking 6 grams (3 grams taken twice daily) has been shown to double blood plasma levels in just a few weeks.

**Lecithin** is known to lower the levels of LDL cholesterol and, at the same time, increase HDL cholesterol. Recently the focus has been on using lecithin to help prevent atherosclerosis by lowering the blood plasma levels of homocysteine. This is usually accomplished by using vitamins B6, B12, and folic acid. However, the choline provided by lecithin has the same effect. Choline is metabolized into betaine, which in turn lowers homocysteine levels.

According to recent research, **Grapefruit Pectin** at about 15 grams per day is showing some promising results in actually reversing atherosclerosis.

**Vitamin K2** has been shown to inhibit calcification of the arteries.

## Athlete's foot (tinea pedis, tinea pedum)

Athlete's foot is a contagious fungal infection of the skin. It causes scaling, flaking, and itching of the affected areas. The fungi require warm, moist areas, i.e. communal showers and swimming pools.

Although the condition typically affects the feet, it can spread to any area of the skin that is kept hot and moist with body heat and sweat. When it spreads to the body or limbs, it's known as tinea corporis. When the groin is affected it's known as tinea cruris (jock itch).

Preventive measures include keeping the feet dry by using socks made of synthetic materials, changing socks frequently, wearing sandals when walking through public areas such as locker rooms, showers, etc., and using antifungal powder. 30-40% of cases of athlete's foot will resolve spontaneously without medication.

The following treatment has proven to be very successful. Soak the foot/feet in a basin of water with a few teaspoons of oregano oil, or rub the diluted oil (1 drop of oil in a teaspoon of olive or coconut oil) on the nails/skin. Follow up by mixing 2 drops of Melaleuca essential oil with 1 ounce of coconut oil and rub on the bottoms of the feet. Do this at least twice daily until resolved.

## Back Pain

Having treated thousands of patients for almost 40 years, I have found that there are three primary causes of back pain. These are: direct trauma, micro-trauma and stress. Direct trauma is easily understood. A fall, a motor vehicle accident, a blow to the back, lifting wrong or lifting too much are examples of direct trauma. Micro trauma is much more complicated and harder to explain. Sitting at a desk or watching TV without proper support, bending to weed the garden, reaching to paint above the head, slumping while sitting, twisting the neck to see are all examples of micro-trauma. It may not be anything more than an "ache" at the time. But later that "ache" along with the accumulation of other "aches" can lead to a severe back pain. The patient generally enters the office and says, "I didn't do anything" or "I just coughed" or "I just bent over" or "I rolled over in bed." That's the accumulation of micro-trauma.

The last of my three categories of causes of back pain is stress. This can manifest in the low back, upper back or neck. Emotional stress causes muscles to contract. Then any aberrant movement that causes muscles on one side of the spine to contract without a similar contraction on the other side can result in a vertebral subluxation. A vertebral subluxation is movement of one bone (vertebra) in a joint in relation to another vertebra in that joint that doesn't return to its normal position when that motion has ceased. In the spine, the abnormal movement and resultant fixation usually results in a compression of the contents of the intervertebral foramen (IVF), a small opening between the vertebrae. Among those contents are nerves that lead to the muscles or internally to organs. If the nerve flow is interrupted, something downstream has to give. If the nerve goes to an organ, there will surely be some malfunction. If it goes to muscle or a superficial area on the body, there will usually be pain and/or numbness.

If the pain is from acute trauma, an ice pack will help keep the area from swelling. Crushed ice in a baggie wrapped in a towel or a commercial ice pack or even a frozen bag of corn or peas will accomplish the task. Studies have shown that oftentimes more damage is done by the inflammation and resultant swelling than is done by nerve irritation. Ice packs or cold compresses will help keep that from happening. Twenty to thirty minutes per hour for the first day depending on the severity of the sprain/strain. If there is doubt as to whether to use cold or hot or if it's been over 24-48 hours since the injury, alternate hot and cold packs in this order: Hot, cold, hot, cold, hot – five minutes each. Always beginning and ending with hot. Then gently stretch the area while avoiding pain.

If the pain is chronic or long standing, heat is recommended. Apply a heating pad, hot rice bag or hot wash cloth in a baggy wrapped in a thin towel to the area for 15-20 minutes each hour.

Ultrasound therapy is often used to reduce swelling and inflammation in an injured area. The unit is turned up to just within patient tolerance for five minutes. The sound head should be kept moving at all times to avoid the sensation of being burned or muscle contraction. If this occurs, the ultrasound unit should be turned down a notch or two to remain within patient tolerance. We often use laser therapy on the affected area if the pain is intense and there's evidence of considerable inflammation.

Chiropractic adjustments are generally indicated when a spinal misalignment is present, however, only a chiropractor can make that determination based on his/her training and experience.

Exercises are beneficial in keeping the affected segement(s) in alignment. For the neck we recommend slow, gentle range of motion (flexion, extension, lateral bending left and right, and rotation left and right), followed by shrugging the shoulders while taking a shower. The warm water relaxes the muscles while the stretching increases flexibility. We suggest that during the day doing the cervical range of motion against the hand (isometric) for five seconds in each motion with five seconds rest in between will increase muscle tone and decrease the frequency of misalignment.

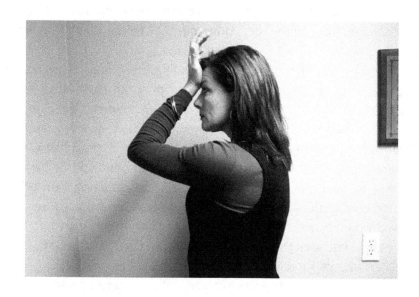

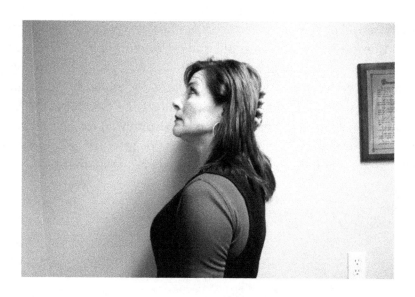

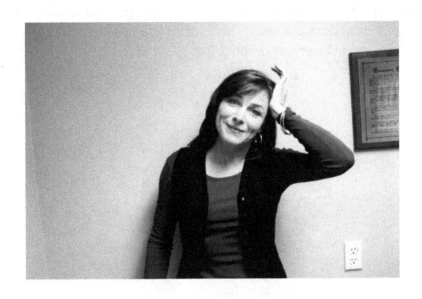

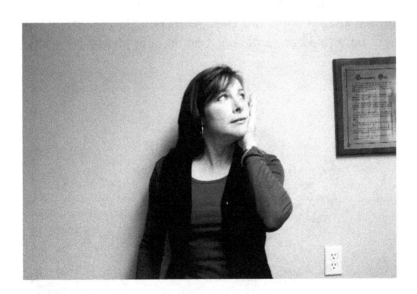

I have found that five exercises for the low back are the most beneficial. First, stand on your hands and knees. As you arch your back up, lower your head down. Then reverse that maneuver – drop your abdomen toward the floor as you raise your head up as to look up at the ceiling. Repeat this 10-20 times.

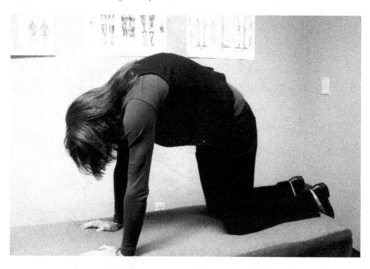

Second, remain in the hands and knees position while you bring one knee toward the chest and then slowly extend the leg straight back to a horizontal position. Repeat this 10-20 times.

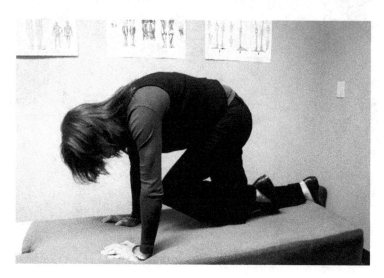

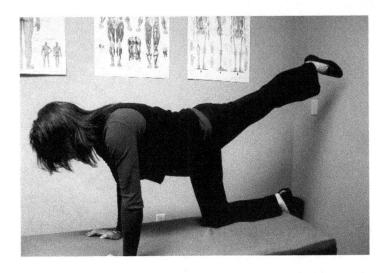

Third, lie on your stomach and raise one leg at a time as high as you can without causing pain. Repeat that 10-20 times with both legs.

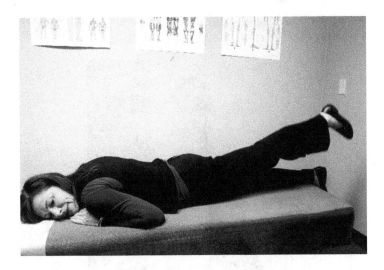

Fourth, do a baby pushup (leave the abdomen on the floor). When you reach full arm extension, tighten your bottom. Hold that for 5 seconds. Repeat 10 times.

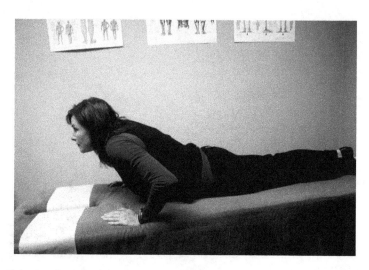

Fifth, and probably the most effective low back exercise, especially for the SI joints, is to stand upright and slowly kick the leg backwards with the knee locked. The motion should come from the hip area. To be most effective, do this maneuver against resistance by using surgical tubing or stretchy bands. Three sets of 10 are preferred alternating legs between sets.

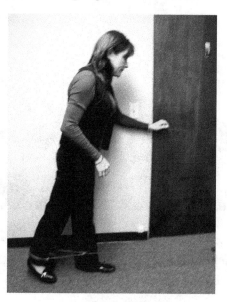

## Bacterial Infection

Antibiotics have become the most over prescribed medicines in the medical world today. Even though the AMA advised doctors years ago to reduce the prescribing of antibiotics and even though research studies have shown that bacteria are mutating due to the over prescribing of antibiotics, the trend continues. Digestive systems have been ruined and immune systems have been compromised because for years doctors have prescribed antibiotics for everything from colds to hang nails. Like so many other conditions, nature has provided an alternative way of dealing with bacteria without harmful side effects. Below are four of the most powerful natural antibiotics that we have found.

- **Garlic** – Garlic is a powerful antibiotic, antiviral, antimicrobial and antifungal herb. It has been used for centuries to treat infections and even the plague. It's a natural antioxidant that supports a strong immune system. Allicin is the key component that wards off bacteria.
- **Oil of Oregano** – Oregano kills pathogenic bacteria without affecting beneficial bacteria. It is also antiviral and antifungal. It affects bacteria without encouraging mutation. Carvacrol is the key component causing antibacterial action.
- **Echinacea**–Echinacea has been used for hundreds of years to treat many kinds of bacterial infections including blood poisoning and diphtheria. Along with garlic and oil of oregano, Echinacea is used in this office to stop colds and influenza in their tracks. It's also effective in destroying the dangerous bacteria staphylococcus aureus which causes MRSA.
- **Colloidal Silver** – This effective antibiotic has been used for centuries to rapidly kill microbes like MRSA, SARS, and the bird flu.

## Bad breath (Halitosis)

Bad breath can be the source of embarrassment and many anxious moments. Friends may back away as you speak and little children may embarrass you by blurting out about your bad breath. Some foods (i.e., onions, garlic), some habits (i.e., smoking, drinking, not brushing teeth or rinsing the mouth), and some health conditions (i.e., bacterial infection, gum disease) can cause bad breath.

Bacteria in the mouth can cause chemicals and gases to be produced that lead to halitosis. One of the best ways to eliminate this condition is a procedure called "oil pulling." The procedure is as follows:

- Scoop 1-2 tsp. of coconut oil into the mouth. Start swishing when it melts.
- Swish the mouth for 20 minutes.
- After 20 minutes, spit the oil into a trash can, not the drain.
- Rinse the mouth with warm water.
- Brush the teeth well, best with all natural non-fluoride toothpaste.

Digestive enzymes – 1-2 with meals
Probiotics – one per meal
Charcoal tablets – between meals – absorbs toxins
Hydrogen peroxide – gargle and rinse mouth
Oil of oregano – 2 capsules three times a day
Green drinks - daily
Cloves – suck on one to two clove buds for a few minutes and then discard
Vitamin B6 2 mg (children), 2.6 mg (pregnant and lactating women) Therapeutic dose: up to 1,000 mg
Anise (Pimpinella Anisum)
Rosemary tea – as a mouthwash

Honey and Cinnamon – gargle with 1 tsp. of honey and cinnamon
powder mixed in hot water first thing in the morning.
One drop of Peppermint essential oil on the tongue helps.

## Baker's Cyst

Also known as a popliteal cyst, a Baker's cyst is a benign swelling of the popliteal bursa behind the knee. The causes range from arthritis to cartilage tear to overuse. Any trauma or continued aggravation of the bursa and surrounding area can lead to inflammation and swelling. The swelling causes pain behind the knee and often to the top of the calf muscle (gastrocnemius). If the cyst bursts, medical attention, including ultrasonography, should be sought to rule out anything more serious.

Treatment for a Baker's cyst is very safe and effective. If the area feels hot to the touch, using cold packs (cryotherapy) for 10-15 minutes every hour should help. A bag of frozen peas works well too. If it has been a long standing problem, some use a heating pad for relief. However, a heating pad can increase the inflammation and resultant swelling. If in doubt, alternate hot packs every 5 minutes. Always begin with heat and end with heat. I use my hand to demonstrate to a patient. Pointing at each finger as I go: "hot-cold-hot-cold-hot." Then I hold up my hand: "For 5 minutes."

A knee brace should be worn, especially when squatting, kneeling, climbing or heavy lifting. Those activities should be avoided if possible. Walking should be kept to a minimum and always with the brace on. Resting with the affected leg elevated whenever possible is most advisable.

Once the swelling has receded, gradually increasing the above activities will avoid aggravating the area. Exercises for strengthening the are suggested but with caution not to aggravate the knee.

## Balance problems

As we get older it seems we find ourselves losing our balance more often. It can be very frustrating and even dangerous if we fall. One of the worst things that people do is to attribute this to "old age" and resign themselves to just living with it. However, like many conditions, this too can be changed for the better.

When we were children we played and did things that honed our skills. We threw balls and rocks. We skipped and ran. We climbed and jumped. We walked on curbs and railroad tracks. We didn't realize that these activities were making us stronger and more well-rounded people. But as we "matured" we stopped doing most of those activities and as the old saying states: "If we don't use it, we lose it." Such is the case with our balance. Granted there are other factors that can be involved, but for the most part we don't practice balancing anymore. Here are a few exercises we can do to regain some of the balance we lost. It's okay to hold onto something or have a partner assisting with balance while you do these exercises.

1. Heel to toe walk or tightrope walk: Stand with your arms stretched out horizontally to the side, parallel to the floor. While looking straight ahead, walk 10-20 steps in a straight line. A variation to this would be to touch your heel to the toes of the opposite foot while walking forward.
2. One leg stand (flamingo stand, Karate Kid stand): Stand facing a wall with arms outstretched in front and hands touching the wall. Lift one knee until the upper leg is horizontal. Hold for 5 seconds then gently lower the foot to the floor. Repeat the same movement with the other leg. Do this exercise 5-10 times with each leg (alternating). Repetitions can increase as proficiency increases. A variation to this can be accomplished as balance improves. Try doing this exercise without holding onto the wall. Do not attempt this unless you are confident in your balance.

3. Lateral rocking: Start by standing with the feet shoulder width apart. Rock side to side putting weight on one foot while taking the weight off the other foot. Then do the same with the other foot. Repeat 5-10 times. A variation would be to lift one foot off the floor for 10 seconds and then repeat with the other foot. Again repeat 5-10 times.

4. The grapevine walk: Stand upright and, while looking straight ahead, cross the right foot over the left and then bring the left foot to join it. Then cross the right foot behind the left and then move the left foot to join the right. Repeat this by starting with the left foot. Repeat this series 5-10 times.

5. Balance step: Use a chair or railing to hold on to for support while doing this exercise. Using a 2-4 inch step, slowly step up using the right foot and then bring the left foot up to join the right. Slowly step down with the right foot first followed by the left. Repeat this 10 times while alternating the lead foot.

6. Side step: Laterally step over a small object with one foot and move the other to it. Repeat going the other way. Repeat 10 times with each foot.

## Bee Stings

Being stung by a bee doesn't happen very often, but when it does it can be a very traumatic event. Always look for a stinger and if one is present, remove it. Immediately after a bee sting, tape a penny on the sting for 15 minutes. The pain will decrease almost immediately and will not return.

## Bell's Palsy

The exact cause of Bell's Palsy is unknown. Theories abound as to it being caused by inflammation, virus, bacteria, trauma and stress. Bell's Palsy is also known as idiopathic unilateral facial nerve paralysis – meaning paralysis of the facial nerve (Cranial nerve VII) on one side for unknown reasons. It displays a rapid on-set and is usually self-limiting.

Some of the possible causes include:
- Stress
- Multiple sclerosis
- Diabetes
- Lyme Disease
- Chemotherapy
- Bacterial infection
- Viral infection
- Trauma
- Tumor
- Anything that causes facial nerve compression

Symptoms of Bell's Palsy include, but are not limited to:
- Sudden onset of facial paralysis
- Drooping and inability to move the muscles on one side of the face
- Loss of control of blinking, closing or tearing the affected eye
- Inability to raise the eyebrows, smile or frown
- Loss of taste on anterior 2/3 of the tongue
- Pain and/or headache
- Changes in hearing

A thorough examination, including blood work, should be done to differentially diagnose the condition. Stroke, herpes and other viral infections, Lyme disease and others need to be ruled out prior to treatment. A House-Brackmann score is used to de-termine the degree of nerve damage in a facial nerve palsy. It's a measurement of the mid eyebrow upwards and of the lateral an-gle of the mouth laterally.

Again, Bell's Palsy is generally self-limiting. The more severe the case, the longer it takes to resolve it. Likewise, the more quickly it's addressed, the better the results. There are several approaches to treating Bell's Palsy including acupuncture, massage, hyperbaric oxygen therapy and vitamin therapy. We have found that EAV testing and treatment, NAET treatment and supplement therapy helps resolve the condition more quickly than other therapies.

Cayenne pepper (Capsicum) improves blood flow but may increase blood pressure

Echinacea, Goldenseal, Olive Leaf are anti-viral

L-Carnitine – is anti-inflammatory and reduces free radical damage

Methyl-Sulphonyl-Methan (MSM) – 500 mg 3 times per day – anti-inflammatory

Vitamin B therapy – A B-complex plus B-12 helps in 60-70% of the cases

Here are some B vitamins that are helpful:

B-1 – 50 mg 3 times per day – increases circulation

B-2 – 50 mg 3 times per day

B-6 – 100 mg 3 times per day

B-12 – 100 mg 2 times per day (or 1 mg 3 times per week by injection) Methylcobalamin is recommended over cyanocobalamin B-12 promotes nerve growth and maintenance and helps repair the myelin sheath (the insulation layer around the nerve)

## Bladder Infection

Cystitis, urethritis, and UTI's (urinary tract infections) are all names for a bladder infection. Symptoms such as pelvic pain, an extreme urgency, a burning sensation during voiding, frequent but minuscule urinations, incontinence and bloody urine are the results of bacteria growing in the bladder. At the first sign of urgency or burning, drink a glass of water every hour to avoid a full blown bladder infection.

Once an infection is established, the following items can be used to minimize pain and expedite recovery:

- **Cranberry Juice** (unsweetened). One glass to 1 quart per day for acute infections. Substances in cranberry juice kill bacteria and make the bladder wall so slippery that bacteria can't attach and thrive there.
- **Cantharis,** a homeopathic remedy, can soothe scalding urination.
- **Uva Ursi** is good for strengthening the bladder and ending chronic bladder infections. The preferred dose is 1 cup of infusion; 10-30 drops of tincture; or 1 tablespoon of vinegar – 3-6 times per day, then 1-3 times per day for 7-10 days.
- **Yarrow** is not only a urinary disinfectant but is also antibacterial and an astringent. One cup of an infusion, once or twice per day for 7-10 days will help tone bladder tissues.
- **The most effective** urinary tract infection remedy that we have found to date is an equal part combination of Juniper berries, Licorice root, Uva ursi leaves, Couch grass root, and Marshmallow root. The combined elements can be made into a tea or put in capsules and taken orally. Since everyone is different, start slowly and build to a point of relief (usually within 2-3 days).

Women who wash their vulva with soap and water, use douches, bubble baths, tampons, nylon underwear and pantyhose are more likely to get vaginal and bladder infections. Urinating after intercourse flushes out bacteria and cuts down on UTI's. Urinating before intercourse increases the risk.

Alcohol, black tea, cayenne, chocolate, citrus juices, coffee and sodas are known bladder irritants.

For more information, see under Urinary tract infections.

## Blood Pressure, High

See High Blood Pressure

## Blood Pressure, Low (hypotension)

Blood pressure is considered low when the systolic (first and higher number) pressure is less than 90 mm Hg and/or the diastolic (second and lower number) pressure is less than 60 mm Hg. In practice, though, blood pressure is only considered low if a low reading is accompanied by symptoms. Severely low blood pressure can deprive the brain and other organs of oxygen leading to dizziness and fainting. If prolonged, low blood pressure can lead to much more serious disorders.

Symptoms of low blood pressure include: lightheadedness, dizziness, fainting, seizures, chest pain, back pain, shortness of breath, irregular heartbeat, indigestion, diarrhea, vomiting, fever and more.

Some causes of hypotension are dehydration, blood loss, heart and/or endocrine problems, poor diet, infection, some medications, and allergies.

A simple home test can determine certain types of hypotension. Gravity will cause blood to pool in the legs when a person stands from a sitting or lying down position. In compensation, the body will react by constricting blood vessels and increasing the heart rate. That will increase the blood flow (and oxygen) to the brain. If, however, the person has low blood pressure, this mechanism will fail and the blood pressure will drop. When it drops, the aforementioned symptoms will occur.

Because there are several reasons for low blood pressure, there are several remedies for it that have worked. As with anything else, not all of these suggestions will work for everyone.

- Licorice root blocks the enzyme that breaks down cortisol and supports healthy adrenal function. If low levels of cortisol is the cause of LBP, steep one teaspoon of licorice in a cup of boiling water for five minutes. Take daily for a few days. If capsules are preferred, 400-500 mg per day for a few days is sufficient.
- Caffeinated beverages (coffee, cola, hot chocolate) can give temporary relief. One to two cups in the morning and one with each meal can be very effective.
- For many years an Ayurvedic remedy for HBP has been raisins. After soaking 30-40 raisins overnight, eat them on an empty stomach. The water they soaked in can be consumed to increase the benefit.
- Salt water is known to increase LBP. One half teaspoon of salt in a glass of water will help stabilize low blood pressure.

We generally start with an Asyra test to help determine the cause of the condition. Any blood tests that the patient has had done are discussed. Iron and iodine deficiencies are often discovered. The EAV test report is discussed and a plan of action is proposed.

## Body Odor

Besides poor hygiene, a body odor can often reveal the condition of an organ inside. The following list of five body odors will reflect the possible imbalances or irregularities of associated internal organs. With this information, one can be more aware of other signs that may lead to a proper diagnosis.

| Odor | Organ Pair |
| --- | --- |
| Oily, Fatty | Liver/Gallbladder |
| Burnt | Heart/Small Intestine |
| Fragrant, Sweet | Spleen/Stomach |

| | |
|---|---|
| Fishy | Lung/Large Intestine |
| Rotten, Putrefying | Kidney/Bladder |

Deodorants and all other fragrant alternatives only mask the bad body odor problem. Bad body odor is a clear and immediate sign that internally you need to get your health in order. Very often men with a body odor problem will also show signs of toxic buildup when "ring around the collar" and under arm stains begin to appear on their shirts.

Detoxification is the key. There are several ways to accomplish this:

- Coffee hydrocolonic therapy or enemas
- Ionic foot baths
- Epson salt and baking soda baths
- Nature's Tea (a combination of herbs that cleans the colon)

## Boosting the immune system

Here are some helpful hints to boost your immune system:

1. **Diet** – Eat lots of <u>fruits and vegetables</u>. They're rich in antioxidants which combat free radicals (known to suppress the immune system).

   Take <u>omega-3-6-9 fatty acids or krill oil</u> (helps production of compounds involved in regulating immunity), <u>garlic</u> (virus and bacteria fighting properties), and <u>ginger</u> (natural anti-inflammatory).

   Drink plenty of water (flushes out the system).

   Vitamins A, B complex, C and D are helpful immune boosters. Zinc increases T-cells to fight infections.

   Echinacea and Aloe vera have many immune-boosting properties.

   Avoid a diet high in sugar and fats as they tend to suppress the immune system.

2. **Exercise** – <u>Moderate exercise</u> (brisk walking for 30 minutes daily) mobilizes T-cells and helps guard against infection. Intense exercise, however, may weaken the immune system.

3. **Hygiene and Sleep** – <u>Washing hands</u> for 15 to 20 seconds with warm water before eating or preparing food or touching the face helps ward off illness, especially after coughing, sneezing, using the bathroom, or touching public surfaces. Getting <u>sufficient sleep</u> each night helps regulate the immune system.

4. **Reduce Stress** – Prolonged stress tends to wear down the immune system. Meditation, yoga, deep breathing and tai chi have all been shown to reduce stress. This may be easier said than done but with a little effort, any of these can be added to a daily routine.

## Breast Conditions

In recent years breast conditions have become a greater concern to our patients than it had been in the past. Therefore I decided to include a section on breast conditions to answer some of the most frequently asked questions in our office.

Before getting into conditions, it is helpful to know some basic anatomy of the breast. The **size and shape** of each breast is determined by the underlying tissues: Pectoralis muscle, fat tissue, ligaments and glands. Support for the breast is provided by the pectoralis major muscle and Cooper's ligament, a fibrous band from the collarbone and chest wall to the skin of the areola that provides upward support for the breast. To transfer milk from the **milk glands** to the nipple, small tubes called **milkducts** are provided. If they become plugged, a condition called **mastitis** occurs (see Mastitis). Tiny holes with sphincters in the nipple are called **milk duct orifices**. Just before going into the nipple, the ducts widen. This area is called the **ampulla or frontal ducts**. The area surrounding the nipple is usually darker than the surrounding tissue is called the **areola**. The small bumps on the areola can either be **Montgomery's glands** or hair follicies. Montgomery's glands provide lubrication during breastfeeding. If blocked, a cyst may form. It does not increase your risk for breast cancer. Hair follicles around the areola are quite common. Pulling the hair out can lead to infection, therefore, clipping is better.

Nipple discharge is normal during lactation, however, if not pregnant or breastfeeding, a discharge should be carefully evaluated. A bloody discharge is never normal, as well as a discharge in one breast and not the other without squeezing or stimulation. Repeated squeezing for discharge can actually worsen a condition. Normal nipple discharge can occur from pregnancy, stopping breastfeeding or stimulation, i.e., rubbing on a bra while exercising or running.

Causes of abnormal discharge may include:

- **Intraductal papilloma**. These non-cancerous growths in the ducts are the most common cause of abnormal nipple discharge. If the ducts become inflamed, a bloody or sticky discharge may result.
- **Mammary duct ectasia**. This second most common cause of discharge is typically seen in women who are approaching menopause. If this occurs, the inflammationmay cause a possible blockage of the ducts underneath the nipple. An infection may develop resulting in thick, greenish nipple discharge.
- **Fibrocystic breast changes**. Development of fibrous tissue and cysts may cause lumps or thickenings in the breast which may cause pain and itching. These can cause yellow, white, green or clear nipple discharge.
- **Infection**. Any discharge that contains pus may indicate an infection. This condition, mastitis, is generally seen in women who are breastfeeding. The breast may also become sore, red, or warm to the touch.

- **Galactorrhea.** This simply describes a condition in which a woman's breast secretes milk or a milky nipple discharge though she is not breastfeeding. There are several causes for this including: Hypothyroidism, illegal drugs, including marijuana, certain medications, including some hormones and psychotropic drugs, some herbs such as anise and fennel, and pituitary gland tumors.

If the discharge is accompanied by a lump or mass within the breast, there is a possibility that some form of breast cancer may be evident. Paget's disease is a rare form of breast cancer that can result in nipple discharge. This condition moves to the nipple from the ducts and may cause the nipple to bleed or ooze. Paget's almost always occurs with another form of breast cancer. In both cases, a medical specialist should be contacted without delay.

The skin of the breast should be checked regularly for puckering or dimpling. These can be caused by old scar tissue from surgery or an infection. This condition usually does not require treatment, however, a health care provider should be called. If the skin is warm, red, or painful it is almost always due to an infection and not cancer. If the skin is itchy, flaky, or scaly it is usually a sign of eczema or a bacterial or fungal infection. Herbs for bacterial infection such as Oregano can help alleviate the condition. Nipples that are itchy, flaky, or scaly can be a sign of Paget's disease. A health care provider should been seen soon. If the skin looks like an orange peal (called peau d'orange), with large pores and thickened skin, it could be an infection or an inflammatory breast cancer. A specialist should also be seen in this instance too.

A lump in the breast can bring up all kinds of fears and suspicions. There are three kinds of benign breast lumps (cysts, fibroadenomas, and pseudolumps) and one type of malignant breast lump.

- A **cyst** is a benign fluid-filled sac of tissue within the breast. It feels smooth and squishy with some give to it when pressed. A cyst can move around with palpation and can change size during the menstrual cycle. It may be tender due to pressure on surrounding muscles. A simple needle aspiration with a syringe will usually solve the problem. It normally does not return. This is more common in women between 30 and 60.

- A **fibroadenoma** is a benign group of cells made up of fibrous and glandular tissue. This lump is round, firm or hard, can move around during examination, and is generally tender due to pressure on the surrounding tissue. Fibroadenomas are harmless but can be removed by lumpectomy or laser ablation and biopsied to rule out cancer. This condition usually appears in teens and younger women and is the most common of breast tumors.

- A **pseudolump** is a benign condition that may be due to scar tissue, hardened silicone, dead (necrotic) fat, or a rib pressing into the breast. It's generally firm, tender, and does not change shape. It may or may not be moveable depending on its composition. An ultrasound examination should be done and a needle biopsy performed if there is any doubt as to its origin.

- **Intraductal papillomas** are small growths in the lining of the mammary duct near the nipple and can produce bleeding. Women between 40 and 50 are more susceptible.

- **Traumatic fat necrosis** is a benign condition that occurs following a traumatic injury to the breast. The injury may or may not be recalled by the woman. The lumps are generally single, round, firm or hard, and painless.

Generally speaking, if the lump is tender, movable, and the edges can be determined upon palpation, the lump is benign. However, if the lump is not movable, tender to the touch, and the edges can't be found, there is a strong possibility that it is something more serious. A specialist should be consulted.

Cancer is a malignant lump made of abnormal breast tissue cells growing in an uncontrolled way. This lump is usually hard with a pebbly surface and no definite shape, or possibly an irregular shape, and the edges can't be easily determined. It usually doesn't change in size or shape during the menstrual cycle. It is not normally moveable, however, depending upon the composition, it may have some give to it.

The common medical approach to breast cancer evaluation and treatment is to do a mammogram and/or a biopsy, surgically remove the tumor, and if suspected, remove the lymph glands. Radiation and chemotherapy are often required of the patient regardless if "they got it all" or not. Often elaborate "scare tactics" are used to ensure compliance. Those are generally effective because a Minor Diety (MD) has said so and the patient is scared to death (and of death) to begin with. Mammograms and biopsies have their own inherent problems with spreading the cancer during the investigative phase.

There are several alternative options available. Some have a much higher success rate than the standard medical approach and at a fraction of the cost. Thermography is a highly successful procedure that is simple, pain-free, and accurate. Many doctors are turning to this as their primary tool for information. However, any new paradigm is met with resistance. In this case it contends with the mammogram money machine.

## Bronchitis

The bronchi are the airways that carry airflow from the trachea into the lungs. When the mucous membranes of those airways become inflamed, it's known as bronchitis. There are two categories associated with bronchitis: acute and chronic.

Acute bronchitis is often (90%) caused by viruses as from a cold or influenza. These viruses infect the epithelium of the bronchi. As the infection grows, the amount of resulting inflammation mucus secretion is produced. A cough generally follows. Common symptoms include: Cough, sore throat, nasal congestion (coryza), runny nose, nasal inflammation (rhinitis), malaise, increased sputum, and possibly a low-grade fever and pleurisy.

Chronic bronchitis (a type of chronic obstructive pulmonary disease or COPD), on the other hand, is characterized by a productive cough that persists for three months or more per year for at least two years. The most probable cause can be given to chronic airway irritation caused by inhaled irritants such as cigarette smoke, air pollution and occupational exposure to irritants. Common symptoms include: a productive cough, shortness of breath, wheezing, failure to take a deep breath without coughing and may have yellow or green colored sputum sometimes streaked with blood.

Medically, this condition is treated symptomatically with corticosteroids, bronchodilators, and anticholinergics. But once again, these only help relieve symptoms and don't address the cause. To address the cause one has to thin the phlegm and remove it, as well as reduce the inflammation.

Our first line of attack, whether it be acute or chronic, is to do an Asyra test and then balance whatever markers that are found. **Isotherapy** is then performed using NAET procedures. It sometimes takes two or three treatments to resolve the problem depending on the severity and/or chronicity of the condition. In the meantime, we ask the patient to breathe steam. To loosen the secretions in the lungs, a hot shower or breathing steam from a pan of hot water helps. To make it more effective, add a few drops of eucalyptus or pine oil to the water. By adding a quarter cup of 3% hydrogen peroxide to one pint of water in a humidifier helps thin the mucus.

Milk products stimulate the production of mucus in the upper and lower respiratory tract and in the intestines. By avoiding milk and milk products part of the problem can often be eliminated.

Two to three cups of mullein leaf tea per day or taking mullein leaf capsules (1,000 -2,000 mg) per day will help loosen and expel mucus from the body. Similar action is found with N-acetyl cysteine, a form of the amino acid cysteine, by taking three 600 mg doses per day between meals.

## Bruises

A bruise is also known as a contusion or minor hematoma of tissue in which small capillaries are damaged by trauma. When a capillary is broken, blood can seep into the surrounding tissues and cause discoloration and discomfort. The blue or purple appearance is what gave rise to the term "black and blue." Bruises are named based on their diameter, i.e., petechia (less than 3 mm), purpura (3 mm to 1 cm), and ecchymosis (1 to 3 cm).

Treatment is usually confined to RICE (rest, ice, compression, elevation). Light exercise, gentle massage, heat to encourage blood flow, and Grape Seed Extract help absorb the interstitial blood and quickly absorb the bruise. Cell salts 5, 9 and 12 also help absorbing the bruise. These remedies should be applied 2-3 days following the initial damage.

Bruising can also occur as a result of rigorously exercising, thinning of the skin due to age, blood thinning medications and vitamin C deficiency. Taking 2,000 mg of vitamin C can help prevent bruising.

## Burning Feet

Sometimes the feet burn, almost like they feel when they wake up from being asleep. It can be just irritating or it can be painfully hot. The feet can look quite red if the condition is strong enough. Most of the time it goes away but sometimes the burning and tingling lingers. It's very concerning and can actually interfere with sleep.

Some diseases can cause burning feet syndrome, such as kidney disease, neuropathy, Guillain-Barre syndrome, Sarcoidosis, erythromelagia, vasculitis, HIV/AIDS, and Lyme diease. However, there are usually other symptoms that would cause you to seek medical advice and treatment. However, other conditions may cause similar reactions;conditions such as low thyroid, vitamin B12 deficiency, heavy metal poisoning, hypertension, infections and inflammation of the feet. Pounding of the feet in vigorous exercise routines can cause the feet to burn and turn red.

For immediate relief, we recommend:
1.  Alternate the feet between cold (not ice), water and warm water. Continue for 3-5 minutes.
2.  Massage the feet with a mixture of ginger, thyme or Apple Cider Vinegar in water or olive or coconut oil. Continue this procedure for 10-15 minutes.
3.  As a preventative, add vitamins B1, B3, B12, Hawthorn, Chromium, Thyme, and Turmeric to your vitamin routine.
4.  Among the many uses of Apple Cider Vinegar, adding 1-2 tablespoons of ACV to water or juice every day helps digestion, eradicates infection, kills fungus and helps balance the body's pH level.

## Burning Mouth Syndrome
**(Burning tongue, glossodynia, orodynia, glossopyrosis)**

This condition is characterized by a burning or tingling sensation on the lips, tongue or the entire mouth. Possible causes range from nutritional deficiencies, chronic anxiety, stress, or depression, medications, underactive thyroid, vitamin and mineral imbalance, type 2 diabetes, menopause, disorders of the mouth such as thrush or dry mouth, and nerve damage (especially cranial nerve C7 – the facial nerve). This is most common in people over 60 and more frequently in women. It can last for weeks or even years.

The most effective treatment found to date is a combination of gabapentin (GABA) and alpha lipoic acid (ALA). By taking 600 mg/day of ALA and 300 mg/day of GABA, a recent double blind study showed 70% of the participants gained relief within two months.

## Burns

Burns from fires, boiling water, etc. can cause a great deal of damage both externally as well as internally. To minimize or eliminate the damage, as soon as possible from the time of the burn, place the area under cold water to decrease the inflammation. Then mix or beat egg whites (the number depends on the size or area of the burn) and spread on the affected area. If on the hands or feet, the egg whites can be placed in a bowl and the burned hands or feet placed in the bowl. Apply for at least 15 minutes at a time. This can be repeated throughout the day.

## Cancer

See Appendix 4 for some successful therapies that tend to be beneficial for most cancers.

The following article sums up the holistic approach to cancer in a few lines. This article was given to this office with no author's name attached. It was so close to what we have been preaching for years that I decided to share it here.

AFTER YEARS OF TELLING PEOPLE CHEMOTHERAPY IS THE ONLY WAY TO TRY AND ELIMINATE CANCER, JOHNS HOPKINS IS FINALLY STARTNG TO TELL YOU THERE IS AN ALTERNATIVE WAY.............

(Ironically, health care practitioners in the holistic health care arenas have been telling their patients this for years.)

1.   Every person has cancer cells in the body. These cancer cells do not show up in the standard tests until they have multiplied to a few billion. When doctors tell cancer patients that there are no more cancer cells in their bodies after treatment, it just means the tests are unable to detect the cancer cells because they have not reached the detectable size.

2.  Cancer cells occur between 6 to more than 10 times in a person's lifetime. Cancer researchers for years have maintained that a 70 year old person has had 5-6 full bouts of cancer in their lifetime and not known it. Their immune systems have simply taken care of the problem.

3.  When the person's immune system is strong the cancer cells will be destroyed and prevented from multiplying and forming tumors.

4.  When a person has cancer it indicates the person has multiple nutritional deficiencies. These could be due to genetic, environmental, food and lifestyle factors.

5.  To overcome the multiple nutritional deficiencies, changing diet and including supplements will strengthen the immune system.

6.  Chemotherapy involves poisoning the rapidly growing cancer cells and also destroys rapidly growing healthy cells in the bone marrow, gastro-intestinal tract, etc., and can cause organ damage, like liver, kidneys, heart, lungs, etc.

7.  Radiation, while destroying cancer cells, also burns, scars, and damages healthy cells, tissues and organs.

8.  Initial treatment with chemotherapy and radiation will often reduce tumor size. However, prolonged use of chemotherapy and radiation does not result in more tumor destruction.

9.  When the body has too much toxic burden from chemo-therapy and radiation, the immune system is either compromised or destroyed, hence the person can suc-cumb to various kinds of infections and complications.

10. Chemotherapy and radiation can cause cancer cells to mutate and become resistant and difficult to destroy. Surgery can cause cancer cells to spread to other sites.

11. An effective way to battle cancer is to STARVE the can-cer cells by not feeding them with foods they need to multiply. Cancer cells feed on:

a. Sugar is a cancer-feeder. By cutting off sugar it cuts off one important food supply to the cancer cells. Note: Sugar substitutes like NutraSweet, Equal, Spoonful, etc., are made with Aspartame and is, therefore, harmful. A better natural substitute would be Manuka honey or molasses, but only in very small amounts. Table salt has a chemical added to make it white in color. A better alternative is Bragg's Aminos or sea salt.

b. Milk causes the body to produce mucus, especially in the gastro-intestinal tract. Cancer feeds on mucus. By cutting off milk and substituting with unsweetened coconut milk or almond milk, cancer cells will starve.

c. Cancer cells thrive in an acid environment. A meat-based diet is acidic. It is best to eat fish and a little chicken rather than beef or pork. Meat also contains livestock antibiotics, growth hormones and parasites, which are all harmful, especially for people with cancer.

d. A diet made of 80% fresh vegetables and juice, whole grains, seeds, nuts and a little fruit help put the body into an alkaline environment. About 20% can be from cooked food including beans. Fresh vegetable juices provide live enzymes that are easily absorbed and reach down to cellular levels within 15 minutes to nourish and enhance growth of healthy cells. To obtain live enzymes for building healthy cells, drink fresh vegetable juice and eat some raw vegetables 2-3 times per day. Enzymes are destroyed at temperatures of 104 degrees Fahrenheit and above. Be sure the vegetables are GMO free.

e. Avoid coffee, tea, and chocolate, which have high caffeine. Green tea is a better alternative and has cancer-fighting properties. It's best to drink puri-fied or filtered water to avoid known toxins and heavy metal in tap water. Distilled water is acidic and will rob the body of minerals. Avoid it. The best would be a filtered alkaline water.

12. Meat protein is difficult to digest and requires a lot of di-gestive enzymes. Undigested meat remaining in the intes-tines will become putrified and leads to more toxic buildup. After 25 our bodies don't have all the enzymes necessary to digest food as well as we did when we were younger. With putrified material in the gut, toxins will be taken into the blood stream along with good nutrients.

13. Cancer cell walls have a tough protein covering. By refrain-ing from or eating less meat, it frees more enzymes to at-tack the protein walls of cancer cells and allows the body's killer cells to destroy the cancer cells.

14. Some supplements build up the immune system (Essiac, vitamins, minerals, EFAs and many other anti-oxidant sup-plements) to enable the body's own killer cells to destroy cancer cells. Other supplements like vitamin E are known to cause apoptosis, or programmed cell death, the body's normal method of disposing of damaged, unwanted, or unneeded cells.

15. Cancer is a disease of the mind, body, and spirit. A proac-tive and positive spirit will help the cancer warrior to be a survivor. Anger, unforgiving and bitterness put the body into a stressful and acidic environment. Learn to have a loving and forgiving spirit. Laughter is healing.

16. Cancer cells cannot thrive in an oxygenated environment. Exercising daily and deep breathing helps to get more oxy-gen down to the cellular level. Oxygen therapy is another means employed to destroy cancer cells.

# Candidiasis (Yeast Infection, Vaginitis, Candida)

Vaginal yeast infections are most-often caused by unhealthy forms of fungus that grow in the warm, damp environment of the female genitalia. The most common form is Candida albicans.

Symptoms can include:
Extremely uncomfortable rectal or vaginal itching
Burning and pain
Vaginal infections, urinary infections
Smelly discharge
Irritability, anxiety, mood swings, depression
Fungal infections of the skin and nails
Chronic fatigue
Bloating, constipation or diarrhea
Eczema, psoriasis, hives or rashes
Seasonal allergies
Possible autoimmune disease such as Hashimoto's thyroiditis
Difficulty concentrating, poor memory, lack of focus, brain fog
Sugar and refined carbohydrate cravings
And more.....

The cause of a candida infection can range from a diet high in refined carbohydrates and sugar, oral contraceptives, alcohol consumption, high stress lifestyle to taking too many antibiotics.

Men can have yeast infections but it's mostly dormant in the male body. However, he can pass it on through sexual transmission. That's why we treat both partners when Candida is found. We use a simple lab test and EAV to determine the yeast infection. There's a simple home test that can be used to initiate the process of eliminating the candida infection. Upon awakening in the morning (before putting anything in the mouth, fill a clear glass with room temperature water. Spit some saliva into the water. Every 15-20 minutes, check the water an hour or so. If there are strings flowing downward like a jelly fish, or if the saliva is cloudy and sinks to the bottom, or if the water is cloudy with suspended specks, there is a strong probability that candida is present. We begin our treatment with the EAV results and then beginning treatment by using simple NAET procedures. Along with that, we recommend the following:

**Borax**(Boron) – Mix 1/8 tsp (500 mg) of the concentrated solution (see Borax in the mineral section) in one quart of good quality water and drink throughout the day. Heavier individuals can increase the dosage to ¼ tsp (1,000 mg) per quart of good quality water. Always begin with a low dose. For vaginal thrush, fill a large capsule with borax and insert it at bedtime for 1-2 weeks. The condition should resolve in that period of time.

**Apple Cider Vinegar Douche** – We suggest Bragg's Apple Cider Vinegar. To soothe a yeast infection, mix 3 tablespoons of Bragg's ACV with 1 quart of water. Add to a douche apparatus and use.

**Probiotics** – If you have recently taken, or are currently taking an antibiotic, especially tetracycline, you are feeding the fungus. Probiotics help restore the natural gut flora that prohibits fungal infections from forming.

**Wear loose, organic clothing** – Remember yeast fungus loves a warm, moist environment. By wearing tight fitting clothes, you're perpetuating the problem. Loose-fitting clothing and underwear will keep oxygen moving and help prevent the fungus from growing. Try wearing organic cotton. It seems to help.

**Organic Yogurt** – Organic plain yogurt can be used topically and vaginally to reduce a yeast infection. It helps restore flora and pH balance. Insert 1 to 2 tablespoons into the vagina and rub some on the affected area externally. Leave for several hours before washing. The yogurt should be free from any added sugars, fruit or other ingredients. Another way is to soak a tampon in yogurt and insert it for 2 hours, then remove.

**Tea Tree Oil** – Place a few drops of organic tea tree oil, a natural antifungal, on a natural tampon and insert it into the vagina for 4 hours. An application in the morning and again in the afternoon should be sufficient. Symptom relief should be experienced within two days. Do not sleep with it inserted.

**Organic Oregano Oil** – Another way to reduce yeast and candida infections is to place 9 drops in a capsule and swallow 2-3 times daily after meals on a full stomach.

**Garlic** – Garlic is known as a natural anti-fungal, as well as a natural antibiotic (anti-bacterial). There are many benefits from taking garlic on a regular basis but in this case, it will help resolve the problem. Taken regularly, it will help prevent a yeast infection.

**Organic Cranberries** – Cranberries are well known for use with bladder infections but they also help with yeast infections. By drinking the unsweetened juice you can help restore a healthy pH balance in the vagina and thus fighting off a fungal infection.

**Essential oils** have been very useful and very safe for relief of vaginal yeast infection. Mix 2-3 drops of Lavender and 2-3 drops of Melaleuca oils with 1 ounce of coconut oil. This mixture can be applied internally without side effects. Another method would be to refrigerate the above mixture until solid. Slice with a knife and insert as you would a tampon before retiring for the night.

**Avoid harsh "Feminine" products** – There is a very delicate pH balance in the vagina. This balance helps prevent yeast infections. Many feminine products such as soaps, hygiene douches and sprays and perfumed products interfere with and reduce the natural protective oils. These products contain harsh chemicals and alcohol which alter the natural pH of the vagina leaving you susceptible to infection. It's best to use only natural organic hygiene products.

Some more positive actions to take include:

Avoid sugars (all forms), refined carbohydrates, sweet fruits and vegetables, processed foods and gluten (wheat, rye, barley, oats).

Avoid soy and soy products.

Avoid trans fats – use coconut oil.

Take good, organic, non-GMO supplements including a multi-vitamin and mineral, omega 3 and 6, extra vitamins C, B complex, D3, K2 and E.

The digestive tract is very important for good health. We recommend taking a small amount of ACV or Betaine HCL before eating a meal. Then by taking a multi amino acid a multienzyme and a probiotic with or shortly after a meal will help restore a healthy digestive tract.

## Canker Sores

See Fever blisters

## Carpal Tunnel Syndrome

The median nerve supplies feeling and movement to the hand. When pressure is applied to the nerve, it can lead to numbness, tingling, weakness, wrist or elbow pain with movement, or muscular damage in the hand and fingers. The diagnosis of this condition is called Carpal Tunnel Syndrome.

The median nerve travels through a group of bones in the wrist called carpal bones. A natural opening or canal through these bones is called the carpal tunnel. The nerve supplies innervation to the thumb, index finger, middle finger and half of the ring finger. The wrist bones (carpal bones) can shift and compress the nerve leading to dysfunction. Over use of the wrist or repetitive motions can cause the wrist bones to shift and encroach upon the median nerve. Commonly typing, writing, sewing, assembly work, repetitive use of hand tools and many other wrist activities can lead to a compression of the median nerve.

Nerve conduction tests, electromyography and x-rays can determine if there is any damage to the nerve or carpal bones. Surgery to remove the pressure is the common treatment for this condition. However, surgery leaves scar tissue which can grow and harden and again cause encroachment on the nerve. Wrist supports or splints have been used to reduce the movement of the wrist. Some doctors will prescribe nonsteroidal anti-inflammatory drugs (NSAIDs) or give corticosteroid injections into the wrist to reduce the symptoms.

A conservative, painless and more effective way of eliminating the cause of Carpal Tunnel is to manipulate the wrist. Some chiropractors are trained in extremity manipulation. A quick "snap" of the wrist is often all it takes to eliminate the problem. It may take two or three treatments to eliminate CTS, but no more than that should be required. Sometimes ultrasound therapy prior to manipulation is used to reduce inflammation and soften the tissues.

If surgery has already been performed, ultrasound therapy is helpful to soften the scar tissue and reduce the possibility of further encroachment of the nerve.

## Cataracts

The eye is a protein membrane ball full of water. The membrane, acting as a filter, allows fluids to flow through. The membrane cleans out harmful particles so that the eyes can be clear and vision good. When membranes become tough, fluids get trapped and particles accumulate. Over time the vision will decrease and be like looking through a frosted glass. This condition is known as cataracts.

The only alternative treatment that we have found to be successful for humans as well as pets is a combination of MSM and flax seed oil. Make a 15% solution of MSM and a saline solution (1 tsp. of MSM to one ounce of solution). Administer two drops of the flax seed oil solution to a corner of the eye (can go directly into the eye). This solution will help soften the tissue. After 10-30 minutes, administer two drops of the MSM solution, preferably to a corner of the eye. This may cause some temporary stinging but it will subside. Repeat this procedure 4 times a day. After 3-4 days a white substance will appear in the corner of the eye. This white substance is from the cataract. Repeat until the substance no longer appears.

The MSM will sooth and soften the membranes and allow nutrients to pass through. It also helps stabilize the pressure in the eye, repairs any damage, clears red spots and removes floaters in the eye. The flax seed oil is rich in omega 3 fatty acids, vitamin E and the antioxidants beta carotene and carotenoids. It also helps lower cholesterol (part of the clouding of the lens).

## Celiac Disease
## (celiac sprue, gluten sensitive enteropathy)

About 3,000,000 people in the United States are affected by Celiac disease each year. The medical establishment portrays the condition as a horrible disease when in fact it is easily treatable and completely curable. Recovery depends upon the severity of the case and determination of the patient.

In the intestinal tract there are good bacteria, called flora, and harmful bacteria, called candida (ie. Yeast). The flora keeps the yeast in check. When there is too much candida (yeast overgrowth) in the intestinal tract, the immune system begins attacking the intestinal tract itself because it has been detected as dangerously toxic. Celiac disease is this panic response by the immune system. Celiac disease is a misnomer in that the body's immune system is doing exactly what it's designed to do. The autoimmune system is protecting the vital organs from toxins and pathogens.

When gluten (from wheat, barley, or rye) is ingested, the body produces antibodies that attack the small intestine, in particular, the villi. The villi are hair-like projections that siphon nutrients into the blood stream.

Some common symptoms include, but are not limited to: Abdominal cramping and/or pain, diarrhea or constipation or a combination of both, bloating, gas and mucus in the stool.

The cause of celiac disease is 'officially' unknown, but it is typically triggered by physical stress such as surgery, pharmaceuticals, pregnancy, childbirth, viral infection, and emotional stress which stresses a body's flora and immune system. It tends to run in families. The allopathic approach to celiac disease is a gluten-free diet – for life.

Nutritional changes to stimulate and repair the intestines and intestinal flora will slowly alleviate the problem. Vitamins, minerals, and herbal supplements can help accelerate the healing process.

Dr. Sidney Valentine Haas in the 1940's treated celiac patients with a dietary plan that eliminated processed carbohydrates in grains, sugars, and homogenized milk products. All those products are indigestible to the celiac patient. He demonstrated relief of signs and symptoms within a year. His treatment was very successful until a prominent medical magazine published a report based on only 10 test subjects, and stated that the "real culprit" was gluten protein. Once again, the medical establishment stepped in and discredited their own in favor of a more pharmaceutical approach. Other researchers pointed out that celiac patients who avoided all gluten still continued to demonstrate deformed cells in the intestinal wall, indicating that the body is still out of balance and in a state of dis-ease.

A dietary change is essential for complete recovery. However, other factors can accelerate the process. We have seen dramatic results by:
- Asyra testing and treatment to balance the system
- NAET treatments to eliminate the candida
- NAET treatments to eliminate gluten and grain allergies, and any other allergies
- Taking a food-based multivitamin and mineral, essential

fatty acids (omega 3, 6, and 9) enzymes, amino acids, and a good probiotic
- Eating no processed or canned meats or vegetables
- Avoiding sugar, alcohol, mushrooms, mayonnaise, white flours and white breads, processed foods, sodas, and caffeine
- Limiting yeast and caffeine
- Eating organic plain yogurt – two tablespoons five times per day if possible
- Drinking alkaline water and/or several glasses of lemonade or pineapple juice per day
- Avoiding microwave foods, fluoride, artificial sweeteners, and potato-based foods
- Drink peppermint tea

Here's some helpful tips on killing Candida yeast:
- Stop all hormone therapies (including birth control pills). Candida thrives on high levels of progesterone
- Avoid all products containing soy or canola oil
- Supplements that help are Garlic, Grapefruit seed extract, Cayenne pepper, Chamomile, Wormwood, and of course tiny amounts of extra virgin, cold-pressed coconut oil each day.

Supplements that help heal the intestinal tract include: Licorice root (be careful, it may increase the blood pressure), Aloe vera, MSM, Paprika, and Apple pectin.

## Chocolate cravings

Very often nothing satisfies like chocolate. Studies have shown that a deficiency in magnesium will create a craving for chocolate. By increasing magnesium intake the cravings will subside. Usually 500 – 1,000mg per day is sufficient.

# Cholesterol, High

Cholesterol is not a bad thing. It's a precursor for vitamin D and several very important hormones (estrogen, progesterone, testosterone, and cortisol). It aids in the permeability of the cell membranes. It is transported in the blood by lipoproteins. High density lipoprotein (HDL), referred to as the good cholesterol, transports cholesterol to the liver. Low density lipoprotein (LDL), referred to as the bad cholesterol, transports cholesterol from the liver to the cells of the body. If blood tests reveal elevated LDL and VLDL (very low density lipoproteins), additional studies should be run including a high sensitivity C-reactive protein (which indicates inflammation in the blood vessels) and lipoprotein to determine risk factors for heart disease.

In the medical world statin drugs are the treatment of choice for high cholesterol. But as one chemist noted: "statins make you stupid." What he was referring to was the side effects of statin drugs. Some of the most notable side effects include headaches, memory loss, burning feet, muscle aches, bloating, nausea, liver toxicity, abdominal cramping, and depletion of coenzyme Q10.

The most effective way to reduce cholesterol is by way of dietary modification.

- Avoid saturated fat and "trans" fatty acids (margarine, hydrogenated vegetable oil)
- Reduce fats from red meat, dairy products, processed foods
- Avoid refined sugar including high-fructose corn syrup
- Avoid processed foods and soda pop
- Eat more non-GMO fruit, vegetables, nuts and seeds
- Supplements that help include niacin (300 mg three times daily), omega-3 fatty acids (1 gram daily) and omega 6's (200 mg daily). Studies performed at OHSU found that by taking 1000 mg of omega 3's per day, the participants

dropped 30 points in 30 days.
- Red yeast rice contains lovastatin that has been shown to help lower cholesterol. 1200 mg per day is recommended, however this should only be used under the direction of a holistic healthcare physician.
- Taking garlic with parsley 3 capsules/day for 2 weeks, expect a 30 point drop.
- Bergamot (1,000 mg daily) has been shown to dramatically decrease cholesterol.

## Chronic Fatigue Syndrome

See Adrenal Exhaustion

## Chronic cough

A chronic cough can be frustrating, painful and embarrassing at times. If it is more than the cough from the common cold, determining the cause of the cough should be the first step. Through EAV testing and specific blood tests, an attempt should be made to rule out any disease patterns.

Chronic coughing associated with bronchitis, whooping cough and smoker's cough can be reduced or eliminated by taking Mullein. Mullein contains Vitamins A, D and B-complex, as well as iron, magnesium, potassium and sulfur.

I generally recommend:
Mullein - 2-4 capsules per day. If only taking 2, do so in the afternoon or evening
Vitamin C – 2,000 – 6,000 per day
Cell Salt Kali Mur (Potassium Chloride) – 8 tablets spread out through the day

## Common Cold (nasopharyngitis, acute rhinopharyngitis, acute coryza)

Now this is a condition that we all can relate to. At one time or another, everyone seems to "catch" a cold. Typically, the symptoms include a cough, low-grade fever, runny or stuffy nose, itchy or sore throat, sneezing, watery eyes, and mild fatigue. (Compare these symptoms to symptoms of the flu.) The primary cause is an infection by rhinoviruses and/or coronaviruses. The symptoms may last from 7 days to 3 weeks. There is no known medical "cure" for the common cold and cold medicines have been proven to have no curative effect. Avoiding areas where people are coughing or sneezing, frequently washing hands, and avoiding touching the mouth or face help in preventing the viral spread. It's important to keep the immune system at its peak by taking a good **multi-vitamin and mineral, garlic, Vitamin C, lecithin, and zinc.**

We treat colds and the flu very aggressively. Besides taking the above nutrients, we recommend taking as much **vitamin C** as possible (gradually increasing to 500-1,000 mg per hour up to 10,000), or just short of getting diarrhea, throughout the day. **Olive leaf extract**, two capsules with each meal and two before bed for a total of 8 per day, helps shorten the episode. Olive leaf extract is a very strong anti-viral. Take a 23 mg **zinc gluconate** lozenge every two hours. We recommend citrus-flavored Cold-EEZE since zinc has a bad taste and for no more than one week. Excessive zinc can lead to a copper deficiency and weaken the immune system. **Vitamin A** (not beta carotene) can be taken up to 100,000 IU per day for two days if taken with plenty of water.

We then treat the patient with isode therapy. Regardless of the name of the virus, the patient is carrying the offending virus. By using the patient's own saliva and nasal mucus, we treat using **NAET** procedures. The symptoms of a cold or the flu, reportedly, have been mostly, if not entirely, eliminated by the next day. Rarely will a second treatment be necessary.

Other nutrients that have been reported to help:

**Elderberry Extract** (Sambucol, Sambucus nigra) is a powerful anti-oxidant that stimulates the immune system by increasing the production of lymphocytes. Dosage is: 2 tsp. daily for children under 1year old; 1-2 Tbs. or 2 lozenges daily for kids 1-6; for children 6-12 - 2-3 Tbs. or lozenges daily; and for anyone over 12 years old – 4 Tbs. or lozenges daily. Take Sambucol following meals due to its acidity.

**Eucalyptus Oil** can be toxic if taken internally. Due to potent bactericides, breathing the fumes can knock out infections. Put 8-10 drops of EO on a handkerchief and keep it close to your nose and inhale the fumes or 10-15 drops added to a vaporizer and inhale.

**Active hexose correlated compound (AHCC)**, a mushroom extract stimulates the body's immune system by aiding the body's natural killer (NK) cells. AHCC is nontoxic and increases NK cells by 300%, as well as increasing T-cells and B-cells. In the acute phase, take 3 grams per day. But as you begin to feel better, drop back to a dose of 1 gram per day. Take ½ dose in the morning and ½ dose in evening.

**Castor Oil** has been an effective treatment for viruses, bacteria, yeasts, and molds for many years. Castor oil packs seem to be the most effective use of CO. Here's how:

1. Place a heading pad on a flat surface and turn it on high.
2. Lay a piece of thin plastic (garbage bag or similar) on top of the heating pad.
3. Place two or three 12-inch squares of flannel that have been soaked in one-half cup of cold pressed CO on top of the plastic.
4. Place the entire pack against your body with the oil-soaked flannel next to your skin. Be careful to not get oil on your bedding. Lay on a large bath towel if necessary.
5. Turn the heating pad to the highest temperature you can tolerate and relax for an hour.

6. After removing the pad, massage the remaining oil into the skin or clean it off using a quart of warm water mixed with two tablespoons of baking soda.

To reuse the flannel, place it in a plastic container in the refrigerator. Warm it before using it again and refresh it with one to two tablespoons of fresh castor oil.

**Echinacea** (Echinacea angustifolia) taken as liquid (5-10 drops in ¼ cup of water and taken 5 times daily) increases certain immune responses and inhibits viral activity.

**Vitamin D**: At the first sign of a cold or flu, increase your maintenance dose to 1,000 IU per pound of body weight per day for no more than one week. Then scale back to your normal maintenance dose.

**Ginger root** helps alleviate the symptoms of a cold or the flu.

The herb **Pleurisy Root** is an excellent expectorant for colds, bronchitis, flu, and other lung issues.

The cell salt **Kali Mur** is a remedy for sluggish conditions and for thick, white fibrinous discharges. When alternated with **Ferr. Phos**, Kali Mur will help alleviate inflammatory conditions affecting respirations such as colds, flu, sore throats, bronchitis, and tonsillitis.

## Cold Sores

See Fever Blisters

## Colic (infantile colic)

By definition, colic involves episodes of crying for more than three hours a day for more than three days a week for three weeks in an otherwise healthy child. This usually occurs in infants two weeks to four months old. This is present in up to 25% of newborns. Generally the cause is unknown. Colic has been known to last up to one year. With prolonged cases there are side effects, mostly with the parents. Cases of tension, depression, breastfeeding failure, excessive doctor visits, relationship problems, spousal abuse and even child abuse have been reported.

Common symptoms include crying, especially in the evening, for no apparent reason and for extended periods of time, legs pulled to the chest, hands clenched, flushed face and wrinkled brow. The cry is normally high pitched and unlike crying when wet, hungry or upset.

Possible causes include: Allergies, lactose intolerance, acid reflux, constipation, migraine headaches, subdural hematomas, and anal fissures.

If the condition persists, consulting with a holistic doctor is advisable. If one is not available or the doctor wants to place the child on meds, here are some alternative therapies that have worked.

Identify and treat any allergens found. Often more are found than are suspected. NAET procedures will help eliminate the allergies without disturbing the baby.

As with ulcerative colitis, reduce, or better yet, eliminate refined carbohydrates (sugar) from the diet. The sugars can create an abnormally high pH problem in the lower intestine. This acidic condition disrupts the normal (good) bacterial flora in the colon. Sugar also feeds certain forms of bacteria and yeast-like fungi like Candida.

An old therapy that has worked for many young families is: 8 oz. sterile water, 1 tbsp white Karo (corn syrup), 1 tsp brandy, mix the ingredients and warm. One drop at a time until ½ oz. Lay baby on mother's chest, skin to skin, helps relax baby's bowels.

Cell Salts 2,9,10 have been shown to help.

## Colitis (Ulcerative colitis)

Colitis, also known as ulcerative colitis or colitis ulcerosa, is categorized as an inflammatory bowel disease (IBD). Unlike Crohn's disease that affects the entire gastrointestinal tract, colitis affects only the large intestine. The onset is gradual but leads to ulcers, or open sores. The main symptomis usually constant diarrhea mixed with blood. That's why it is often misdiagnosed as irritable bowel syndrome. Other symptoms may include: Abdominal cramping and/or pain, rectal bleeding, feeling of urgency but unable to have a bowel movement, and weight loss. According to mainstream medicine, drugs are prescribed for pain relief and anti-inflammation, but outside of performing a total colectomy (i.e., removing the entire large intestine), there is no known cure.

However, in the alternative world of health care, much can be done to relieve the symptoms and promote healing.

1.  Determine if allergies and sensitivities are causing the irritation. Asyra testing or NAET testing can help to accurately determine what is irritating the system. Often, with a few life-style modifications, and eliminating the allergies by using the NAET system, the bowel system will heal.
2.  Eliminate gluten and sugar from the diet. The sugar can create an abnormally high pH problem in the colon and it disrupts the normal bacterial flora.
3.  Take high doses of multiple vitamins, enzymes, and amino acids to support good digestion and nutrition without irritation. Two capsules of the protolytic enzyme Bromelain with each meal helps stop E coli and its ensuing infection and helps resolve ulcerative colitis symptoms.
4.  Increase the intake of omega-3 oils as they help reduce the inflammatory process.
5.  Probiotics are effective in stopping the action of unfriendly microorganisms.
6.  Drink water free from chlorine and other additives found

in public drinking water. Purified alkaline water is desirable.

7. The herb Boswellia has been shown to have an 82% remission of symptoms rate if taken three times per day.

8. Aloe vera and American ginseng help prevent ulcerative colitis and helps reduce the symptoms. Aloe vera helps improve the microscopic structures of the colon tissue.

## Conjunctivitis (Pink Eye)

The white part of the eyeball is called the conjunctiva. When it becomes inflamed or infected, the increased blood in the blood vessels become more apparent. The whites of the eyes become pink or reddish in color, therefore, the term pink eye for conjunctivitis. Other symptoms include a watery drainage (tearing), infects one and sometimes both eyes and a crust may form during the night around both eyes.

This highly contagious condition is commonly caused by a bacterial or viral infection, allergic reaction or incompletely opened or blocked tear duct (in babies). The latter two are not contagious and not treatable with meds. However, bacterial infection is treated medically with antibiotics and the viral infection is treated with immune system support.

According to the CDC, conjunctivitis is self limiting. However, during the recovery time, the condition remains highly contagious and painful. The most effective treatment we have found to expedite recovery and relieve symptoms is as follows:

Dissolve ¼ teaspoon of pure, natural locally grown honey and a pinch of salt (optional) into ¼ cup of warm distilled water. Place 1-2 drops in each eye with a clean dropper every few hours as needed.

The most effective way to resolve conjunctivitis that we have found is to skim the whey (the liquid part) off of plain, organic yogurt. Using a sterile dropper, drop 1-2 drops of the whey into the corner of each eye. The conjunctivitis should be resolved by the next morning.

To reduce pain, the discharge should be removed from each eye. With a clean warm or cold washcloth, make a compress for the eyes. A different washcloth should be used each time.

Some have found that dissolving one half teaspoon of salt into one cup of distilled water and dropping the cool solution into the eyes with a clean eye dropper, has relieved the symptoms. The eye can be rinsed with the cooled salt solution with similar effects. A new solution is made each day until all symptoms are gone.

Prevention is by assuring that a good amount of vitamin A and B-complex (especially B2) is available from food or supplementation. If there are pre-existing eye conditions, a weakened immune system, moderate to severe eye pain, blurred vision, photophobia (increased sensitivity to light), symptoms get worse or the redness of the eye won't subside, a health care provider should be sought.

## Constipation

The medical definition of constipation is infrequent or difficult evacuation of the feces. It takes eaten food approximately 1-5 minutes to pass through the stomach, four and a half hours to pass through the small intestine and up to 24 hours to pass completely through the large intestine (colon). In other words, it takes food about 24 hours to pass through the entire alimentary canal (digestive system). All of that is assuming the digestive system is working properly. Without sufficient stomach acid, digestive enzymes, amino acids and bacteria, the movement can be stalled or even stopped. Even though the length of time may vary from person to person, the longer the person goes without a bowel movement the harder the stools become and the more difficult to pass.

The diagnosis of constipation is given when two or more of the following symptoms have been experienced for at least 3 months:

Two or less bowel movements per week
Straining 25% of the time during a bowel movement
Hard stools 25% or more of the time
Incomplete evacuation 25% or more of the time

There are many causes for constipation such as, but not limited to: Neurological conditions, traveling, inadequate water or fiber intake, stress, hypothyroidism, antacid medicines, pain meds, antidepressants, eating disorders, irritable bowel syndrome and many more.

Several remedies have been suggested, and may work for some people: Drink more water, take magnesium, eat prunes, eat more fruit and vegetables.

Our greatest success has come with the use of an herbal tea. Each bag contains: Senna Leaf, Buckthorn Bark, Peppermint Leaf, Stevia Leaf, Uva Ursi Leaf, Orange Peel, Rose Hip Fruit, Marshmallow Root, Honeysuckle Flower, and Chamomile Flower. The tea is called Nature's Tea from Unicity International. The flavor is light and sweet without adding anything to it.

## COPD (Chronic Obstructive Pulmonary Disease)

COPD most commonly describes the overlapping of chronic bronchitis and emphysema. Sometimes asthma and bronchiectasis fall into that same category. These progressive and debilitating lung diseases often lead to lung tissue damage, obstructed air flow and difficult breathing. It's estimated that over 12 million people have COPD and over 3 million have emphysema. It is now the fifth leading cause of death worldwide. Any of the following conditions, separately or in combination, can lead to a diagnosis of COPD. However, most often the diagnosis is based on a combination of emphysema and bronchitis.

ASTHMA is a chronic lung disease that results in narrowing of the airways caused by inflammation. Unresolved allergies can lead to asthmatic conditions.

## CHRONIC BRONCHITIS

Chronic Bronchitis is a chronic inflammation of the bronchial tubes (the small air passages leading in and out of the lungs). Constant coughing, shortness of breath, wheezing and fatigue are classic symptoms of bronchitis.

A person with EMPHYSEMA, because of the distruction of the alveoli (small air sacs), finds it difficult to breathe. The distruction results in holes in the air sacs which results in diminished gas exchange.

A severe lung infection, repetitive infections or an injury can result in damaged airways. The airways can widen and become flaccid resulting in a chronic lung disease called BRONCHIECTASIS. This condition too can cause difficulty breathing, shortness of breath and fatigue.

Some of the most common symptoms of COPD include:
   Chronic cough
   Fatigue
   Shortness of breath, especially during or after performing routine activities
   Wheezing while breathing, audible and sometimes leading to coughing
   Tightness in the chest even with simple activities
   Abnormally excessive amount of mucus or phlem produced especially in the morning

Some even more serious symptoms can occur if the condition is not addressed or allowed to progress.

According to Western medicine there is very little that can be done. Most often the patient is told that the disease is progressive, irreversible, incurable and ultimately fatal. A variety of drugs are often prescribed in an attempt to help breathing. But this is admittedly palliative and not curative.

However, turning back to nature's medicine, researchers have found that a course of treatment with vitamin A, specifically all-trans-retinoic acid (ATRA), regenerated the ability of test animals to produce alveoli. There are some disadvantages of taking a synthetic vitamin A, or beta carotene, as a supplement as opposed to taking it as a food. People working around asbestos, smokers and former smokers face the risk of lung cancer when taking large doses of beta carotene. The safest way of taking vitamin A is by eating food rich in vitamin A. The following is a list of foods high in beta carotene in descending order.

- Baked sweet potato     23,018 mcg per cup
- Cooked carrots     12,998 mcg per cup
- Cooked spinach     11,318 mcg per cup
- Romaine lettuce     2,456 mcg per cup
- Green leaf lettuce     1,599 mcg per cup
- Red leaf lettuce     1,259 mcg per cup
- Butternut squash (cooked)     9,369 mcg per cup
- Pumpkin (mashed)     5,135 mcg per cup
- Cantaloupe     3,575 mcg per cup
- Sweet red peppers     2,420 mcg per cup
- Apricots (dried)     2,812 mcg per cup
- Peas (cooked)     1,000 mcg per cup
- Broccoli (cooked)     725 mcg per cup

Some ways to minimize or eliminate the symptoms include:
1. Improve breathing by practicing diaphragmatic breathing, also known as pursed-lip breathing. Take a deep breath through the nose, purse the lips and exhale through the mouth. This is very similar to playing a brass instrument, i.e., trumpet, French horn.
2. Exercise helps strengthen the respiratory muscles and thus breathe easier. If cardiovascular exercise or interval training seems too difficult, try brisk walking.

3. Avoid an environment that would irritate or inflame the lungs, such as a smoky room, campfires, burning leaves or wood, air pollution, etc. Avoid smoking of any kind.

4. As with many conditions, good nutrition is very important. Milk is a mucus producer so avoiding milk and milk products is very important. Eliminate sugars, additives, processed foods and preservatives from the diet. Drink abundant amounts of pure water. Taking Turmeric, vitamin C and omega 3 supplements will help control the inflammation. The essential oils Melaleuca, Helichrysum and Frankincense have been used topically with a carrier oil or inhaled have been shown to help reduce inflammation.

## Cramps

See muscle cramps or menstrual cramps

## Cravings

Chocolate cravings have been linked to magnesium deficiency. Reseachers belive that women's bodies scream for chocolate during PMS. That strong desire for chocolate before and during menstruation is due, they believe, to magnesium deficiency. Studies have shown that over 75% of Americans are deficient in magnesium.

Refer to the chapter on vitamins for detailed descriptions of overdose and deficiency symptoms.

Sweet cravings are generally associated with a deficiency in chromium, vanadium, carbon, phosphorus, sulfur or tryptophan. By taking a multi-mineral supplement or adjusting the normal diet to include higher quantities of chicken, beef, poultry, broccoli, nuts and fresh fruits should lessen the craving for sweets.

Cravings for unusual foods (called pica), such as dirt, paper, ice, sand or paint, especially in children, is often associated with iron deficiency.

Alcohol cravings are usually associated with deficiencies of several vitamins and minerals, protein, glutamine, potassium or calcium. By taking supplements or increasing the consumption of meat, seafood, poultry, broccoli, granola and oatmeal in the daily diet can help get rid of alcohol cravings. A test for candida or yeast infection should be done as candida often causes a craving for alcohol, especially beer or wine.

A craving for cheese often indicates a need for EFA's (essential fatty acids), proteins and amino acids.

Other cravings include:
Salt – need for water and/or minerals.
Spicy foods – need for vitamins and minerals, especially zinc.
Ice – This person may be anemic. There is a need for iron, folic acid, B6 or B12.

Cravings for non-food substances, i.e. dirt, clay, soap, paint chips, etc. are generally deficient in minerals. A metal toxicity can lead to this disorder. A thorough evaluation, as with an Asyra system, should be performed to determine the extent of deficiencies and toxicities.

## Crohn's Disease (ileitis, ileocolitis, regional enteritis)

Crohn's disease is a chronic inflammatory bowel disease that affects the entire digestive system. The inflammation causes swelling and then deep sores or ulcers can develop. The most common sites are the last part of the small intestine and first part of the large intestine.

Symptoms include: loss of appetite, chronic diarrhea or loose bowel movements, abdominal pain, and weight loss. If left untreated rectal bleeding, bowel blockages, anal fissures and anal fistulas can develop.

Enteritis (inflammation of the small intestine) is usually caused by bacteria or viruses. A very similar condition is ulcerative colitis which involves only the colon. Both conditions are considered chronic and incurable by the mainstream medical profession.

The mainstream medical approach is with a variety of medications, often several at a time, for the reduction of symptoms. When necessary, surgery is always an option.

We have found that Asyra testing for allergies and then NAET treatment for those allergies, helps to heal the intestinal walls. We advise that a complete detoxification regime be accomplished along with NAET treatments. Part of the detox treatment would include coffee colonics or enemas. By doing this the liver, as well as the intestinal tract, can be detoxed at the same time. In the gut, the bad bacteria and fungus (disease causing organisms) are killed to be replaced by healthy organisms through probiotics. By giving the bowel system a rest with a liquid diet for a short time, the inflammation and ulceration in the intestinal tract can heal. The Asyra test can point to nutritional deficiencies and hormonal imbalances which can then be addressed. And a TFT for emotional components can provide useful healing. In many cases candida overgrowth is a complicating factor. If present, that issue should be addressed as well.

Nutritional support is a major factor in resolving Crohn's disease as well as many other intestinal dysfunctions. Food avoidance, diarrhea and/or a lack of absorption of nutrients make this vitally important. Here are a few suggestions:

- A high quality, full spectrum multi-vitamin and mineral is the foundation for all other supplements. However, many with Crohn's cannot tolerate capsule or tablet vitamins. In that case, a high quality liquid multi is preferred. If a person can't afford or can't tolerate any other vitamins, a good multi is essential.
- 3,000 to 6,000 IU of vitamin D3. A blood test to determine one's need is desirable. Best taken with Vit. K2
- Cod liver oil – 2 teaspoons or 2-4 capsules.

- CoQ10 – one mg per pound of body weight.
- Vitamin C –2,000 mg in non-GMO ascorbate form. Ascorbic acid form will cause loose stools or diarrhea.
- Slippery elm, either by capsule or one teaspoon two times per day, will help heal the intestinal tract. The powder version can be flavored by adding cinnamon and sugar.
- Peppermint oil capsules can help relieve the spasmodic component of an inflammatory bowel disease. Peppermint candy helps with an upset stomach.
- Identify and eliminate emotional causes of Crohn's disease. Over 60% of the body's neurotransmitters are located in the gut. There is now a specialty, called neurogastroenterology, devoted to the effects of emotions on the digestive system. The body won't heal fully as long as it's dealing with emotional problems. The most effective therapy we've found is Thought Field Therapy (TFT).
- Take a non-GMO, organic multivitamin and mineral, essential fatty acids (omega 3, 6, 9), multi enzymes, multi amino acids and a good probiotic.
- Eat no processed or canned meats or vegetables.
- Limit yeast.
- Avoid caffeine, sugar, alcohol, mushrooms, white flours and breads (any made with wheat, rye or barley), soy products, microwaved foods, fluoride, artificial sweeteners, food additives, milk, and potato-based foods.
- Drink pure, non fluoridated, non chlorinated, alkaline water, if possible.
- Ensure all master hormonal glands are balanced. Use Barnes temp. test.

## Dementia

Dementia is a general term for a set of symptoms that clouds a person's memory and thinking. It is often associated with aging.

The condition usually begins with forgetfulness, difficulty keeping track of time, and location disorientation. Dementia usually progresses with time. Forgetfulness gets worse and then the person becomes more confused and upset. Names and faces become more difficult to remember. Personal care declines as well as decision making abilities. Often the person will ask the same question over and over. When riding in a car, they will repetitively read signs and billboards. As the condition progresses, the above symptoms increase to the point that they are unable to care for themselves or recognize familiar people and places. They become more confused and aggressive which often leads to depression.

Too often dementia is caused by toxins and/or deficiencies. Toxins can come in the form of chemicals in medicines, herbicides, pesticides, food, water and air contamination and allergies.

Medically there is no cure. However, the effects of dementia can often be minimized or eliminated by a healthy lifestyle. Eliminating allergies, balancing the hormones, eating organic, non-GMO fruits and vegetables, eating meat free from hormones, antibiotics, pesticides or herbicides, drinking pure water free from chemicals, abundant rest, exercise, playing mind testing games and/or learning a different language or a new instrument are all helpful in keeping the body youthful and alert. This takes a great deal of effort. However, the rewards are well worth it.

In our office we do an EAV test to find allergies, toxicities, hormonal imbalances and deficiencies. We first balance the system. Then we eliminate any allergies using NAET procedures. We address the hormonal system, especially the thyroid and adrenal glands to insure they are functioning properly. Exercises are based on the person and their lifestyle. Nutrition and supplementation is discussed.

*Jeanie brought her father in because he and she had noticed that he was having some difficulty remembering people's names or the directions to some familiar places. He was becoming confused and frustrated. He was tested and we began eliminating his allergies (he thought he had none). After doing an at-home thy-*

*roid test, he was given a natural thyroid supplement. He was instructed in a detoxification program to eliminate any mercury, lead, or heavy metal poisoning, as well as chemical poisoning. He was encouraged to exercise (at least walking) 30 minutes each day and set aside some time for relaxation. He was encouraged to take a multivitamin and mineral supplement along with a vitamin B complex, extra vitamins B3, B6, B12 and folate, vitamin C, vitamin D and an omega3, 6, and 9 supplement. He was encouraged to avoid sugar, glutens, and transfats (fast foods, margarine, and baked goods). He was also encouraged to use coconut oil for cooking and take a small amount every day. After one month of faithfully following these suggestions, he was back to his old self again – quick and sharp witted. His mind was as sharp as a tack.*

## Depression

Depression is a mood disorder caused by the body's inability to produce the neurotransmitter Serotonin. This chemincal helps regulate mood, metabolism, and appetite. Serotonin is produced in the intestinal system by the enterochromaffin cells.

Depression can affect how one feels, behaves and even thinks. There are two accepted forms: mild depression and severe depression or clinical depression. A depressive episode, whether mild or severe, may range in severity and may include:

- A feeling of sadness or hopelessness or worthlessness
- Inability to concentrate or make logical decisions
- Outbursts of anger or frustration
- Restless anxiety or agitation
- Difficulty remembering things
- Fatigue, loss of energy
- Changes in appetite and sleep patterns
- Loss of interest or pleasure and blaming oneself for it
- Thoughts of suicide

Antidepressant medications have given some help to cases of moderate to severe depression. However, the side effects in many cases are unbearable. Some alternative remedies that help lift depression include:

- Exercise
- Meditation
- Acupuncture
- Light therapy
- Support groups, church groups
- B complex vitamins (especially B12), omega-3 supplements
- St. John's wort and SAM-e

We have found the fastest and most long lasting treatment for depression is Thought Field Therapy. We have seen dramatic improvements in cases involving pain, loss of a loved one, rape, anger, guilt, loss of a job, deadlines, addictions, panic attacks, phobias (including heights, bridges, animals, water, closed spaces), depression, anger, rage, obsessions, guilt, and more. An explanation of this therapy can be found in the Miscellaneous Therapies Section.

## Diabetes (Diabetes mellitus)

Diabetes is a condition in which a person has high blood sugar either because the body doesn't produce enough insulin or the cells don't respond to the insulin produced. Some classical symptoms include: increased thirst (polydipsia), frequent urination (polyuria), and increased hunger (polyphagia). There are threeprimary types of diabetes:

**Type 1** diabetes (insulin-dependent and juvenile diabetes) is a result of the body's failure to produce insulin.
**Type 2** diabetes (adult onset diabetes) is a result of cellular resistance to insulin.

**Gestational** diabetes occurs frequently during pregnancy and is usually resolved following delivery.

There are other forms of diabetes but these are the most common. To date, medical science has not found a cure for diabetes. However, in the case of type 2 diabetes, many have, in effect, eliminated the problem by diet modification, exercise, weight loss, detoxification and allergy elimination. Even those with Type 1 diabetes have found that the need for insulin can be reduced by following the same protocol.

Vitamin B1 (Thiamin): 2-10 mg.
Biotin: 8-16 mg.
Vitamin C: 1-2 grams
Chromium: 1,000 mcg. (can use 3,000-4,000 mcg.)
Cinnamon: ½ tsp.
Magnesium: 400-800 mg.
Zinc: 25 mg.
Omega-3 fatty acids: 2-3 grams (balanced with 250-500 mg. omega-6 fatty acids, like GLA from evening primrose oil (or take a basic essential fatty acid supplement).
Alpha lipoic acid: 250-1,000 mg.
Low-carbohydrate and/or high-fiber diet
Exercise: five days a week
Cook with coconut oil

Note all doses are daily in pill or capsule form unless otherwise noted.

For immediate help, some have gained relief from cutting the ends off a few stalks of okra. Soak them in a cup of water overnight. The next day remove the okra and drink the water. This may not work for everyone, but it has helped many for a long time.

## Diarrhea

A person who eats two to three meals a day should experience one or two normal, well formed bowel movements each day. However, if a person experiences more than three bowel movements with loose, watery stools, that's considered diarrhea. Most people experience one or two bouts of diarrhea each year. But there are those who suffer with this condition chronically. Symptoms may include cramps, gas, nausea and vomiting. Food poisoning, allergies, bacterial and viral infections and some medications can cause the condition.

Very often an Asyra test will reveal toxins or deficiencies that may lead to diarrhea. Very often addressing those concerns with a good probiotic, (either by supplement, yogurt, or kefir), and by keeping well hydrated, the condition will quickly subside.

One area often overlooked in either a constipation or diarrhea situation is the ileocecal valve. This small but very important valve lies between the small intestine and the large intestine. Generally speaking, it allows the contents of the small intestine to move to the large intestine without backing up. If the valve "sticks" open, liquid can flow into the large intestine without being regulated. Excess fluid can lead to a loose, watery stool. Vice versa, if the valve "sticks" closed, stools become hard and less likely to move along in a normal manner. Usually a symptom of an ileocecal valve problem is pain in the lower right abdominal quadrant half way between the hip bone (anterior superior iliac spine) and the umbilicus (belly button). By massaging that area laterally and inferiorly, the valve will be more likely to open. By massaging medial and superior, the valve will tend to close.

## Diverticulitis

In the lining of the colon are small, bulging pouches known as diverticula. When these pea size pouches bulge outward, a condition known as diverticulosis (condition of the diverticula) develops. These pouches sometimes become infected and inflamed. Then the condition is called diverticulitis. Generally these develop in the lower large intestine (descending colon and sigmoid colon) and can become large especially if straining during a bowel movement is common. The exact cause is still unknown. However, repeated, long term use of antibiotics can destroy much of the good bacteria. Without good bacteria, parasites, viruses, yeast (candida albicans), and bad bacteria can thrive.

Sometimes a person experiences no symptoms at all. However, for most the symptoms may include:

Abdominal pain or tenderness (usually severe and quick onset)

Constipation or diarrhea

Nausea

Fever

Bloating

Occasionally a person may experience rectal bleeding, blood in the stools, frequent and painful urination and vomiting.

The standard medical approach is symptom relief with medications and eventually, if no permanent relief is found, surgery becomes the logical option. Too often surgery is suggested during the initial phase.

A natural, alternative approach to alleviating diverticulitis is to begin by identifying any deficiencies, toxicities and allergies. We use the Asyra to quickly provide a picture of what we will be dealing with. We use NAET procedures to eliminate allergies and Dr. Hulda Clark's procedures to eliminate parasites.

It's best to give the bowel system a rest for a few days. Some like to do a fast while others enjoy a liquid diet. When doing a liquid diet, we recommend adding aloe vera juice to the liquid for healing of the intestinal walls. While giving the colon a rest we recommend taking two coffee enemas followed by a yogurt enema. The coffee enemas will eliminate the bacteria in the colon (good and bad), and the yogurt enema provides good bacteria back to the colon. Colonic hydrotherapy is often recommended in place of enemas. Following those procedures, a regular regiment of probiotic supplementation is recommended. Usually 7-10 billion CFU (colony forming units) per day is sufficient.

Supplements that help restore good intestinal health include:
    Multi vitamin and mineral
    B-complex – 100 mg 3 times daily
    Vitamin C - 4,000 to 8,000 mg daily (reduce if it causes diarrhea)
    Multi enzymes and multi amino acids with each meal
    Garlic – 2 capsules three times daily
    Alfalfa – 2,000 mg daily
    Aloe vera juice – ½ cup three times daily

To help prevent diverticulitis, the following suggestions are given:
    Avoid alcohol and smoking
    Exercise moderately
    Drink plenty of water – at least 1 quart or liter daily with lemon juice and shavings mixed in
    Avoid indigestible roughage such as celery and corn
    Eat fresh, organic, non GMO fruits and vegetables high in fiber
    Avoid processed foods, sugar products, gluten products and spicy foods
    Refrain from straining during a bowl movement

## Dry Skin (Xeroderma)

Dry, itchy skin can be unpleasant and sometimes embarrassing. It generally occurs on the arms, hands, lower legs, knuckles, scalp and sometimes on the thighs and abdomen. The causes are varied: genetics, age, allergies, frequent showers and/or baths, daily swimming in a swimming pool, washing soaps and powders, household chemicals, certain medications, vitamins A or D deficiency and sunburn.

Prevention can come from without and within. Eliminating allergies, avoiding harsh chemicals, i.e. wear gloves when working with chemicals inside or outside of the house, eat organic, non-GMO foods, take a full spectrum of supplements, etc.

We have found that using the Asyra to identify toxins and deficiencies, a course can be plotted for each individual need and then treated accordingly. Allergies respond well by using NAET procedures. A hot 30 minute bath with 1 cup of baking soda or a handful of cornstarch will relieve the itching and dry skin. Olive oil or coconut oil applied as a skin cream can help relieve the immediate problem and act as a preventative. A good, high quality multi-vitamin and mineral, from a health food store and not a supermarket or discount store, is essential for a foundation for proper nutrition. Adding extra vitamins A, C, and D, along with essential fatty acids will help insure soft, moist skin.

## Ear Infection

Ear infections can be very painful and frustrating, especially in children. The child may complain of ear pain. He/she may grab or pull at the ear in an effort to relieve the pain. Often we take the child to a doctor who looks at the ear, diagnoses ear infection and prescribes an antibiotic. Is it an ear infection or the fact that fluid is not draining well through the eustacian tube? If fluid is present, a swab culture will confirm if it's viral or bacterial. The American Academy of Pediatrics tells us that most ear infections are viral in nature. Therefore, if it is a viral ear infection, antibiotics will have no effect. And most ear infections clear up without any treatment. However, if pus is coming out of the ear, don't put anything in it and contact a holistic pediatrician. The tympanic membrane (ear drum) may be perforated.

One of the best remedies that we've found for ear infections involves garlic. If an immediate need arises, break open and mix some garlic oil pearls or caps. Mix with some olive oil. Put two or three drops twice daily in the ear that aches. Seal the ear with a cotton ball soaked in the same mixture. It's best to do this in the evening and at night. Results should be seen within a day or two.

You can prepare your own garlic oil by peeling 4-8 ounces of fresh garlic and mincing it. Put it into a jar. Pour cold pressed olive oil over the minced garlic until it's covered. Tightly close the jar and place in a cool dark area. Shake it daily to mix the ingredients. After it has been allowed to set for three to five days, strain the particles off and pour into a dark, glass bottle. Use it as necessary. In a Washington State University study, they found that garlic is 100 times more effective than two of the most popular antibiotics at killing bacterial strains related to foodborne illness. They also found that it worked in a fraction of the time.

Another fact that makes garlic so effective is that it contains allin and allinase. When crushed and combined they form allicin, a natural anesthetic. So, pain relief is attained rather quickly.

Two or three drops of the above garlic/olive oil combination mixed with mullein oil gives quick, soothing relief from the pain. With a dropper, put two to three drops of warm oil in the ear. Allow it to penetrate for 30 seconds. Do this six or more times per day until well.

Essential oils have been effectively used to help reduce pain and eliminate the infection. Combine 3 drops of either Basil or Melaleuca oils with 1 ounce of coconut oil or olive oil. Rub behind the ear and around the opening of the ear but never inside the ear. Apply this mixture several times per day if possible. If not possible, at least first thing in the morning and last thing at night.

Chiropractic adjustments performed by a chiropractor well versed in treating children helps flush lymph fluid from congested areas. It also relaxes the tight cervical muscles associated with the pain of an ear infection. Also according to the University of Maryland Medical Center, elderberry may have anti-inflammatory and antiviral properties. As a syrup, this can be taken in conjunction with the above treatment.

## Ear Wax (Cerumen)

Believe it or not, there is a purpose for ear wax. It not only lubricates the outer ear but it also protects from dust, dirt and bacteria that can cause us harm. However, if it builds up too much it can cause an ear infection or hearing loss. It's best to avoid an accumulation before it begins. Poking in the ears with a cotton swab or bobby pin is very dangerous. And if the doctor wants to clean the ear with a metal probe, I'd run for the door.

Two methods that we recommend are:

Mix 4-5 drops of Lavender essential oil, 4-5 drops of Thyme or Melaleuca essential oil with 1 ounce of coconut oil. Warm slightly. Drop 5-6 drops of that mixture into the affected ear. (Tilt head away from the affected ear.) Insert a cotton ball gently into the ear. Leave in the ear for 1-2 hours or over night. The wax should dissolve and wash away.

Method two would be to use the same mixture and instead of leaving the cotton in for hours, remove it and while using a child's nasal syringe, flush the wax out by forcing water into the ear. The syringe should be held at an angle pointing to the top of the ear canal. Carefully squeeze warm water into the ear. Be careful to not insert the tip too far into the ear. The wax will either dissolve into a film or come out as a glob.

## Eczema
## (atopic dermatitis, atopic eczema, infantile eczema)

This skin disorder is characterized by red, scaly, dry or leathery skin and often itchy rashes. Occasionally there is oozing and crusting. Most commonly theses areas appear around the knees and elbows, sometimes on the cheeks (usually in children). The condition will often persist or flair up if the person is exposed to stress, chemical irritants or allergies.

There are many "cures" available on the internet, however, most are like many drugs, just bandaids – covering up the symptoms. Again, common sense and using what we have been naturally provided, will alleviate the problem.

Remember, the skin is the largest organ of elimination of the body. Toxins within the body will find their way to the skin. If not eliminated, we end up with a whole host of problems. So first of all, **improve your diet**. Eliminate as many processed and gluten foods as possible. Change the diet to include more fruits, nuts, seeds and vegetables. Be sure they are natural, organic and GMO free. Raw is better than processed. Eat meat that has been grass-fed and without hormones or preservatives.

**Eliminate milk and dairy products.** Most milk bought in stores today is full of hormones and chemicals. Coconut milk, almond milk and rice milk are good substitutes for cow's milk.

**Choose skin care products that are non-irritating.** Avoid antibacterial and antiperspirant products. Avoid shower gels and soaps with perfumes and dyes in them. If you can't say the chemical name, avoid it. Don't put anything on your body that you wouldn't put in your body. Parabens and many sulfates are irritating and drying to the skin. Prolonged exposure can lead to much more serious conditions.

**Use natural, biodegradable washing detergents.** Wear smooth-textured clothing such as cotton, silk and bamboo.

**Minimize stress.** Do whatever is necessary to reduce stress that we face every day. Visualization, meditation, prayer, hypnotherapy, soft music are all forms of de-stressing techniques.

No matter how well we eat, we still need to **supplement our diet** with vitamins, minerals, enzymes, amino acids and probiotics. For eczema, Omega 3, 6, and 9 fatty acids help reduce inflammation and relieve dry skin. Vitamins A, D and E boost collagen production, protects the skin from free radicals, retains hydration and improves texture. Supplements containing gamma-linolenic acid (GLA) as found in evening primrose oil, borage oil and blackcurrant oil, help balance lipids in the skin and relieve inflammation.

Topically there are several **creams and gels** that have helped.

**Aloe vera**–the sap has been used for thousands of years for wounds, burns and many other skin conditions. There are no known side effects.

**Chamomile and licorice creams and gels** have been used to reduce redness, swelling, itching and inflammation. Chamomile essential oils can be massaged into the skin or drop a few drops into a warm bath. Holding a compress soaked in chamomile for 10-15 minutes on the affected area oftentimes helps. The same can be done using licorice oil. Some people can be allergic to chamomile so try just a little at first or test to see if you are allergic to it.

**Calendula oils**, lotions and salves can be used topically to reduce inflammation and pain. There are no known side effects when used topically.

**Coconut oil** – organic, cold pressed, virgin coconut oil for many people works better than store-bought creams. Cold pressed means that it was processed at temperatures below 116 degrees. By processing this way the oil's nutrients, enzymes and minerals are preserved. The list of healthy uses of coconut oil goes on and on.

## Emphysema

Emphysema is a form of chronic obstructive pulmonary disease (COPD). One of the key characteristics of emphysema is damage to the air sacs in the lungs. With the damage, air flow is limited and patients find it difficult to breathe. Smoking and air pollution are two of the most common factors leading to emphysema.

Some common symptoms include:
- Shortness of breath
- Coughing
- Wheezing
- Chest tightness
- Decreased physical activity

- Excessive mucus discharge
- Fatigue
- Poor appetite
- Weight loss

The medical world offers no cure for emphysema although there are many pharmaceuticals available to temporarily mask some symptoms. The current medical opinion is that the condition is irreversible and progressive. However, there have been rebels who have not accepted the medical/pharmaceutical line of thinking and have done extensive research into this condition and what can be done to reverse it.

Because the condition is so progressive, even in the face of strong medications, the hypothesis was made that something is growing or proliferating inside the lungs. The thought was that it might be a pathogen introduced by ingesting chemicals from smoking or pollution. Based on that theory the "rebel scientists" attacked the condition as if a pathogen was the cause. As in many disease conditions, including cancer, pathogens thrive in sugar. By removing sugar and simple carbohydrates from the diets, patients with cancer and other debilitating conditions tend to improve remarkably. It is believed that such a diet starves the pathogen that causes emphysema or COPD. Many patients show improvement within the first two weeks.

Along with starving the pathogens, we recommend an Asyra evaluation and resultant treatment to balance the patient's systems and begin detoxifying. Further detoxification procedures via baking soda baths, ionic foot baths and colonics are recommended.

A strong immune system is necessary for improvement. Supplements to boost the system on a daily basis include:

- A high quality multi vitamin and mineral
- Multiple enzymes
- Multiple amino acids
- Probiotics

- EFA's including omega 3, 6 and 9
- CoQ10 – 1 mg/pound of body weight
- N-acetyl-L-cysteine (NAC) 500mg-800mg
- Alfalfa 600-700 mg
- Caprylic acid 600 mg
- Beta-1,3/1,6 Glucan 250 mg
- Oregano
- Olive leaf extract
- Vitamin C 2,000 mg

## Endometriosis

This chronic and often painful condition in which the tissue (endometrial cells) that normally lines the uterus (called the endometrium) starts growing outside the uterus. The most common locations are the fallopian tubes, ovaries, or the pelvic lining. In some cases it can spread outside the pelvic area. It's estimated that over 5.5 million women in the U.S. and Canada are affected. About 90% of women who experience pelvic pain have endometriosis.

Signs and symptoms include:
- Painful periods. This pain can begin several days before the period and last for days after. Lower abdominal pain, low back pain, and sciatica have been noted.
- Fatigue
- Heavy menstrual periods or bleeding between periods
- Sharp, deep pain during ovulation, sexual intercourse, bowel movements, and/or urination
- Indigestion, diarrhea, constipation, and nausea
- Infertility caused by adhesions that trap the egg

Some natural treatments include:
- Reduce chemical intake such as dioxins and polychlorinat-

ed biphenyls (PCBs) by reducing animal fat, especially high-fat dairy, red meat, and fish. These chemicals accumulate in animal fat. By eating more fresh fruit and vegetables the risk can be reduced. Eating a healthy diet of low refined carbohydrates and limiting caffeine, sugar, preservatives, additives, red meats and processed foods has been shown to be helpful.

- Plant chemicals called flavones can inhibit aromatase, the enzyme that converts androgens to estrogens. Good sources are celery and parsley. Indoles found in broccoli, cauliflower,cabbage, kale, brussel sprouts, and bok choy help improve estrogen metabolism.

- Natural progesterone cream is not considered a cure, but it may improve symptoms. Natural progesterone has the molecule diosgenin extracted and converted to a molecule exactly like human progesterone and added back to the cream. Caution: Too much progesterone can cause side effects such as mood changes, depression, water retention, weight gain, and absent or abnormal menstrual bleeding. The goal is to balance estrogen with progesterone.

- Omega-3 Fatty Acids, as found in salmon, mackerel, sardines, and anchovies, are best taken by capsules. The compounds EPA and DHA can relieve pain by decreasing levels of an inflammatory chemical called prostaglandin E2. Fish oils have been shown to slow the growth of endometrial tissue. We recommend Omegas 3, 6, and 9. Omegas are also used to control mood swings and depression.

- By reducing stress the hormone Cortisol can be reduced. Cortisol is needed to make hormones such as progesterone. Reducing Cortisol may reduce the available progesterone and aid in hormone balance.

- Contrast sitz baths have been used as a remedy. A cycle of three minutes in a tub of hot water followed by one minute in a tub of cold water repeated three times has helped alleviate symptoms.

- Ginger tea has been shown to relieve nausea.
- Herbs that have been helpful in relieving endometriosis include blue cohosh, cranberry, plantain, St. John's wort, peppermint, valerian, dong quai, false unicorn, evening primrose oil, chasteberry/vitex, black cohosh, uva ursi, couchgrass, red raspberry, yam, and white willow.
- Acupuncture helps restore and balance the body's energy flow. Chiropractic adjustments, especially to the lumbar and lower thoracic regions, help relieve back pain.
- Exercise stimulates the release of endorphins and helps reduce stress, pain, and depression.
- It has been shown that there's a strong connection between endometriosis and candida yeast overgrowth. Studies have shown that 80% of women treated for candida significantly reduced endometriosis symptoms within two months.

In our office we use the Asyra to help balance the patient's system and NAET to eliminate the candida. By modifying the diet, encouraging an exercise routine, and taking high quality supplements, endometriosis can be virtually eliminated. We suggest a high quality multi-vitamin and mineral, B-complex, vitamin C, omega 3, 6 and 9, digestive enzymes, and amino acids.

## Epstein-Barr Virus (EBV)

Epstein-Barr virus is a common, highly contagious virus that sometimes causes what is known as mononucleosis. The virus is transmitted through the saliva of an infected person, thus the distinction of being called the kissing disease. However, it can be transmitted by kissing, sharing a drink, or simply touching something with an infected person's saliva on it and then touching your mouth. Symptoms most commonly attributed to EBV are: Fever (usually around 102 degrees), sore throat lasting up to a couple of weeks, swollen lymph nodes in the neck, groin, and arm pits, fatigue, malaise, and occasionally an enlarged spleen, although there may not be any symptoms for several weeks. The incubation period is usually 7-14 days in children and adolescents and up to 30-50 days in adults.

EBV is a virus and therefore antibiotics have no effect. It is generally self limiting (1-2 weeks) provided the infected person rests and doesn't re-infect himself or herself. Therefore, the common medical treatment is bed rest.

We've found that a NAET treatment for virus infection, EBV and immune deficiency helps shorten the recovery time. If we employ isodetherapy, we can further enhance recovery. It is generally suggested to the patient to take 2,000 to 6,000 mg of vitamin C and two capsules of Olive Leaf Extract four times per day for 2-3 days.

The best thing to do is to keep one's immune system tuned so as to avoid infection in the first place.

## Eye Mucus (Rheum)

The eye discharge that is sometimes seen in the morning is actually a combination of mucus, oil, skin cells and particles that have accumulated from the air and have been lodged in the eye. The body is simply flushing out the eye.

Symptoms may include: blurred vision, sensitivity to light (photophobia), and eyes that are bloodshot, dry, watery, sore, burning or itchy. If the discharge is yellow or green in color and the vision is blurry or light sensitive, it could be a sign of an eye infection or disease. An ophthalmologist should be consulted to determine the root cause. Sometimes dirt or an eye lash can get into the eye and become gritty, irritated, red and/or itchy. The discharge then can be white, yellow or green. A clear, watery discharge with a white or light yellow tint can be a sign of viral conjunctivitis. A thick, sticky pus-like (purulent) discharge with a yellow, green or even gray tint can indicate a bacterial conjunctivitis. The latter two conditions are highly contagious, so great care should be taken.

Usually a warm wash cloth gently rubbed across the closed eye is sufficient to rid the eye of the discharge. Contaminated make-up is a leading cause of recurrent infection. So, throw it away. Proper care or replacement of contact lenses can prevent reoccurrence. Washing the eyelids with baby shampoo or a very mild soap in a downward motion to remove excess oil will help prevent reoccurrence.

## Fever blisters

Fever blisters, cold sores, and canker sores are considered Herpes Simplex Virus #1. Genital Herpes are considered Herpes Simplex Virus #2. L-lysine displays an inhibitory effect on herpes virus growth while L-Arginine accelerates growth.

Since allergies and stress are major contributors to a herpes breakout, we first do an EAV allergy evaluation. Allergies are addressed using NAET procedures and dietary changes are discussed. The patient should refrain from Arginine containing foods. Some of the most popular foods containing Arginine are peanuts, peanut butter, cashews, chocolate, Cocoa, almonds, pecans, sesame, and cakes and breads containing bleached flour. Lysine containing foods should be emphasized. Among those are cheeses, chicken, eggs, fish, milk, organ meats, turkey, potatoes, and yogurt. This anti-herpes diet should continue for 3 months to assure the herpes will remain in remission. 1,000-1,400 mg. of Lysine should be consumed as a maintenance dose. As a rule of thumb, 10 mg. of Lysine should be consumed perpound of body weight. Echinacea and Golden Seal can be taken as cleansers. Vitamins E and F (safflower oil) are needed as skin regenerators.

Once an eruption has occurred, directly applying Lysine to the site will hasten recovery. If stress is suspected, Pantothenic Acid (Vitamin B-5), Potassium, and sodium will nourish the adrenal glands. Citrus foods should be avoided as they will irritate the outbreak. Avoid cantaloupes, grapefruit, lemons, oranges, pineapples and tomatoes. Alfalfa and Royal Jelly capsules can be taken to re-place nutrients burned up by an outbreak. We often recommend cell salts #5 (Kali. Mur) and #9 (Nat. Mur) to expedite healing.

Another tried and true remedy is to place garlic on the erup-tion. Gently place a finely chopped garlic clove on the cold sore/fever blister. Let it remain on the site for 10 minutes and then rinse with lukewarm water. It may sting at first but the relief will be almost instantaneous. The process can be repeated several times per day if necessary. In many cases the cold sore has been shown to be gone or mostly gone within a day.

## Fibroid Cyst (Uterine Fibroid, Myoma, Leiomyoma, Fibromyoma)

Uterine fibroids are non-cancerous fibrous tissue that grows on the uterine wall generally during a woman's reproductive years. They tend to shrink or disappear after menopause. It's been estimated that 25% of women over 30 are affected. They can be so small that they are hardly detectible. But they have been known (rarely) to weigh as much as 100 pounds. Fibroids are generally classified into three categories: Suberous (outside the uterus), Intramural (confined in the wall of the uterus), and Sub-mucous (inside the uterus).

The young lady may be symptom-free or she may experience abdominal pain, back ache, constipation, urinary problems, bloat-ing and digestive problems. If the fibroid distorts the uterine lin-ing, abnormally heavy vaginal bleeding (menorraghia) may occur or irregular bleeding outside of normal periods (metrorraghia).

Several options are available when faced with this painful condition. A common medical approach is to wait and see how the patient reacts to her normal change in hormonal levels, i.e. the effects of a normal period. There is a belief that by altering the progesterone and estrogen levels will shrink the fibroids. However, the hormonal imbalance leading to uterine fibroids has not yet been proven.

Often surgical removal of the uterus (hysterectomy) is suggested, especially when excessive bleeding cannot be controlled. If the woman is of childbearing age, a priority is the preservation of reproductive capacity.

An encouraging alternative treatment is MR guided focused ultrasound treatment (MRgFUS). At this point it is the only non-surgical treatment for fibroids approved by the FDA. The fibroid is located by magnetic resonance and then ultrasound waves are focused on the target to destroy the tissue. This procedure does not affect the surrounding tissue. This is an outpatient procedure with minimal recovery time.

Another alternative medical treatment is by using magnetic imaging to guide very fine needles into the fibroid. Thermal energy is introduced into the fibroid by laser fibers attached to the needles. Some minor side effects have been noted. They include: minor skin burns, shorter and lighter periods and urinary tract infections.

The following remedies have been shown to be effective in reducing or eliminating painful symptoms and eliminating some fibroid tumors:

Probiotic – Helps the liver create an enzyme breakdown of estrogen

Chasteberry, dandelion, milk thistle and yellow dock – helps balance estrogen and progesterone and helps eliminate excess estrogen

Natural Progesterone cream to help balance progesterone and estrogen

Vitamin E – Helps improve estrogen metabolism

EFA's – To reduce inflammation

B Complex – Assists the liver in hormonal balance

Spirulina – Helps liver break down estrogen

Red clover, wormwood, black cohosh, dong quai, red raspberry and evening primrose have been effective in eliminating fibroids. These can be used as teas, tinctures, compresses or essential oils

The Barnes Thyroid Temperature Test is helpful to determine the status of the thyroid gland and therefore other hormonal glands. An Asyra test is usually performed to determine toxicities, deficiencies, hormonal imbalance and allergies. NAET procedures are used to eliminate complications caused by allergies.

A low fat, organic diet is recommended. To avoid unnecessary hormonal interference, red meat and dairy products should be eliminated. Avoid birth control pills as they contain estrogen. Avoid tampons and napkins bleached with chlorine because they can mimic estrogen. Warm castor oil packs placed over the lower abdominal area can help reduce the pain. Adequate supplementation should be maintained with emphasis on the digestive system. By taking apple cider vinegar with each meal to help the stomach digest more efficiently, amino acids and digestive enzymes to assist in digestion in the small intestine, and a good probiotic for the large intestine, will ensure proper nutritional maintenance. Digestive enzymes should be taken on an empty stomach.

## Fibromyalgia

Fibromyalgia is a chronic condition characterized by widespread pain in the muscles, tendons and ligaments. Some of the symptoms include: wide-spread aches and pains, neck pain, rib pain, low back pain, thigh pain, tension headaches, chronic fatigue, depression, lethargy, irritability, anxiety, weight gain, sleep disruption, vulvar pain syndrome, myofascial pain syndrome, immune deficiency syndrome, restless legs syndrome, irritable bowel syndrome, TMJ disorders, digestive problems including IBS, brittle nails and hair, concentration problems and sugar cravings. These symptoms may vary from person to person and can, be misdiagnosed. If an obvious cause cannot be found or the practitioner is frustrated by the symptoms, it is easy to simply diagnose the condition as Fibromyalgia and send the patient on their way with either an anti-depressant or a pain pill, or both. That can be very frustrating for the patient in that the cause has not been addressed nor a definite plan for its elimination presented.

It's estimated by the American College of Rheumatology that fibromyalgia affects over 8 million people in the United States. It is more common in women than men, especially between the ages of 30 and 50. It's estimated that 4.3% of all women and .5% of all men in the United States suffer from fibromyalgia. Women with this condition tend to be tense, depressed, stressed, anxious, and striving. However, not all patients are considered type A personalities.

Because there is no specific one thing that causes fibromyalgia that's why it's been shrouded by mystery and disbelief. Adding to that is the fact that there is no specific test for fibromyalgia, therefore fibromyalgia patients suffer with no foreseeable relief. They are left with trial and error prescriptions that often lead to further complications. Some have postulated that genetics, stress, sleep disturbance, past physical trauma, hormonal changes, viruses, and dysnutrition (wrong chemicals induced into the body) play a role in the cause of fibromyalgia. Yet none have been proven to be an ultimate cause.

Since there are no tests specifically for fibromyalgia, the diagnosis is based on ruling out other conditions. The patient must have had widespread body pain for over three months affecting all four quadrants of the body. The patient must have 11 of 18 specific pain spots. The patient must feel sharp pain with just 8 pounds of pressure applied. Only 3 or 4 spots suggests myositis and 10 spots suggests polymyalgia.

The points are on both sides of the body. The points include: above the eyebrow (frontal bone), base of the neck above the clavicle, below the clavicle, upper position of the fold of the elbow, inside of the knee, back of the head, top of the shoulder, between the shoulder blades, upper part of the buttocks and lateral side of the buttocks.

Drug treatments, including cortezone, appear to have had no effect on this condition. Aspirin, Tylenol and Ibuprophen have had only a slight, short-lived effect for some. Anti-seizure medication has shown some relief for some as well. However, in most cases, the side-effects are often worse than the original condition.

Stretching and exercise have shown significant benefit for those with fibromyalgia by increasing circulation and mobilizing tight muscles. This has shown the most immediate improvement over any other therapy.

Those suffering from fibromyalgia, chronic fatigue, chemical sensitivities, etc., have been shown to gain a great deal of relief from detoxification and metabolic elevation. An Asyra evaluation, followed by NAET treatments for sensitivities are good starting points for relief. Liver and colon detoxification leads to proper metabolism, digestion and elimination.

We also suggest the following nutritional approach:

Vitamin C – 1,500 to 12,000 mg/day
Lecithin (phosphatidyl choline) – 5-10 grams/day to balance nerve function
Omega 3, 6, 9 – 1.5-3 grams/day
Calcium – 2,000 mg/day
Magnesium – (citrate or malate) - 1,000 mg/day
Vitamin D – 5,000 IU/day
Valarian – before and after exercise and before bedtime
Ashwagandha – 6 capsules per day
Boswellia – 2 capsules three times per day
Protein – consume 60-120 grams per day
Vivex (Shacklee) – 1-3 tsp/day
Melatonin – 3 mg at bedtime
5-HTP – 100 mg 3 times per day
SAMe – 800 mg/day

We also recommend mild exercise (swimming or walking), reducing stress, getting more sleep, simplifying life, and keeping a positive attitude to reduce pain and overcoming this devastating condition.

## Fingernail Fungus

See Nail Fungus

## Flu (Influenza)

Every year the airwaves are filled with warnings about the up-coming flu epidemic with exhortations nearing threats to "get your flu shot." The media would have you believe that if you didn't get your shot, you might die. They cite statistics relating to deaths related to the flu. The fact is, according to the CDC (Centers of Disease Control and Prevention), influenza related deaths "are deaths that occur in people for whom seasonal influenza infection is LIKELY a contributor to the cause of death, but not necessarily the primary cause of death." Again according to the CDC, "many seasonal related deaths occur because the person may develop a secondary infection or because seasonal influenza can aggravate an existing chronic illness." In other words, getting the flu along with having a severely depressed immune system or a chronic illness can severely compromise a person's ability to fight off another attack.

Flu symptoms (including the H1N1 virus) are virtually the same as those of the common cold, but much more severe.

- Runny of stuffy nose
- Sore throat
- Coughing
- High fever
- Fatigue
- Body aches
- Headache
- Chills
- Vomiting or diarrhea

We have two approaches to treating the flu; both have proven successful in eliminating the symptoms within 1-2 days. The best time to start is at the first sign of a cold or flu.

1.  Taking 2 Olive leaf extract capsules and one Oregano capsule four times per day (breakfast, lunch, dinner, and at bedtime), along with high doses of vitamin C(4-10 grams per day), Vitamin D3 (up to 10,000 IU), zinc, Echinacea, and garlic can stop the flu within one day. Repeat this formula the following day if any stray symptoms persist. The amount should be modified for children.
2.  Our 'secret weapon' for eliminating the flu is isode therapy using NAET. It's always recommended that the patient follow the above recommendations to insure it's completely eradicated. Then the patient is given a NAET treatment using homeopathic vials of influenza, viruses, bacteria, rhinitis, complete sinus membranes, lungs and bronchi. Along with those, the most important ingredient we add is the patient's own mucus and saliva. By spitting into a tissue and blowing the nose into a tissue, we have now captured whatever is causing the condition. It matters not what the name is, we have it in tissues and placed in a plastic bag. A NAET treatment is performed as per normal procedures. Normally the patient's symptoms are relieved within hours.

## Fluid Retention (Edema)

The lymphatic system is a network of tubes that drains fluid (lymph) from tissues and empties into the bloodstream. When fluid isn't removed from the tissues, a condition known as edema (fluid retention) occurs.

There are many causes of edema. Some of the most common include:

Certain medications including high blood pressure meds, cor-

ticosteroids and nonsteroidal anti-inflammatory drugs (NSAIDs).
Pregnancy
Gravity– standing for long periods of time
Oral contraceptives
Dietary deficiency – especially of protein or vitamin B1 (thiamine)
Hot weather
Burns

Symptoms may include:
Swelling – especially of the feet and ankles
Joint stiffness
Rapid weight gain and often fluctuations
Pitting edema – skin indent for a few seconds after being pressed
Non-pitting edema – skin doesn't indent with pressure

Some medical conditions have been known to cause fluid retention. Among those are allergic reactions, thyroid disorders, arthritis, liver, kidney or lung diseases, heart failure, and others. A holistic doctor can order blood tests, urine tests, as well as, liver, kidney and heart function tests.
Some suggestions to reduce fluid retention:
Eliminate food and environmental allergies
Reduce salt intake in the diet
Avoid tea, coffee and alcohol
Treat any underlying thyroid condition
Increase supplementation, especially – vitamin B6, B5, calcium, magnesium, manganese, and evening primrose oil
Drink cranberry juice
Try herbal diuretics such as dandelion leaf, corn silk, horsetail, parsley, fennel seeds, lemon juice, nettle
Epson salt bath – 2 cups per bathtub, soak for 15 minutes
Apple Cider Vinegar – one teaspoon per glass of water 2

times per day

Exercise

Drink plenty of water

## Food Allergies/Sensitivities

See Allergies and/or NAET

## Food Poisoning

Although this condition is rarely seen in the office, the question of what to do if one encounters food poisoning arises often enough to warrant inclusion in this section. Food poisoning can be caused by bacteria, viruses or other toxins in food. Most often we are unsuspecting until it's too late. According to the Centers for Disease Control (CDC), the four most common contaminants include *Campylobacter* (from cutting raw chicken on the same surface as vegetables or undercooked poultry),*Salmonella*(from food handlers' contamination), *E. coli* (from undercooked beef or unclean handling), and norovirus (from unwashed hands).

The symptoms may develop within an hour after consumption or up to days later. Symptoms may include nausea, vomiting, headache, dizziness, sweating, tearing eyes, dry mouth, confusion, abdominal cramps and diarrhea. In most cases the condition is self limiting. Simply let nature take its course and it will resolve itself. However, if you are in the middle of dealing with food poisoning, that's not what you want to hear. If there is prolonged abdominal pain, bloody stools, a fever, or dehydration, a holistic healthcare provider should be contacted.

Depending upon what's available or what's palatable, the following home remedies have proven successful in giving relief from the symptoms and expediting recovery.

- **Drink plenty of fluids** to counteract the dehydrating effects of vomiting and diarrhea. Into one liter of water, add one teaspoon of lemon juice, a pinch to a teaspoon of sugar and a pinch of salt. This will add electrolytes that have been lost back into the system.

- **Activated charcoal** acts like a magnet to toxins in the system. Mix 1-3 ounces of activated charcoal to 8-10 ounces of water. It will also act as a magnet to any medicines or supplements taken 2-3 hours earlier. Charcoal has a tendency to turn stools black.
- **Apple Cider Vinegar**, although acidic, has an alkaline effect on the digestive system. It can soothe the gastrointestinal lining and kill bacteria. Simply mix two tablespoons of ACV in warm water and drink for relief. Alternatively, mixing 2-3 teaspoons of ACV to water, apple juice or grape juice helps relieve symptoms. This can be taken daily as a preventive to sooth and help regulate the digestive system.
- **Ginger** can stop the heartburn and pain caused by food poisoning. Either drink a cup of ginger tea or mix a few drops of ginger juice to one teaspoon of honey and swallow.
- **Peppermint** tea or even sucking on a piece of peppermint candy will help digest food, expel gas and reduces stomach contractions.

## Fractures

There are several types of fractures, all involving a disruption of the cancelous or outside layer of bone. And there are three phases of fracture healing. The reactive phase occurs immediately after the fracture. Almost immediately the surrounding tissue begins to inflame then granulation tissue forms. This begins the healing process. During the reparative phase a cartilage callus begins to form and calcium is drawn to the area. This callus is like a bridge of repair that can even be seen on an x-ray. Sometimes, as in the case of ribs, a fracture cannot be seen on x-ray for two or three days. But when the callus appears it is quite obvious where the break was. Finally, there is the remodeling phase. New bone is now being laid down in the original bone contour.

If an x-ray system is not available or if there's a question about whether a bone is either broken or not, there's a simple test that's almost 100% effective in determining whether to have an x-ray or not. By striking a tuning fork (preferably in the key of C) against the heel of the hand and then placing the base of the fork on the same bone but slightly away from the possible fracture site, the result will either confirm or deny the need for x-rays. The reaction is a sharp, severe pain at the site of the suspected fracture. If fractured, there will be no doubt that it should be x-rayed. At the site of the break the two pieces of bone are slightly separated. When vibrated, the periosteum (nerve rich covering around a bone) gets pinched between the segments and the pain is immediate. If that occurs, a holistic doctor or orthopedist should be contacted. If the apposition or alignment is good, the bone will simply be wrapped.

Complete healing may range from months to years. We have found that **comfrey** taken daily will expedite the recovery process. Comfrey (also known as the knitting herb) helps direct calcium to the site of most need – in this case, the fracture. Comfrey can be taken anytime during the day either by way of a tea or in capsule form.

## Fungus, Nails (Onychomycosis)

Fungus, once it invades the toenails or finger nails, may cause them to become thick, discolored, misshapen, or brittle. It can become painful and, in rare cases, more serious. It generally takes some time for the affected nail to grow out for complete resolution.

Here are some treatments that have worked for our patients:

1. Soak the nails for 20 minutes nightly in Pao d' arco tea.
2. Mix equal parts of DMSO (a sulfur compound) and SSKI (a saturated solution of potassium iodide). Rub this compound on and under the affected nail(s) 2-3 times per day.

Be sure to get a 75-90% pure DMSO. The DMSO is a carrier that allows the SSKI (a strong antimicrobial) to penetrate the nail and skin. The SSKI may discolor the skin and clothes.

3. Apply Tea Tree Oil to the nails daily.
4. Wet the hand(s) or foot (feet). Rub Borax power over the affected area(s). Do this daily until the condition has disappeared – usually 1-2 weeks. It also works well for athlete's foot.
5. First thing in the morning and last thing at night apply a mixture of 3 drops Melaleuca essential oil and 1 ounce coconut oil to the affected area.

These are safe and inexpensive and can be purchased at a health food store.

## Gallbladder Problems and Gallstones

The gallbladder is a small hollow organ located just below the liver (right upper abdomen). It's an inactive organ that supplies bile to the digestive tract to emulsify fats and oils. Stress, excessive amounts of fats, oils and spices, and very cold liquids are believed to contribute to gallbladder damage.

Gallbladder attacks can be extremely painful and frightening. I've heard my patients tell me that child birth and passing kidney stones have no comparison to the pain of a gallbladder attack. The most common phrase I hear is that "you just want to die." Some of the most common symptoms include:

- Mild to severe pain under the right side of the rib cage
- Pain often radiates to the back between the shoulder blades
- Nausea
- Indigestion after eating fatty or greasy foods
- Fatty stools

- Bloating
- Gas
- Burping or belching
- Constipation

According to Dr. Jonathan Wright, M.D., there is a method of eliminating gallbladder pain by removing a small group of foods from your diet. Eggs (93%), pork (64%), and onions (52%) were the most common culprits. Following that were fowl (35%), milk (25%), coffee (22%), oranges (19%), corn (19%), beans (19%), and nuts (19%). The % is the percent of the time this food was involved.

However, eliminating foods from the diet does not address the cause of the condition. Fat allergies are often at the root of this condition. By using NAET to eliminate the fat allergy (the cause), we can now concentrate on eliminating the results (symptoms).

If you have stones, gallbladder pain or an ultrasound shows a "thickened" gallbladder wall, the following supplements will help. Vitamin C and lecithin can reduce the tendency of bile to crystallize. Iron deficiency increases the tendency for cholesterol to form stones. The majority of individuals with stones have been shown to be deficient in stomach hydrochloric acid (HCl). There are several supplements available to increase bile production and inhibit the formation of bile crystals. We have also successfully used Magnesium, Methionine, Cysteine, and Taurine.

A low-fat, low-cholesterol diet is suggested to prevent the occurrence of gallstones. Weight loss, reduction of refined sugar, and elimination of transfats are all important in preventing or eliminating gallbladder problems. There is a higher incidence of gall stones in people with celiac disease. Therefore, eliminating gluten from your diet may help prevent the development of stones.

Another treatment that has shown to dissolve stones and prevent their recurrence is vitamin B6, magnesium and the South American herb called Chanca piedra. This herb is known for its ability to dissolve and prevent both kidney and gallbladder stones. It has been shown to increase the urinary excretion of uric acid, helpful in managing gout and hyperuricemia. Therefore, the following protocol seems to be the most effective.

Magnesium - 100 mg three times a day

Pyridoxine (vitamin B6) – 10 mg once per day

Chanca piedra – 2 grams daily

Culver's root extract – 10-25 frops in ¼ glass water, 3 times daily

GB Plus – NutriWest – as directed

## Ganglion Cyst

Ganglion cysts are usually found on the back of the hand or top of the wrist. They are sometimes unsightly and uncomfortable but harmless. Think of the bump as a small balloon under the skin. The bump didn't just appear out of nowhere. There is usually an opening through which fluid is allowed to accumulate. The opening closes off and traps the fluid inside. In olden times, people smashed the bump with the family Bible (largest book in the house). However, there is a better way. First, apply a thin layer of Apple Cider Vinegar to the area. Let it dry. Mix 10 drops of Oregano essential oil and 10 drops of Frankincense essential oil with 2 ounces of virgin coconut oil. Rub 2-3 drops onto the cyst – massaging the area 30 seconds to a minute. By attempting to reverse the flow of fluid, a reduction in size should be seen within a few days.

## Gastritis (Stomach ache)

Gastritis is an irritation or inflammation of the lining of the stomach resulting in a swelling of the tissue. Acute gastritis can be for a very short time but chronic gastritis can last for months or even years. Certain medications, excessive alcohol consumption, bacterial infection (Helicobacter pylori) and extreme stress are the most common causes of gastritis. Other causes might include trauma, food poisoning, allergies, insufficient food or gastric hydrochloric acid, or an over abundance of food. Some common symptoms may include loss of appetite, nausea, vomiting and pain in the upper part of the abdomen. Sometimes the gastritis becomes so severe or long term that a person can vomit blood or pass black stools. If the pain is accompanied by nausea, vomiting, abdominal distention, fever and signs of shock (rapid heartbeat, low blood pressure, irregular breathing), the most common cause is appendicitis. Immediate medical attention should be sought. If the pain is not accompanied by the above symptoms, it is probably benign.

If the condition persists, blood work would be in order. A complete blood scan, including a CBC (complete blood count) should be performed to check for anemia. When having blood work done, ask that they test for H.pylori. This will rule out a bacterial infection. We've found that endoscopic examinations and stool testing are unnecessary in most cases. Question the motives for doing the tests.

Medical treatment includes antacids, H2 antagonists (Pepsid, Tagamet, Zantac, Axid), and proton pump inhibitors (Prilosec, Nexium, Prevacid, etc.). However, each one has its own set of adverse side effects.

A comprehensive analysis using the Asyra can reveal amino acid deficiencies, digestive maladies, enzyme deficiencies, dietary concerns and inflammatory patterns. By narrowing the areas of concern, the practitioner can better determine the course of treatment.

We have found that 1 teaspoon of baking soda mixed with 1 cup of water will, in most cases, relieve an upset stomach.

Dissolving peppermint candy in the mouth will soothe an irritated stomach.

If convenient, add one teaspoon of cinnamon powder to two tablespoons of honey and ingest slowly.

Finally, if the above two are not convenient, measure two finger widths above first wrinkle in wrist closest to the palm. With two fingers of the opposite hand, lightly rub that spot in a clockwise motion.

If, in fact, testing finds the H.pylori bacteria present, a different approach can be taken to treat and remedy the infection. This bacterial infection can be spread through food, water, saliva, vomit and fecal matter. It's very easily spread but most often occurs in children. Symptoms include nausea, burping, vomiting, burning abdominal pain and bloating.

The most successful remedies that we have found involve a combination of the following:

Apple cider vinegar (ACV)
Coconut oil (VCO virgin coconut oil)
Aloe vera
Lemon water
Baking soda
Oil of oregano
Manuka honey

Here are some combinations that work:

1. 1 teaspoon of virgin coconut oil 3 times per day plus 5-6 drops of ACV
2. Mix equal amounts of VCO, ACV, aloe vera and manuka honey.

Take 1 teaspoon 3 times per day.

## GERD

See Acid Reflux

## Gout

The immediate cause of gout is an excessive accumulation of uric acid in the body. When uric acid in the body increases and excretion decreases, uric acid can build up in the body in the form of uric acid crystals and cause pain, swelling and even lead to arthritic and kidney destruction. Gout generally shows up in the big toe but can also attack the wrist, ankle and thumb joints. High Fructose Corn Syrup (HFCS) is a leading cause of excessive uric acid in the system. Avoid it like the plague.

Treatment: Eat red cherries or drink red cherry juice – without sugar or HFCS. At the first sign of an attack, drink 32 ounces of tart cherry juice without sugar added.

Drink plenty of water from a reverse osmosis system.

Develop on a <u>good</u> vitamin and mineral program.

## H. pylori (Heliobacter pylori bacteria)

See Gastritis

## Hair Loss (Alopecia)

There are many causes of hair loss, just as there are many remedies. The following is a partial list of causes.

- Genetics –the mechanism is not fully understood
- Hypothyroid – low thyroid
- Infections – ringworm, fungus, mites
- Medications – cancer, arthritis, depression, heart conditions, high blood pressure, diabetes, hormone replacement, cholesterol, steroids, acne, mycotic infections, chemotherapy, radiation therapy
- Nutritional deficiencies – especially biotin, zinc, iron, protein
- Hormonal – pregnancy, childbirth, menopause
- Trauma – pulling hair with force, i.e., pony tails, cornrows, vigorous brushing

The most common cause that we have addressed over the years has been hypothyroidism. Most of the other causes have a definite focal cause. With a low thyroid, the onset is gradual and very subtle.

See "Hypothyroidism" for an effective treatment.

# Halitosis

See bad breath

# Hammer Toes

See Trigger Finger

# Headache (cephalgia)

There are over 200 types of headaches. Some are very minor in nature and some are very serious. Primary headaches are recurrent, benign headaches not caused by a disease or structural problem. Migraine headaches and headaches caused by turning the head wrong, sleeping wrong, coughing, sneezing are all primary headaches. Secondary headaches on the other hand, are caused by injuries, tumors, infections and diseases.

Most headaches are classified as primary. Symptoms include sensitivity to light and/or sound, head pain, neck pain, nausea, eye pain, tearing and fatigue. Secondary headaches can include the above plus visual disturbances, taste disturbances, vomiting, irritability, depression, diarrhea and/or constipation, etc.

Headaches that are benign and low-risk generally have the following in common:

- Under 30 years old
- Have a history of headaches
- No abnormal neurological problems
- No new history or accidents that present concern
- No disease patterns

Concerns that identify secondary headaches include:
- Onset after 40 years old
- Sudden onset

- Positive neurologic signs and symptoms
- Systemic disease or symptoms

Patients with secondary headaches are referred to a lab or a primary holistic physician for diagnostic testing to rule out serious, life threatening conditions.

Most primary headaches can be resolved by eliminating allergies through NAET procedures and identifying toxins and deficiencies through Asyra testing and then reducing those. But most of the time headaches can be resolved by using chiropractic adjustments to the cervical spine.

*Joan had been an RN for over 20 years. She was the head of her department at the local hospital. She came to the office with a severe headache that she had had for weeks. She had tried medication. She had tried physical therapy. She had tried biofeedback. Nothing seemed to make a difference. She awoke with the headache and went to bed with it. Blood tests and CT scans were negative. She came to our office as a last resort. Before the examination she got in my face and said, "I don't believe in you. This is all quackery and it's going to be a waste of my time." At that I told her she was free to leave now without charge and without hard feelings. She said that she had tried everything and, at this point, had nothing to lose.*

*After the first treatment she returned stating that her headache had subsided a bit, but that it probably would have anyway. After the second adjustment, her headache was completely gone. A few days later the headache returned but very mild this time. Her neck was adjusted again and she was not seen for over a month. When she returned she was overjoyed and thankful for stopping her headaches. She said, "I don't know what you did, but it works." From that point she became a great advocate for conservative care.*

# Heartburn

See Acid Reflux

# Heel Fissures

There are many causes for cracked heels but one of the most common causes is from within. Deficiency of zinc and omega-3 fatty acid is the prime cause of this condition. They generally don't cause a problem unless the fissures become deep or wide and begin to bleed. That can lead to infection and then we get into a more complicated condition.

Some proven remedies for heel fissures include:
1. Apply coconut oil on dry and cracked areas after washing the feet clean. Wear a pair of thick socks overnight and you should see results in a few days.
2. Apply the pulp of a ripe banana on the dry or cracked area. Leave it on for 10 minutes and rinse it clean.
3. Soak the feet in lemon juice for about 10 minutes. Do this weekly until you see a change.
4. At the end of the day, soak the feet in warm soapy water for about 15 minutes. Rinse the feet and pat dry. Make a healing mixture comprised of: one teaspoon Vaseline and the juice of one lemon. Rub this mixture onto the cracked heels until it is thoroughly absorbed. Do this until results are visible.
5. Regularly apply a mixture of glycerin and rosewater until results are visible. You should see results in 10 days.
6. Melt paraffin wax and mix it well with a little mustard oil. Apply this mixture on the dry or cracked area of the heels. Rinse it off in the morning. Doing this nightly should achieve the desired results in 10-15 days.
7. Mix butter with baby powder and bicarbonate of soda. Apply to the feet at night. Wear thick socks. You should

see results after 10 days.
8. Apply Benocoolen Virgin Coconut Oil Cracked Heel Repair Cream nightly. You should see results within two months.
9. Soak feet in crystal sea salt or Epsen salt and then apply Aloe Vera, Tea Tree Oil or coconut oil.

To help curb the deficiencies, a diet rich in vitamins, minerals and zinc is necessary. Omega-3 fatty acids are not produced in the body, so they have to be obtained by supplements. Since it is not always financially possible or physically possible to eat all the right foods and in the amounts necessary to get all our required nutrients, it's a good idea to supplement our diets with GOOD vitamins, minerals, omegas, amino acids and enzymes.

## Hemorrhoids (Piles)

Hemorrhoids are very painful and embarrassing. However, they usually aren't dangerous. Hemorrhoids are inflamed blood vessels in and around the rectum and anal canal. As the vessels engorge, they displace the surrounding tissues causing pain and irritation. Some common symptoms include: bleeding, itching, protrusion, lack of complete evacuation, constipation, and difficulty keeping oneself clean after a bowel movement. The causes of hemorrhoids varies from person to person. Localized weakness due to age, digestive problems like diarrhea and constipation, poor diets, obesity, heavy lifting, rough sports, pregnancy, and hypertension are a few common causes of hemorrhoids.

There are two classifications of hemorrhoids: Internal and external. External hemorrhoids are more painful than the internal and, of course, more visible. They are tender to the touch and often bleed with bowel movements. Internal hemorrhoids are less painful due to the lack of nerve supply to that area.

Witch hazel is a good herb to use to reduce swelling and inflammation, thereby reducing pain and itching. Witch hazel bark tea can be taken internally to stop hemorrhages and as an enema to stop hemorrhoids from bleeding.

A more permanent and painless approach to the elimination of hemorrhoids is an old procedure called the Keezy Technique. According to Dr. Steven Cranford of the Sandy Boulevard Clinic in Portland, Oregon: "It is the use of a special galvanic electrode that conducts a very low voltage, low amperage, electrical current into the diseased hemorrhoidal tissue causing electrochemical destruction." By non-surgically treating the internal hemorrhoid, the external hemorrhoid shrinks and ultimately disappears. "It is a safe, effective alternative to the painful surgical operation (hemorrhoidectomy)", says Dr. Cranford.

## Herpes outbreak

See Fever blisters or Shingles

## Hiatal Hernia

Hiatal hernia is a condition in which a portion of the stomach protrudes upward into the chest, through an opening in the diaphragm. The cause is unknown but age and obesity are known risk factors. Symptoms include chest pain, heartburn, worse when bending or lying down and difficulty swallowing.

Exercise, good nutrition and losing weight help prevent or reduce a hiatal hernia. Two other methods that we've used in our office that seem to help:

Bend at the waist while holding the two middle fingers just below the sternum. Press internal and pull down while rising to an upright position. Repeat this 7 times twice per day for the first week. Repeat the procedure bowing 3 times once per day for the second week and as often as necessary thereafter.

Another proven exercise to diminish a hiatal hernia is to drink a glass of water and spend 3-5 minutes jumping on a rebounder. The weight of the water in the stomach will help pull the trapped upper part of the stomach below the diaphragm. Eventually the diaphragm will tighten and reduce the flair ups. If you don't have a rebounder, you could do jump rope, do jumping jacks, simply jump up and down for 5 minutes or stand on your toes and drop to your heals.

## High Blood Pressure (Hypertension)

Blood pressure is a measurement of the force of the blood against the arterial walls as it circulates throughout the body. Blood pressure varies from day to day and from hour to hour. It decreases when we rest or are asleep and it rises when we're physically or emotionally active. This "silent" or largely symptomless disease affects almost one-third of the population. If left untreated, it can lead to hardening of the arteries (atherosclerosis), kidney disease, diabetes, blindness, and even congestive heart failure. Some symptoms may include: dizziness, headaches, nosebleeds, fatigue, ringing in the ears, insomnia, and sweating. It is sometimes associated with a lack of potassium or the ratio of potassium to sodium is upside-down from an improper diet. (See the mineral section regarding Potassium.)

There are two parts to the blood pressure reading. The first number is called Systole. It's the measure of the force of the heart when it's contracting. Diastole, the lower number, is the force of the blood when the heart is resting. Diastole, the most important number, actually measures the true condition of the arteries. Years ago, the World Health Organization of the United Nations set the upper limits of blood pressure at 160/90. The United States, after pressure from the large pharmaceutical companies, lowered the numbers to 140/90. Anything over that is classified as Hypertension. Therefore, more drugs could be prescribed and the diagnosis is permanently in your file.

Most doctors don't want to spend the time it would take to learn what's causing the hypertension. Mainstream medicine claims that over 90% of all cases of high blood pressure are "essential," which is a bizarre medical term for "we don't know the cause." So they prescribe the latest and greatest drug as if your blood pressure problem is due to some sort of drug deficiency.

Very often the first drug prescribed is hydrochlorothiazide (HCTZ). It's a water pill that helps your body absorb less salt. But it can cause dry mouth, fatigue, irregular heartbeat, nausea, stomach pain, clay-colored stools and dark urine. It can actually hasten the onset of diabetes. If that drug doesn't reduce the blood pressure to the doctor's standards, then another equally harmful drug will be prescribed.

To reduce hypertension, the medical world will offer drugs (of course), exercise, reduce weight, reduce salt intake (however, only 20% of Americans are salt sensitive), eliminate stress, eliminate birth-control pills and review your prescription drugs. Beyond that, they have nothing to offer.

We have found that there is much more that can be done to reduce blood pressure. We begin by finding any allergies and eliminating them with NAET. Then we recommend the following:

**Exercise** – Simply walking (briskly) 30-60 minutes a day while swinging your arms will help you lose weight, lower your blood pressure and feel better.

**Monitor your salt consumption to about 2 grams per day** (preferably sea salt).

**Vitamin D3** – 4,000 – 6,000 IU per day. This will help normalize your rennin levels. Renin regulates salt and fluid balance. A simple renin blood test can help determine if Vitamin D3 therapy is needed.

**Coenzyme Q10** (CoQ10) strengthens a weak or weakened heart. Statin drugs deplete the body of CoQ10. I recommend 100 to 300 mg per day. A rule of thumb for a good CoQ10 is 1 mg/pound of body weight.
**Garlic** – Take the equivalent of one clove per day. Cook with it or take it as a supplement.

**Grape Seed Extract** – Reduces high blood pressure within one month at 100 mg. three times per day.

**Celery** – A potent diuretic can be taken by eating stalks (4-6 per day), by juice or by celery seed extract in capsule form. It helps with water retention, muscle cramps, arthritis, gout and helps calm nerves.

**Taurine** – An amino acid that helps treat high blood pressure (helps regulate fluid balance and normalize aldosterone levels), heart failure and anxiety. A dose of 2-4 grams daily split into two doses seems to work.

**Bonito Fish peptide** – A fish-derived protein has shown great success in Japan. Vasotensin from Metagenics contains this protein.

**Other things that have worked:**Beet root, Cinnamon and hawthorn have been used for centuries to reduce blood pressure. Magnesium helps relax blood vessels and lower blood pressure. Use 400-1200 mg daily from magnesium citrate, orotate, malate or fumurate. Take in the evening for better sleep (calmative). Magnesium oxide is poorly absorbed and can cause diarrhea. Celery and carrot juice for temporary reduction of BP.

**Dark Chocolate,**for all of us chocolate lovers, helps reduce blood pressure a tiny amount. However, it's loaded with calories.

**Hibiscus tea** –Three cups daily for 4-6 weeks has been shown to significantly reduce systolic blood pressure

## High Cholesterol and Triglycerides

See Cholesterol section and Triglycerides section
## Hives (Uticaria)

Hives is a common skin condition caused by the body reacting to a stimulus. They may appear as small, swollen (angioedema), itchy, red areas on the skin, singularly or in clusters. These patches may last a few minutes to a few weeks. Acute uticaria is the diagnosis given if the hives last for less than six weeks. Chronic uticaria means they have lasted over six weeks. When small cells in the skin called mast cells release histamine, a chemical that causes tiny blood vessels (capillaries) to leak fluid, it causes the leaked fluid to accumulate in the skin. That accumulation appears as small swellings that we call hives.

There are several causes of hives. Allergies, obviously, are the number one cause. These can include food or environmental allergies and sensitivities. Other causes include: Sudden exposure to cold, hot showers, vaccines for flu or tetanus, prescription medications, infections, parasites, alcohol, excessive sweating, insect stings, emotional stress, contact items such as perfumes, laundry detergents, makeup, new clothes, new carpet, and the list goes on.

Symptoms include: Swelling of skin, airways, eyelids, severe itching, erythema (redness of the skin) and airway obstruction from swelling of the airways.

We have found the most effective way to combat hives is to find the source of the allergic reaction. We first do an Asyra test to determine which items may be the causative factor. The offending items are listed in an order to be treated by NAET procedures. By eliminating the allergies and sensitivities, the hives disappear and the chances of them returning is decreased or eliminated.

To expedite recovery, a cold compress will temporarily reduce the itching and swelling. For some people herbal teas can reduce the symptoms temporarily. These might include green tea, goldenseal tea, Devil's claw tea, and chamomile tea. Ginger taken by capsule, tea or applied locally as a salve has been shown to be effective. Applying aloe vera topically to the skin on and around the hives helps the skin heal quicker.

## Hot Flashes

The most common, and most irritating, symptom of menopause is hot flashes. It's estimated that 50-85% of women in the US experience hot flashes as they journey through menopause. About half of those ladies experience symptoms severe enough to seek medical help. The hot flashes can become so severe as to cause excessive sweating, especially at night. Simply put, the cause is an imbalance between estrogen and progesterone. Many approaches have been made to help balance the hormones without harmful hormone replacement therapy. Once again, one approach is not going to work for everyone. Here are a few ideas that may help:

- If overweight, studies have shown that for each 11 pounds lost, there is roughly a one-third decline in frequency and severity of hot flashes.
- Regular aerobic exercise everyday for 30 minutes has been shown by studies to reduce hot flashes by 50%.
- Acupuncture by a qualified, experienced acupuncturist has been shown to help.
- A diet low in refined carbohydrates, processed and heated fats, empty foods and sugars help balance hormonal levels. Eat more non GMO, organic vegetables.
- Herbs such as Wild Yam, Black Cohosh, and Dong Quai help treat hot flashes as well as mood swings and irritability.
- Supplements added to a high quality multi vitamin and mineral such as vitamin D and omega-3 fats help minimize hot flashes.
- EFT has helped many ladies overcome the symptoms of menopause.

## Hypoadrenia

See Adrenal Exhaustion

## Hypoglycemia (Low Blood Sugar)

## Hypothyroidism (Low Thyroid)

Hypothyroidism, or underactive thyroid, is a very common problem and often misunderstood and misdiagnosed. Blood tests generally provide normal or low normal readings. Some of the causes can be traced back to elevated toxin levels in the system, drinking fluoridated and/or chlorinated water, and eating brominated flour, both of which cause a displacement of iodine in the system. A major causative factor, and usually overlooked, is stress. I call people with underactive thyroid glands pushers. They tend to push themselves to the limit. They strive to be best at everything they do. Therefore they overtax their thyroid glands.

For years, Dr. Broda Barnes was the international expert on the thyroid gland. His research and books are well known by doctors who are serious about working with the thyroid gland. The Barnes Temperature Test is found in an appendix at the end of this book. Dr. Barnes felt that the temperature test was more accurate than the blood test.

Iodine is used to maintain the health of the thyroid. A daily dose of 12 to 14 mg of iodine is sufficient to maintain good thyroid health. Iodine is important for breast health in ladies in that it combines with a lipid to form molecules that actually kill new breast cancer cells. Iodine has also been used successfully for fibrocystic breast disease. In this case, 2-3 mg of iodine will be sufficient.

Symptoms of low thyroid include:

| | |
|---|---|
| Fatigue | Irritability |
| Concentration problems | Decrease in libido |
| Depression tendencies | Mood swings |
| Memory lapses | Dry skin |
| Constipation | Weight gain |

Accumulation of fluid in the ankles

Thinning of the outer margins of the eyebrows

We have found the most effective treatment for low thyroid is a procedure established by Dr. Barnes years ago. It involves using a natural thyroid from specially grown cattle in New Zealand. It's the purest form of natural thyroid found to date. The patient is placed on a specific schedule of consumption for six weeks. Then a maintenance dose is recommended. The maintenance dose can be varied according to symptoms without harm or regression. Overdose symptoms include hyperactivity and hot flashes. If this occurs the patient is instructed to refrain from taking thyroid supplements for 1-2 days and drink plenty of water. Then begin taking the supplement again at a lower dose. Symptoms could disappear within three days or it may take up to two months. The temperature test is more gradual in reflecting a change.

We have used this test very successfully for over 35 years. To improve the T4 readings in the blood test, taking L-Tyrosine along with iodine will help. We have found that using the same procedure for hyperthyroidism is very effective.

## Indigestion

See Gastritis

## Influenza (Flu)

Influenza, commonly called "the flu," is ordinarily a short-lived respiratory viral infection. It is very contagious and spread by droplets from sneezes and coughs. The illness lasts from 4-5 days but its effects can last for weeks. The common symptoms are: rapid onset, weakness to the point of excessive fatigue, fever, head pain, pain in the muscles, back and joints and sweating. If vomiting or diarrhea are present it's often diagnosed as intestinal flu.

Rest and isolation are important. Avoid those who are sneezing or coughing if possible. Repeatedly washing the hands and avoid touching your face or mouth will help. When out in public, shopping or dining, assume that the last person to touch that door knob, shopping cart, or merchandise, had spread their germs to those items. Rest and avoid strenuous exercise.

During the flu season, it is important to build your immune system. Increase your dosage of vitamins C and D3. Flu vaccinations tend to lower the immune system leaving the victim more vulnerable to the flu and with a false sense of security.

When a patient enters our office with symptoms of the flu, we treat them with a modified allergy elimination procedure. The patient holds vials of homeopathic influenza mix, respiratory mix, lung mix, bronchial mix, and a sample of their own sputum and nasal discharge. Twelve acupuncture control points are stimulated on either side of the spine while the patient inhales and hold, exhales and hold, hyperventilates and then breathes normally. The patient then lies on their back while nine acupuncture points called the "gates" are stimulated. The patient rests for 20 minutes while holding the vials and samples. The final procedure is to use the EAV system to stimulate the patient's meridians and organs. We have found this procedure to be very effective in eliminating a patient's flu symptoms within a day.

It's recommended that the patient rest for 24 hours and absolutely avoid any strenuous activity, especially exercise. Supplements that help accelerate recovery include:

Vitamin C – 2,000 mg minimum
Vitamin D3 – 4,000 – 6,000 IU
Garlic – 2-3 tablets
Oregano – 1 capsule four times per day
Olive Leaf Extract – 8 capsules per day

The Oregano and Olive Leaf should be taken at breakfast, lunch, dinner and just before going to bed.

## Ingrown Hair (Pseudofolliculitis barbae)

This condition doesn't come up often in our office, but when it does it is usually very worrisome for the patient. However, it doesn't have to be. An ingrown hair is simply a hair that has grown back into your skin instead of breaking through the skin to the surface and rising from it. For whatever reason, dirt or dried skin, the hair follicle can become clogged and prevent the hair from surfacing.

An ingrown hair can irritate the skin, produce an inflamed, raised red bump and can fill with pus and look like a pimple. They are usually itchy and uncomfortable. The problem can affect any-one but is more common in people with course and/or curly hair. In men, ingrown hairs can most often be seen on the chin, cheeks or neck. In women, it's common to experience ingrown hairs on the legs, pubic area and armpits. It is very common to see them in areas that have been or are being shaved often.

Often the ingrown hair will resolve on its own. But if it doesn't, it can become infected. A medical doctor may take a scalpel and make a small incision to release the hair. However, there are ways that are less traumatic and less expensive.

1. We generally use a sterile needle and tweezers to free the hair and then gently pull it out from under the skin. We use a warm compress first to bring the hair to the surface. We then cut the hair just above the skin line.
2. Some have dipped a piece of bread in some warm milk and then placed it over the ingrown hair. Leave it on for about 2 minutes. This procedure can be repeated 5-6 times. Sometimes, the hair will rise to the surface making it easi-er to use a needle and tweezers.
3. Exfoliate the area gently. Add salt or olive oil and sugar to assist in exfoliation.
4. Some have told us that they have taken the membrane from inside an eggshell and covered the problem area with

it. It will dry and shrink. Once it has dried, pull the membrane off. The hair should come with it.

## Insomnia (sleeplessness)

Insomnia can be frustrating and even agonizing. You go to bed and spend the next six hours watching the clock wishing that you could drift off into restful sleep. You don't want to take drugs due to their side effects and possible dependency. You know that you will feel drowsy the next day and your thinking and reasoning will be impaired. Your stress hormone, cortisol, will spike the next night which may lower your ability to deal with stress. Your immune system will become impaired. Your blood pressure may rise and you will burn less fat than if you had a good night's sleep.

There are three primary classifications for insomnia. **Transient insomnia** lasts for less than a week. Changes in sleep environment or timing, depression, or stress may lead to a short bout of insomnia. **Acute insomnia** is the inability to sleep well for a period of less than a month. Stress, anxiety, and depression are major factors in this form of insomnia. **Chronic insomnia** is the inability to sleep well for over a month. Causative factors may include depression, high levels of stress hormones, shifts in the levels of cytokines, muscular or mental fatigue. Some other conditions that may lead to insomnia include: anxiety disorders, pain, clinical depression, sleep apnea, hormonal imbalance, nocturnal polyuria (nighttime urination), stimulant drugs and medications, antibiotic drugs, Restless Legs Syndrome, fear, mental disorders, disturbance of the circadian rhythm, certain neurological disorders, parasomnias (nightmares, sleepwalking, night terrors), and physical exercise (especially close to bedtime).

Here's what we suggest in our office:

Drink 8 ounces of **tart cherry juice** in the morning and evening for two weeks. Tart cherries contain a substantial amount of melatonin which will help moderate the sleep cycle.

**Melatonin** is a natural hormone found in the body. Serotonin, produced by the pineal gland in the brain, is converted into melatonin at night when exposure to light decreases. Taken 30 minutes before bedtime has been found to help induce sleep. It should not be used if pregnant, nursing, or diagnosed with depression, schizophrenia, autoimmune disease or other serious illness. It has no known serious side effects when taken for 3 months or less.

**Diet** has a great deal to do with sleeplessness. Avoid caffeine (coffee, tea, soft drinks, chocolate, cough and cold medicine and many over the counter medicines. Avoid sweets as they cause uneven blood sugar levels. Eat foods rich in tryptophan (an amino acid precursor to serotonin which is converted to melatonin). Carbohydrate snacks help promote sleep. Eat foods rich in magnesium. Magnesium is a natural sedative that helps with difficulty sleeping, constipation, muscle cramps or tremors, anxiety, and pain. Magnesium rich foods such as legumes, seeds, dark leafy green vegetables, wheat bran, almonds, cashews, blackstrap molasses, brewer's yeast and whole grains are helpful to relax and induce sleep.

**Valerian** has been shown to be helpful as a remedy for insomnia. Taken one hour before bedtime, it takes two to three weeks to work. It should not be taken for over three months. Side effects may include mild indigestion, headache, palpitations, and dizziness.

Drink 2 grams of **inositol** in water before going to bed.

Having a cup of **chamomile tea** one to two hours before going to bed can help reduce anxiety, calm the digestive system, and relieve muscle tension.

Some success has been noted by placing 2-3 drops of **lavender oil** on a handkerchief and placing it between the pillow and the pillow case.

**Relaxation techniques** such as yoga, muscle relaxation and visualization help to relax when done 20 minutes before bedtime. Soft, gentle music helps improve sleep quality and decrease nightly awakenings.

Regular **exercise**, especially in the afternoon, helps promote a good night's sleep. Exercising in the evening before going to bed increases adrenaline and may make it more difficult to go to sleep.

## Intestinal Parasites

It has been estimated that over 3.5 billion people suffer from some type of parasitic infection. The problem is not limited to third world countries. It's very prevalent in highly developed countries. Some of the infections are so highly contagious that simply casual contact with something that has been handled by an infected person can infect another. It's been said that people who have pets, have parasites. Symptoms and characteristics vary so greatly that after reviewing the symptoms, anyone may think they have parasites. The best way to know is to have laboratory tests performed, but even those tests often miss the presence of intestinal parasites.

Symptoms vary widely, but here are a few:
Acute infection:
Abdominal distress and diarrhea-often urgent with burning sensations and tremendous fluid loss
Gas or bloating
Nausea or vomiting
Fatigue or weakness
Stomach pain or tenderness
Chronic:
Alternating periods of constipation and diarrhea
Abdominal distention and bloating
Sudden urges to eliminate
Weight loss due to malabsorption of nutrients
Passing a worm in your stool
Grinding teeth at night
Trouble sleeping
Skin irritations such as eczema, rashes and eruptions
Mood swings, depression or anxiety
Allergies

Sudden food cravings

Blood sugar fluctuations

Itching in moist areas –nose, eyes, ears, anus

Dr. Hulda Clark spent her career exposing the dangers of parasites. In her book, *A Cure for all Diseases*, she describes the use of a frequency generator and how to make a smaller version she called a Zapper. We have had a great deal of success using the frequency generator. It is very helpful when the patient knows the name of the specific parasite. But the Zapper has also been very successful. The Zapper can be made very easily using Dr. Clark's instructions found in her book. The cost is under $50.

We have found that performing a NAET treatment for parasites and following up with some sessions with the frequency generator, the patient's parasite problems can be resolved within just a few weeks.

## Irritable Bowel Syndrome (IBS)

See Crohn's or Celiac's disease

## Itchy Feet/Hands

Any kind of skin infection can cause an irritation to the skin and can lead to an inflammation. When it occurs on the hands or feet, a mild, persistent itch may occur. The desire to scratch the area is sometimes overwhelming. Most of the time, the triggering mechanism is either bacteria or fungus. The most common cause, for the feet, is wearing socks or shoes that cause the feet to sweat.

If parasites appear to be a problem, a frequency generator or Hulda Clark's "Zapper" can eliminate that problem by using Dr. Clark's protocols.

If a fungal infection is suspected, as in Athlete's Foot, be sure to keep the feet dry and change socks frequently. Soaking the feet/hands in a solution of Pao d Arco added to water and then thoroughly drying the feet/hands and allowed to air for a while will help. Walking barefoot (grounding) helps in many cases.

Other remedies that help are:

Drying the feet with a hair dryer after a bath,

Applying vinegar to the affected area,

Applying hydrogen peroxide to the affected area,

Applying cornstarch or talcum powder sprinkled on the feet before putting on socks.

## Keratosis Pilaris, "chicken skin"

This condition occurs in 50-80% of all adolescents and 40-80% of adults. There is no known medical cure for this condition. The skin resembles goosebumps especially on the back sides of the upper arms (typically) and it can occur on the thighs and buttocks. Rarely, if ever, is it found on the palms of the hands or soles of the feet. These bumps are harmless but tend to get worse during the winter or at times of low humidity.

Treatment: Mixing 10 drops of the following essential oils: Lavender, Lemon and Melaleuca plus 6 drops of vitamin E oil in 2 ounces of coconut oil or olive oil. Apply that mixture directly to the skin daily. The skin should respond very quickly.

Cold laser directed toward the same area repeatedly, helps diminish the bumps.

## Kidney Stones

The kidneys help filter impurities and waste products from the blood and urine and, therefore helps in the detoxification process. Contrary to popular thought, kidney stones are not from taking too much calcium. They form, in fact, from the crystallization of unprocessed minerals and a calcium deficiency. When the kidneys become unable to process minerals, they build up and form stones. The most common type of stone is made up of calcium oxalate. The liver produces the oxalate. Eating soy and drinking beer contributes to the creation of oxalates. Calcium in the diet binds with the oxalate and helps it be excreted in the urine. Some causes of kidney stones include: urinary tract infections, improper protein metabolism, excessive loss of certain amino acids (cystinuria), and calcium deficiency.

Some of the symptoms of kidney stones include:

- Pain in the low back and side, sometimes excruciating
- Pain can radiate to groin and/or abdomen and last up to 60 minutes
- Painful urination
- Foul smelling, cloudy or bloody urine
- Persistent urge to urinate
- Possible nausea, vomiting, fever, chills

Some foods contain high levels of oxalates, besides soy and beer. Eating or avoiding these foods helps reduce the possibility of getting a kidney stone. These foods include: sodas (especially diet sodas), processed foods, processed salt, sugar, chocolate, beets, nuts, pepper, wheat flour, strawberries, rhubarb, spinach and parsley.

If stones are present, the following suggestions may help soothe the discomfort and speed up the body's natural healing process.

- Mix 2 oz of organic olive oil with 2 oz of organic lemon juice. Drink this solution straight then follow that with a 12 ounce glass of purified water. Wait 30 minutes. Then squeeze the juice from ½ a lemon into 12 ounces of purified water, add 1 tablespoon of Bragg's Apple Cider Vinegar. Drink. Repeat the lemon juice, water and apple cider vinegar recipe every hour until symptoms improve.
- Magnesium (300-800 mg preferably before bedtime) has been shown to reduce existing stones and prevent the formation of stones. Too much magnesium will cause diarrhea. Just reduce the amount taken until diarrhea disappears.

- Uva Ursi has proven effective in reducing pain and cleansing the urinary tract. 500 mg three times per day is recommended.
- Again a poor diet is the primary cause of kidney stones. By eliminating sodas, energy drinks, processed foods, fast foods, and alcoholic beverages the body can take care of itself and prevent the formation of stones. Drink lots of water. Keep those kidneys working.

## Laryngitis

Laryngitis is an inflammation of the larynx (voice box). The larynx contains your vocal cords and therefore any inflammation or irritation can cause swelling which leads to hoarseness or even loss of voice.

There are many causes of laryngitis, colds, flu, allergies, chemical irritants, acid reflux, but the most common cause is a viral infection. Some symptoms include: sore throat, dry cough, tickling sensation in the throat, fever and swollen lymph glands.

Common treatments include:
Resting the voice
Sucking on throat lozenges
Drinking at least eight glasses of water daily

Besides the above treatments, we've found that:
Olive Leaf Extract, two capsules four times per day, helps kill the virus
Mullen in tea or lozenge form helps sooth the throat and reduce the inflammation
Slippery Elm in tea or lozenge form can calm irritated or inflamed tissue

## Leaky Gut Syndrome

Leaky Guy Syndrome is a condition of the gastrointestinal system where the lining of the bowel is damaged or altered. A single cell layer of mucous lines the digestive tract from beginning to end. This mucous layer accounts for 80% of the immune system in the form of the single antibody, Immunoglobulin A (IgA). Poor diet, toxins, chronic stress, imbalanced gut flora or certain medications can damage that lining and then a myriad of conditions can occur.

Lining the wall of the intestinal tract are tiny fingerlike projections called microvilli. These microvilli are responsible for secreting the enzymes needed for digestion and absorption of nutrients. If sufficiently damaged, digestion becomes severely impaired and nutritional deficiencies develop. Effects from this damage can be seen throughout the body. It's believed that up to 90% of chronic health symptoms and conditions are the result of poor gut health.

In a healthy gut, there are small gaps between the cells of the intestinal lining. These gaps allow only fully digested nutrients through and into the bloodstream. As the damage continues, the openings enlarge allowing unwanted particles such as undigested food, toxins, parasites, bacteria, and yeast into the bloodstream. Once in the bloodstream, they can cause symptoms such as arthritis, headaches, hyperactivity, anxiety, chronic fatigue, eczema, and depression. Many believe that death begins in the colon. Because the intestinal lining is constantly leaking, the immune system doesn't have a chance to fully recover. Eventually the system becomes so overwhelmed that it begins to attack healthy tissue and organs and thus begins an autoimmune disease.

Now after all that gloom and doom, there are ways to treat Leaky Gut Syndrome.

1. Determine the cause. Most often the cause of the inflammation is food allergies. Right on the heels of allergies is Candida, medications, especially NSAIDs (nonsteroidal an-

ti-inflammatory drugs), parasites, and fungus. NAET is an excellent way to deal with the above causes.

2. Balance the digestive and hormonal systems. Eating a proper diet is essential. Cutting out or down gluten intake, eliminating sugars and processed, canned and fast foods, and eliminating alcohol are just a few ways to improve the gut. If over 25 years old, Betain HCl should be taken with each meal to properly break down food in the stomach. Also a total enzyme and a total amino acid should be taken with each meal to ensure proper digestion in the small and large intestines.

   The diet should primarily consist of fresh meat and vegetables. Animal protein is important. Limit whole grains, nuts, seeds, and fresh fruits.

   The Barnes temperature test should be done to determine if the hormonal system, and especially the thyroid gland, is in balance. (See appendix 4.)

3. Restore balance to the gut flora. We suggest at least three colonics or enemas to clean the colon. The first two should be with coffee and the third with yogurt. The coffee will eliminate the unwanted bacteria and the yogurt will replace it with good and necessary bacteria. Many conditions will improve by doing the colonic hydrotherapy or enemas.

## Lichen Planus

Lichen Planus is an inflammatory autoimmune skin disease that can affect the skin and oral mucous membranes. This disease can affect males or females between the ages of 30-60 but more women are affected than men. The mouth symptoms appear as small, tender (can be asymptomatic or very painful), blue with white spots, papules on the sides of the tongue and inside the cheeks. The lesion lines become a lacy-looking network and will gradually increase in size. The lesions can become very painful ulcers. On the skin, the lesions can be anywhere – arms, legs, genitals, torso. The lesions are usually symmetrical and itchy. They can be in clusters or single. The papules are generally 2-4 cm in size, have sharp borders and can be either shiny or scaly. They can be flat topped when clustered or look like pimples when single. They are generally dark colored and reddish-purple in appearance. They can develop into blisters or ulcers.

Treatment: We first test the patient using EAV. Any allergy found is treated and eliminated. Any organ or system that is weakened or overly stimulated is brought back into balance. A thorough parasite evaluation is made. If parasites are found, the patient will begin a parasite elimination program according to Hulda Clark, N. D. The patient's liver and colon are detoxified using the detoxification procedures. Because stress is an important factor in Lichen Planus, Thought Field Therapy for stress is performed. The patient is sent home with instructions on exercise, i.e., walking, jogging, Tai Chi, Chi Gong, rebounding, etc., and meditation.

## Liver Cleansing

The liver is the largest glandular organ of the body and works 24 hours each day. Everything you eat, drink, breathe or rub on the body is processed through the liver. It's a three pound organ located in the upper right quadrant of the abdomen. It filters about 1.5 quarts of blood every minute. The liver's major functions are:

Producing bile to breakdown fats
Detoxifies the blood, including alcohol, drugs and chemicals
Stores and regulates glucose (sugar) for energy
Converts stored sugar to usable sugar
Stores some vitamins and iron
Breaks down hemoglobin, insulin and other hormones
Destroys old red blood cells
Converts ammonia to urea

Regulates many hormones

Produces and regulates cholesterol

Obviously the liver is a very important organ. Without it our digestion, and ultimately our health, would suffer. With all the filtering and detoxifying that the liver does, it's not surprising that it can get clogged up just like the filter in your car. There are many liver cleansing programs available – some work and some don't. We have found that the safest and most thorough way to cleanse the liver is by doing three enemas or colonics. Colonics are preferred since they can reach places that enemas can't. The first two procedures involve mixing one part water to three parts coffee (regular, strong, caffeinated). The coffee mixture will not only kill all the bacteria in the large intestine, but it also draws toxins from the liver. Therefore, the benefits are double. The third procedure involves mixing one part plain organic yogurt to three parts water. This procedure will replace the bacteria in the colon with good bacteria. With each procedure, the water temperature should be at body temp.

## Low Thyroid

See Hypothyroidism

## Lyme Disease

Lyme disease was originally thought to be spread only by a tick bite. Now it's been found that it can spread by insect bites, especially mosquitoes. According to the Centers of Disease Control (CDC), several hundred thousand Americans are affected every year. Even with that, some medical facilities refuse to admit that the condition exists.

The disease, caused by the bacteria *borrelia burgdorferi,* can appear differently in different people. It generally starts with flu-like symptoms, fever, neck pain, headaches, sweats, chills and muscle and joint pain. A temporary (acute) "butterfly" skin rash can appear where the bite occurred. If it progresses, symptoms of depression, fatigue, forgetfulness, digestive issues, sleep disturbances, mood swings and chronic fatigue can occur. There can be many more symptoms and they can be more or less severe with different people. If a person has a weakened immune system caused by viral or bacterial infection, parasites, mold exposure or allergies the symptoms can become debilitating.

Here are some ideas that have helped our patients that have suffered from Lyme desease.

1. Determine what allergies, toxicities and deficiencies your body is dealing with. We use the Asyra EAV system to begin the process. When necessary, blood tests and urinalyses are used.
2. Once determined, we begin eliminating allergies using NAET procedures.
3. Concurrently we begin eliminating toxicities. We suggest eliminating sugar, alcohol and glutens from the diet. Soda pop and carbonated beverages should be reduced or eliminated. If parasites are involved, we suggest using Hulda Clark's Zapper. It uses frequencies to kill parasites in different stages. Barberry root, wormwood, walnut hull and garlic are also strong parasite killers.
4. Deficiencies are generally addressed by using diet and supplementation. The diet should consist of organic, non-GMO products. At least one salad per day using a variety of vegetables, herbs and spices including garlic, turmeric, pepper, good fats such as avocado and coconut oil. All this can be modified to suit taste. Avoid GMO's, processed foods, foods laced with chemicals, refined foods, breads, cereals and pastas.
5. For supplementation (because we don't get all the vitamins and minerals we need in our food), we suggest a strong base of a high quality multi vitamin and mineral,

vitamin c (2,000 mg/day), vitamin D (5-6,000 IU/day), and a vitamin B complex (enough to turn the urine bright yellow). More can be added depending on the person's condition and desires, i.e. CoQ10 and hawthorn berry for heart conditions, etc. For digestion, a multi amino acid, a multi enzyme and a good probiotic. If over 25 years old, we suggest a boost to the stomach acid by way of Betaine HCL or a capfull of Bragg's Apple Cider Vinegar before each full meal.

A good diet with supplementation, eliminating toxins, deficiencies, allergies and parasites will eventually rid the body of Lyme for most people.

## Lymphedema

Lymphedema (lymphatic obstruction) is a condition of tissue swelling and localized fluid retention caused by a compromised lymphatic system. The lymphatic system returns the fluid between the tissues (interstitial fluid) to the thoracic duct and then to the bloodstream. It is then recirculated back to the tissues. The lymph is a clear fluid that collects bacteria, viruses, and dead cells throughout the body. The lymph nodes strain out these impurities which are then destroyed by infection-fighting white blood cells. The nodes also create a balance of water between the cells so that the cells can exchange nutrients, wastes, and gasses as needed. If these nodes are damaged or removed, lymph can accumulate in the tissues and cause an uncomfortable swelling that's called lymphedema. The damage most often occurs as a result of surgery or radiation, as in cancer treatment.

The most common treatment for lymphedema is manual lymphatic drainage massage (MLD). Not all massage therapists are qualified to do this type of massage. However, the internet is useful in finding a qualified MLD therapist in the local area. Taking the enzyme preparation Wobenzyme as directed on the label along with MLD has been shown to be effective in reducing swelling and pain within two months.

The following has been shown to be effective for most with lymphedema:

- Avoid alcohol and caffeine – both suppress the immune system.
- Detoxification – can include Epsom salt or baking soda baths, ionizing foot baths, and colon hydrotherapy.
- Exercise – since the lymphatic system doesn't have a pump, it needs activity to flow effectively. Exercise such as jumping on a mini-trampoline (rebounder), walking, jumping, swimming, cycling or lifting light weights are all helpful.
- Red light therapy – many studies have shown that red light therapy used at 670 nanometers alternating days three times a week for 10 weeks will reduce swelling, pressure, pain and tightness. Shine the light for 1-2 minutes on each part of the affected limb about an inch above the skin.
- Cabbage leaf packs – Famed Swiss healer Father Thomas Haeberle professed that a poultice of crushed cabbage leaves over the swelling can reduce the swelling over night. It sounds ridiculous, but who knows.
- Nutrients:
  Bromelain, a natural diuretic and anti-inflammatory, 350-450 mg per day on an empty stomach. It's pineapple based so if there's an allergy to pineapple, this might be skipped.
- Diosmin, a citrus bioflavonoid, increases the strength and frequency of the lymph vessels' contractions. Take 1,000 mg per day along with 500-1,000 mg of hesperidin.
- Horse-chestnut extract reinforces connective tissue, vein tone and seals off small pores in the veins. Take 250-500 mg per day.
- Rutin – 400 mg twice per day reduces swelling and strengthens lymph vessel walls.

- Potassium-rich foods reduce fluid retention and act like diuretics. Some foods that help include bananas, figs, sweet potatoes, artichokes, raw almonds, and tomato juice.
- Green power drinks that include wheatgrass, celery and parsley juice, and spirulina are very helpful.

## Macular Degeneration

Macular degeneration is a condition caused by damage to the macula, or center of the eye and resulting in blurry vision or vision loss. This affects the central or center point of the visual field. There are two forms: Dry form (most common) is due to a slow, progressive deterioration of the macula in the back of the eye. Symptoms include the inability to read fine print or street signs, missing areas of vision and distorted letters. The wet form (10% of the cases) has a quick onset caused by blood vessels bleeding in the retina. Some people with the wet form respond to laser therapy. However, a possible side effect in some cases is permanent blindness in the treated eye.

Most experts agree that a lifetime of poor nutrition, poor digestion, poor circulation and inadequate antioxidant defenses can lead to macular degeneration. Until recently, the prevailing viewpoint was that the condition was progressive and irreversible. Recent studies have shown that the condition can not only be prevented, but can actually be reversed. Here are some natural suggestions:

- Avoid foods that cause macular degeneration, including trans fats, hydrogenated fats, grilled foods, sugar, caffeine, alcohol
- Avoid low fat diets
- Avoid high amounts of calcium without balancing with magnesium
- Eat non-GMO spinach, kale, yellow and orange vegetables

– high in vitamin c, lutein and zeaxanthin
- Detoxify the GI tract – coffee and yogurt enemas/colonics, foot baths, baking soda baths
- Take betaine hydrochloric acid or Bragg's apple cider vinegar (one capful) before each meal. Take a multi amino acid and a multi enzyme with each meal.

The following supplements have been shown to reverse macular degeneration:

- Vitamin C 2,000 mg daily – strengthens arteries
- Lutein 15 mg daily – prevents oxidative damage
- Vitamin E 400 IU daily
- Vitamin B12 300 mcg daily
- Magnesium 400 – 600 mg daily
- Selenium (organic) 200 mcg daily
- Bilberry 160 mg 2x/day – antioxidant, improves blood flow
- Fish oil – 1,000 mg minimum daily (600 – 1,000 mg EPA, 400 – 1,000 mg DHA)
- Astaxanthin – 2 mg daily – helps prevent retinal damage
- Zeaxanthin – 6 mg daily – prevents oxidative damage

Essential oils – Frankincense, helichrysum, and cypress have been shown to improve eyesight and improve circulation to the eyes. Applying 3 drops of any of these or 3 drops of an equal mixture of these to the cheeks and lateral to the eyes twice daily helps. Avoid putting any of them in the eyes.

## Mastitis (lactation mastitis, puerperal mastitis)

Mastitis is a common breast infection among lactating women caused by bacteria (most commonly *Staphylococcus aureus*). The bacteria enters a breast through a crack or break in the nipple and then localizes the infection and develops an abscess of pus.

The signs and symptoms of mastitis include:

A painful lump or swollen area in the breast
Red discoloration of the skin due to inflammation
Swelling of a nearby gland in the armpit
Pus discharge (white or bloody) from the affected nipple
Fever (101 or higher) and malaise often accompany other symptoms

Taking drugs while breast feeding is never recommended in that the drugs are passed on to the infant. It doesn't matter if it's legal or illegal drugs, the infant still absorbs them. Too often antibiotics and analgesics are prescribed for just about everything. These too enter the infant through breast milk and will develop antibiotic-resistance in the system of the infant.

There are several natural remedies for mastitis including:

- **Nurse the baby frequently**. Since this condition begins as a plugged duct, nursing becomes the fastest remedy. The down side is that it may be painful during an active infection.
- **Hot showers** with the water hitting the affected breast will reduce the pain and inflammation, as well as help loosen a clogged milk duct.
- **Massage the breast** to loosen the plugged duct. This is especially effective after a hot shower. Always massage from the chest wall toward the nipple.
- **Hot and cold packs** can be effective when hot showers aren't reasonable. Alternate hot and cold packs at 10 – 15 minute intervals.
- **Green cabbage leaves** stuffed into the bra seems quite unusual, however, it's very effective. Cabbage leaves have anti-inflammatory properties. When taken out of the refrigerator and put in the bra, they have a cooling and soothing effect. Repeat this every few hours.

- We recommend **garlic** as a natural antibiotic. There are no negative side effects and is safe to ingest while breastfeeding.
- **Homeopathic** remedies that help include: Belladonna, Bryonia, Silicea and Phytolacca.
- **Acupuncture** points to stimulate for relief include: Stomach 18 and 44, Gallbladder 41, Large Intestine 4, Small Intestine 1, and Conception Vessel 1.
- **Lavender essential oil** – rub 2-3 drops on the affected breast several times per day for best results.
- **Oregano** supplements taken 1 capsule at a time four times per day is helpful in eliminating the bacteria.

## Meniere's Disease

Meniere's disease is characterized by vertigo (world spinning around), tinnitus (ringing in the ears), a pressure or fullness in the ears or head and loss of hearing. The condition may be constant or intermittent. There are many possible causes but no one specific item or condition. Several possible causes have been given: Allergies, viruses, bacteria, chemicals, poor circulation and even stress. Unfortunately, Meniere's is not identified by tests but rather by symptoms.

Medically there is no cure. However, alternatively there have been several avenues that have reported success in alleviating the symptoms.

- Allergies and sensitivities can cause Meniere's symptoms. Food sensitivities and environmental sensitivities can produce symptoms that mirror Meniere's symptoms. Chemicals such as aspartame and MSG have been proven to cause the same symptoms. Many food companies know this and therefore hide their chemicals under another name. By eliminating allergies and avoiding the hidden chemicals in food, many symptoms disappear.

- Olive leaf extract, oregano and colloidal silver have been shown to reduce or eliminate viral and bacterial infections. Ginko Biloba has been shown to be very effective in relieving the symptoms of Meniere's.
- Supplements that have helped include:

  Ginko biloba, CoQ10 (1mg/pound of body weight), vitamin B3 (niacin), MSM, cayenne pepper – improves circulation

  Vitamin C, High quality B complex, extra vitamin B12 – to strengthen and clean the arteries

  Olive leaf extract & Oregano (1 capsule of each with meals plus 1 before bed) and colloidal silver – antiviral and antibacterial

  Calcium – 800 mg daily

  Magnesium – 600-800 mg daily

  Manganese – 50-100 mg daily

  Lipase enzyme – with each meal

  Helichrysum essential oil

## Menstrual Cramps

Many women suffer from monthly premenstrual cramps. Often a simple chiropractic low back adjustment will ease the pain. However, it's not always convenient to see a chiropractor when the pain hits. We have found through the years that a simple stretching exercise can ease the pain or completely eliminate it.

With the young lady (patient) lying on her stomach, a second person (practitioner) stands to her side. The practitioner bends forward and places the inferior hand (hand closest to the feet) on the lower mid back. The superior hand (hand closest to the patient's head) rests on the sacrum (tailbone). The idea is not to push down. The visualization is to spread the sacrum and the lower spine apart. Hold this for 15 seconds. SLOWLY release the pressure. Repeat this procedure two more times. There should be some relief almost instantly. Repeat this whole procedure as often as necessary.

Other remedies that have worked for some:

Buckwheat is high in bioflavonoids, and so are fruits, nuts and seeds. When taken with vitamin C, heavy bleeding can be reduced.

Citrus fruit and apricots are high in iron and can stop the depletion of iron from blood loss.

Drinking cinnamon, fennel, ginger, peppermint or wintergreen tea just prior or during the period can relieve cramps.

Caffeic acid is a known analgesic. Both Thyme and Basil are rich in caffeic acid. By adding 2 tablespoons of leaves of either herb to one pint of boiling water, a tea can be brewed to help relieve the pain from the cramps. Drink ½ to 1 cup an hour until the pain is gone.

By making a ginger tea (2 cups water with 2 teaspoons grated fresh ginger and steeped for 15 minutes) and adding 1 tablespoon of honey, and taken four times per day, the pain should be relieved.

A method that has been used extensively to balance the hormones is:

20-30 drops thyme
20-30 drops clary sage
20-30 drops sandalwood
20-30 drops ylang ylang

Mix with 1-2 ounces of coconut oil or olive oil.
Rub 5-6 drops onto the neck and/or wrists twice daily.

Another method using essential oils for the pain is:

15 drops Clary Sage
15 drops Helichrysum
15 drops Marjoram

Mix with 2 ounces of coconut oil.
Rub 2-6 drops across the lower abdomen twice daily.

## Mercury Poisoning

In today's highly toxic world, heavy metal poisoning is becoming more prevalent. Two of the most common toxins are mercury and lead. The effects can cause severe damage to children as well as adults. Excess levels of lead can cause aggressive behavior, irritability, damage to the brain, nervous system and reproductive system. Lead can be found in just about everything from cosmetics to fruit. Excessive mercury can damage the kidneys, brain and central nervous system. Common symptoms of mercury poisoning are: fatigue, lethargy, depression, blood sugar instability, and female reproductive problems. Two of the most common culprits are: fish (84% of consumable fish have high levels of mercury) and dental fillings. High fructose corn syrup, found in most processed foods, is high in mercury.

Nature has provided us with some natural ways to detoxify our systems. Here are just a few: Garlic, cilantro, chlorella, aloe vera and Brazile nuts. Be sure to use organic, non-GMO, hormone and pesticide-free ingredients. A fun way to detoxify mercury poisoning is to make a salsa from garlic, cilantro, tomatoes and onions.

Supplements that have helped in detoxifying mercury are vitamin E (400 IU daily), selenium (200-400 mcg daily), vitamin C (2,000 – 6,000 mg daily) and MSM (methylsulfonylmethane –½ to 1 grams three times per day).

## Migraine Headaches

We often hear people complain of having a migraine headache. But is it truly a migraine or is it a severe headache? See the section on Headache for a description of some different types of headaches. A migraine headache is defined as a chronic neurological disease characterized by moderate to severe headaches and associated with various autonomic nervous system symptoms. The symptoms may include nausea, vomiting, irritability, depression or euphoria, fatigue, food cravings, constipation or diarrhea, sensitivity to light (photophobia), or sound (phonophobia) or smells.

A prominent feature of a migraine in most cases is an aura phase. This phenomenon may appear minutes or days before the pain. It may present as a distortion of vision in the entire visual field or in one part. It may appear as a halo around an object, a splitting of a line or road in front of the person, zigzagging lines that should be straight, or converging lines that should be parallel. There may be color distortions or field of vision distortions.

Before puberty, migraines are more prevalent in boys than girls. However, after puberty women are much more susceptible to migraines. The frequency, severity and duration is variable. There are phases to a migraine: The prodrome (hours or days before the headache), the aura (generally immediately before the headache), the pain, and the postdrome (the effects after the main body of pain).

We have found that by eliminating allergies, toxicities and deficiencies migraine headaches are less frequent and less severe – some have disappeared entirely. We use the Asyra to help identify problem areas. Once identified, we use the NAET procedures to eliminate the allergies. Detoxification comes in many forms – ionic foot baths, colon hydrotherapy, Epson salt baths and herbal remedies. But the most difficult aid to migraine relief is dietary changes. Until the allergies have been eliminated, avoiding processed foods, fast foods, all GMO foods, glutens and sugars will reduce the symptoms. And of course, chiropractic adjustments for any cervical misalignments will open the nerve flow and blood flow to the brain.

## Morning Sickness

For some ladies during pregnancy morning sickness can be devastating. Some ladies, on the other hand, may not understand the concept of morning sickness. For some the sick, queasy felling may be only in the morning while for others it may last all day. For most, morning sickness lasts until the third or fourth month and yet for others it may last throughout the pregnancy. Symptoms range from an ill feeling, especially with certain smells, to retching and vomiting.

We suggest several things to try to help relieve the symptoms. Since everyone is different, a single item, a combination of items or possibly none at all will help.

- Before getting out of bed, eat some crackers. It's best to eat them while lying down. Rest for 15-20 minutes. This will help absorb the gastric juices.
- Begin the day with brown rice, oatmeal, wheat germ or yogurt.
- Eat 5-6 small meals throughout the day. Avoid three large meals.
- Green leafy vegetables contain magnesium which helps prevent nausea.
- Magnesium (400-500 mg daily), vitamin B6 (25-50 mg three times daily)
- Avoid aspirin and antibiotics
- Acupuncture point Pericardium 6 (P6) is located two finger widths up the arm from the first crease above the palm of the hand. By rubbing that point on both arms for 20 seconds each the nausea should subside within a minute or two.
- Peppermint is noted for soothing the stomach. Ever wonder why peppermints are at the cash registers at some restaurants? Sipping peppermint tea, sucking on peppermint candy or rubbing peppermint oil on the abdomen will often stop the nausea right away.
- Ginger root tea is often the most effective natural remedy for nausea. Ginger root can be taken in several forms - tea, lozenges, gum or capsules.
- There are several homeopathic remedies for morning sickness that help. Here are a few: Asarum, colchicum, ipecac-

uanha, kreosotum, lacticum acidum, nux vomica, pulsatil-
la, sepia and tabacum.

## Mosquito Bites

Mosquito bites can be extremely uncomfortable, itchy and
even painful. Recently it has been found that Lyme disease, as
well as many other blood borne diseases, are carried by mosquitoes. The best action is prevention. The following are some ideas
that may help prevent being bitten by a mosquito. As with course
of remedies, what works for one may not work for another. Fur-
thermore, dosages may vary as well as various combinations.

**2% MgCl Spray** – Marketed as "**Ancient Minerals,**" Magnesium
chloride is a water soluble liquid that feels like an oil when
sprayed on the skin. It's sold as a 16% solution, which means it
needs to be diluted four times. It can be sprayed all over the body
with no toxicity or overdose. It can be used by anyone.

**Essential Oil – Lemon Oil** – This oil can be mixed with olive oil or
almond oil and the appliedto the skin. As with the MgCl, there is
no known toxicity or overdose point.

**Citronella oil**–this can be sprayed directly on the skin without mixing. And again, no OD and no toxicity.
**Vitamin B** – especially **Vitamin B1 (Thiamin)** has been used for
years to keep mosquitoes away. Adults should take 250 mg per
day for a few days before exposure. Children should take a smaller amount. During the mosquito season we recommend that a
person should take this on a daily basis.

Mosquitoes like sweet, smelly things. Being a "thing", as humans are, mosquitoes love us. By reducing our intake of sugar and
sugary things such as candies, sodas, bananas, etc., will help keep
them away. Avoid wearing perfumes, colognes, after-shaves, or

using smelly detergents. If you have to be outside amongst the mosquitoes, try putting a Bounce Fabric sheet in your pocket. They seem to stay away from that aroma.

## Motion Sickness

A person can get motion sickness anytime movement is involved, whether it be on an airplane, boat, car, train or an amusement ride. Most often when the movement stops the motion sickness stops. It can happen when you're riding in the back seat of a car and you can't see the road ahead or when you're in an airplane and not anticipating the next move. It happens when the eyes, inner ear and body send conflicting signals to the brain. It is aided, and sometimes precipitated, by anxiety. Sometimes the very thought that you're going to get sick, maybe because of a past motion sickness or suggestions by others, will lead to symptoms.

Some common symptoms of motion sickness are:
- Nausea
- Cold sweats
- Dizziness
- Increased salivation
- Headache
- Vomiting
- Loss of pallor (pail skin)
- Fatigue

Some actions to prevent motion sickness include:
- Eating light meals or snacks in the 24 hours prior to the event
- Don't smoke or drink alcohol before the event
- Avoid salty, spicy or dairy foods
- Sit in the front seat and keep eyes fixed on the horizon

- Roll the windows down or turn the air vents toward you

When motion sickness strikes there are several things that can be done to neutralize the symptoms:

- Ginger (*Zingiber officianale*) is very effective but very potent so use this with caution. Take a half teaspoon of finely knife-diced fresh ginger and swallow it. Or slice off some fresh ginger and steep it in a cup of hot water for several minutes. Taste this frequently to ensure it doesn't get too strong. A third alternative is to take 250 mg daily in capsule form. Be careful if you are taking blood thinners as ginger increases the risk of bleeding.
- Peppermint (*Mentha piperita*) can be taken as a tea or in capsule form. As a capsule, take one capsule three times daily.
- Black horehound (*Ballotta nigra*) can be taken in capsule form three times daily. However, it can interact with Parkinson's medications. Or it can be taken as a tincture (1-2 ml three times daily) or as a tea.
- To make teas from Peppermint and Black horehound, put about 1 teaspoon of the dried herb into a tea strainer and place it in a cup of hot water. Drink a cup two to three times per day.

Thought Field Therapy (TFT) is very effective when the motion sickness is the result of anxiety. Through TFT (explained earlier), anxiety can be eliminated and, therefore, the fear of getting sick will no longer be a factor.

*Jean became nauseated by the thought of riding in a car on a curvy road or flying on an airplane. After one TFT session she was able to fly across country without getting sick and she now drives on curvy roads to the coast without even the fear of getting sick.*

By stimulating the acupuncture point Pericardium 6, nausea can be relieved very quickly. It is located two finger widths up the arm from the crease closest to the palm of the hand. Gently rub the area for 10-15 seconds.

Several homeopathic remedies have been found very useful. They include: Borax, Cocculus, Nux vomica, Petroleum, Sepia, and Tabacum. When taken as drops, hold the liquid under the tongue for 20 seconds before swallowing. If taken as tablets, hold under the tongue until dissolved. It's best to do either way on an empty stomach at least 5 minutes before eating anything.

## MTHFR (Methylenetetrahydrofolate Reductase)

MTHFR is an abbreviation for Methylenetetrahydrofolate reductase. This enzyme helps make folic acid usable by the body. It is vitally important in converting homocysteine into methionine and later helping create glutathione. All this is important for metabolism. The enzyme also helps convert homocysteine to methionine. Without the above processes the body would be unable to convert folic acid into a form usable by the body. With low MTHFR enzyme levels the body's homocysteine levels will increase. Elevated homocysteine levels have been associated with inflammation, difficulty to detoxify, heart disease, birth defects and increased risk of cancer.

At the time of this writing, there have been over 20 types of MTHFR mutations identified by science. The passing of genes from each parent amplifies the possible scenarios of passing on the mutated gene that can occur. The two most common, and most problematic, mutations are C677T and A1298C. These are identified placement of the mutation on the gene. The following is a brief look at three types:

1. Homozygous: When the same gene is passed on from both parents.
2. Heterozygous: Occurs when one parent passes on one mutated gene (677 or 1298) and the other parent passes on a normal gene.
3. Compound heterozygous: Occurs when one parent passes

347

on one mutated gene and the other parent passes on the other.

The list of possible signs, symptoms and conditions associated with the MTHFR mutation. The following is an abbreviated list of possible symptoms and conditions. Keep in mind that a person may have a number of these symptoms and conditions or none at all.

Symptoms: Abdominal pain, aggression, anemia, asthma, depression, diarrhea, chronic fatigue, diarrhea, decreased immunity, hair loss, hand tremor, headaches, heart attack, hypertension, loss of memory, muscle pain, rashes, tachycardia, stroke and many more.

Conditions: ADD/ADHD, autism, chronic fatigue syndrome, cancer, depression, erectile dysfunction, fibromyalgia, insomnia, irritable bowel syndrome, migraine headaches, Parkinson's, peripheral neuropathy, pulmonary fibrosis, Raynaud's, recurrent miscarriages and more.

As with all conditions in this section, the information presented is for information only and is not intended to treat, diagnose or prescribe in any way. This information is provided to guide you into further investigation. For further, more individualized, information, contact your natural, holistic healthcare provider.

Treatment suggestions:

1. Repair the digestive system. Eliminate the bad flora, including candida, and optimize the good flora. A coffee enema followed by a plain yogurt enema will help flush the liver and clean the colon. See #9 for more suggestions.
2. Don't take supplements that contain folic acid. Avoid cyanocobalamin (synthetic form) and use methylcobalamin instead. 5-MTHF is a good supplemental substitute for folic acid. If you are double homozygous for MTHFR, be very careful with methyl B12 and methyl-folate. Avoid high doses of niacin (vitamin B3). It has a tendency to hinder methylation.

3. Avoid processed foods since most often you can't be sure of the ingredients.
4. Eat at least one cup of natural, organic, non-GMO dark leafy greens each day. See below for a list of some good sources of folate.
5. All meats should be grass-fed and hormone free. The same goes for all dairy products. Eggs should be from organic, free-range chickens.
6. Supplements that should be taken include: Vitamins B2, B6, C, D, E, fish oil, curcumin and probiotics.
7. Avoid exposure to aluminum as in antiperspirants and aluminum cookware. Have mercury amalgams removed by a specially trained biological dentist. Toxins can be removed by using liposomal glutathione.
8. Exposure to toxins in the home can be subtle but cumulatively disastrous. Avoid chemical house cleaners and air fresheners. There are plenty of natural, organic cleaners and air fresheners available.
9. Do a gentle detox regularly. Sweating either by exercise or sauna helps pull toxins through the pores of your skin. Epsom Salt baths, soaking for a minimum of 20 minutes does the same. With both, exercise or the bath, be sure to shower afterward to remove any toxins on the skin. As mentioned above, a coffee enema or colonic (1/3 regular coffee with 2/3 water) will pull toxins from the liver and the colon. Be sure to follow with a plain yogurt enema (1/3 yogurt with 2/3 water) to replace the good bacteria in the colon.

A diet high in folate gives the body more opportunities to create the active form of 5-MTHF. Here are some suggestions from NutritionData (in descending order):

    Beans and lentils
    Raw spinach
    Asparagus

Romaine lettuce
Broccoli
Avocado
Oranges/mangoes

Eating a folate-rich diet has been shown to be as effective as taking a folic acid or 5-MTHF supplement in lowering homocysteine levels.

Vitamins B2 and B6 are very important in metabolizing folate. The following are some suggested sources for:

B2:

Organic, non-GMO almonds
Grass-fed, hormone free beef and lamb
Non-GMO wild oily fish
Hard boiled eggs from organic, free-range chickens
Mushrooms
Non-GMO spinach

B6:

Organic, non-GMO sunflower seeds
Organic, non-GMO pistachio nuts
Non-GMO wild oily fish
Organic, free-range, hormone free turkey, chicken, pork and beef
Organic, non-GMO bananas, avocados, and spinach

Avoid antacids, type 2 diabetes medication Metformin, blood pressure medications, and contraceptives.

For a comprehensive genetic profile, you can purchase a kit for $199 from www.23andme.com. You simply swab the mouth and send it to them. They will return a thorough report with your genetic findings. You can then run your 23andme methylation report through www.geneticgenie.org for free to help explain the findings.

## Multiple Sclerosis

Multiple Sclerosis (MS, disseminated sclerosis, encephalomyelitis) is a chronic, inflammatory, degenerative disease in which the fatty myelin sheaths around the axons (nerves) of the brain and spinal cord are damaged, leading to a demyelization process. Myelin is the insulating substance around the nerves in your central nervous system. When the myelin sheath is damaged, the function of the affected nerves deteriorate over time.

A few of the symptoms of this demyelization process include:

Muscle weakness
Tremors
Loss of coordination or imbalance
Astigmatism and visual disorders
Fatigue
Mood swings
Musculoskeletal pain
Depression
Diarrhea or constipation
Incontinence

Medical science, with its multitude of drugs, has shown very little progress in curing MS. Again, the emphasis has been more on the band aide approach in suppressing symptoms rather than affecting a cure.

Research by Dr. Terry Wahls concerning her own debilitating MS revealed some insights that completely reversed her MS. She found that by switching to a Paleo-style diet focused on fresh raw foods, high in specific nutrients were necessary for proper functioning of myelin and the mitochondria (the source for all cellular energy). Nutrients essential for proper mitochondrial function include animal-based omega-3 fats, creatine, and coenzyme Q10. The myelin itself needs vitamins B1, B9, B12 omega-3, and iodine. Vitamin D is one of the most important preventive against auto-immune diseases like MS.

Based on the research, we suggest to our patients the following:

- Detox the colon and liver. Chlorella and MSM are useful in flushing mercury.
- Eliminate allergies using NAET or a similar technique.
- Eliminate processed foods, grains, and starches.
- Eliminate sugar as much as possible.
- Eliminate pasteurized milk and dairy.
- 3 cups daily of green leaves –high in vitamins A, B, C, K, and minerals.
- 3 cups daily of sulfur-rich vegetables from the cabbage- and onion- families, mushrooms and asparagus.
- 3 cups daily of brightly colored vegetables, fruits and/or berries – antioxidants.
- Wild fish for animal-based omega-3's.
- Grass-fed meat – without hormones, antibiotics, or preservatives.
- Organ meats for vitamins, minerals and CoQ10.
- Seaweed for iodine and selenium.
- Vitamin D – preferably by sunlight or 6,000-8,000 IU's per day and about 35 IU's per day for children.
- Eliminate emotional traumas. We use TFT. It's fast and effective.

## Muscle Aches and Cramps (nocturnal or recumbency cramps)

Muscle cramps can happen with any muscle but most commonly they happen in the legs. They can be incredibly painful and debilitating to the point where you want to move but can't due to the pain. Loved ones will ask to help but you don't want anyone to do anything – just make the pain go away.

Most commonly, muscle cramps during or after exercise are

due to dehydration. The cure is simple – drink more water. Also a good warm up with stretching and a good cool down with stretching will help.

What we see the most are called nocturnal or recumbency cramps. However, muscle spasms or cramps can happen any time. The cause for these cramps is generally caused by electrolyte or mineral imbalance in the body.

We have found that taking magnesium will most often stop the spasms within seconds. We use a granulated magnesium so that it will be absorbed more quickly. Mix ½ teaspoon (1 gram) of magnesium powder in water (1/4 to ½ cup). The cramp or spasm should immediately begin to dissipate. As a preventative, take one to two grams per day before bedtime.

Low potassium levels can also cause leg cramps. By taking 2 teaspoons of apple cider vinegar with water can help relieve cramps. The taste can be softened by mixing 1 teaspoon of honey with it. We prefer Bragg's Apple Cider Vinegar because it's organic with no added chemicals. Two tablespoons of honey can be added for taste.

If you are caught out without magnesium or potassium, we've been told that pinching below the nose and above the upper lip will relieve muscle spasms.

Foods high in magnesium include: Raw chocolate (raw cacao), broccoli, Kale, and almonds. Foods high in potassium include: Apples, bananas, cantaloupe, dried fruits, avocado, mushrooms, spinach, tomatoes, yogurt, kefir, and baked potatoes.

Essential oils Balsam fir (30 drops), Helichrysum (10 drops), Peppermint (5 drops) and Oregano (1 drop) mixed with coconut oil or olive oil and rubbed on the affected area can give relief almost immediately.

## Muscle Atrophy (Disuse atrophy)

Muscle atrophy is a wasting away of muscle mass. The affected muscle or muscle group becomes weak and the use of that muscle or group becomes impaired. Several disease states can lead to atrophy including: Cancer, congestive heart failure, COPD, burns, starvation and kidney failure. Most commonly, disuse atrophy can result from a sedentary job or lifestyle, decreased activity, prolonged bed rest, or simply from prolonged wearing of a cast or support, i.e., low back support. Over 1½% per day of muscle tone is lost when a muscle group is immobilized. That becomes cumulative over time.

We recommend moist heat or whirlpool baths for increased blood flow, pain relief and mobility. Because of the loss of nutrients, 1,000 mg. of calcium as well as 1,000 mg. of magnesium are recommended for repair. As much as possible without pain, resistive or isokenetic exercise using surgical tubing or stretchy bands is highly recommended to increase muscle tone. The cell salt Thallium oxide has been shown to be useful in restoring muscle tone. If there is access to a galvanic muscle stimulating system, ultrasound unit, or TENS unit, a holistic doctor can advise in the use of any of those to make up for the loss of muscle tone.

## Nail Disorders

Nail changes often indicate illness before any symptoms appear. A number of disorders show up in the appearance of nails. The following is a list of appearances of the nails and the conditions they tend to indicate.

**Black, Splinter-like bits** under the nails can be a sign of infectious endocarditis, a serious heart infection; other heart disease; or a bleeding disorder.

**Black bands** from the cuticle outward to the end of the nail can be an early sign of melanoma.

**Brittle, soft, shiny** nails without a moon may indicate an overactive thyroid.

**Brittle** nails signify possible iron deficiency, thyroid problems, impaired kidney function, and circulation problems.

**Crumbly, white** nails near the cuticle are sometimes an indication of AIDS.

**Dark** nails and/or **thin, flat, spoon-shaped** nails are a sign of vitamin B12 deficiency or anemia. Nails can also turn gray or dark if the hands are placed in chemicals such as cleaning supplies (most often bleach) or a substance to which one is allergic.

**Deep blue nail beds** show a pulmonary obstructive disorder such as asthma or emphysema.

**Downward-curved nail ends** may denote heart, liver, or respiratory problems.

**Flat nails** can denote Raynaud's disease.

**Greenish nails**, if not a result of a localized fungal infection, may indicate an internal bacterial infection.

**A Half-white nail with dark spots at the** tip points to possible kidney disease.

An **isolated dark-blue band** in the nail bed, especially in light-skinned people, can be a sign of skin cancer.

Lindsay's nails (sometimes known as "half-and-half" nails), nails in which **half of the top of the nail is white and the other half is pink**, may be a sign of chronic kidney disease.

**Nail beading** (the development of bumps on the surface of the nail) is a sign of rheumatoid arthritis.

Nails **raised at the base with small white ends**, show a respiratory disorder such as emphysema or chronic bronchitis. This type of nail may also simply be inherited.

Nails **separated from the nail bed** may signify a thyroid disorder (this condition is known as onyholysis) or a local infection.

Nails that **broaden toward the tip and curve downward** are a sign of lung damage, such as from emphysema or exposure to asbestos.

Nails that **chip, peel, crack, or break easily** show a general nutritional deficiency and insufficient hydrochloric acid and protein. Minerals are also needed.

Nails that have **pitting** resembling hammered brass indicate a tendency toward partial or total hair loss.

**Pitted red-brown spots and frayed and split ends** indicate psoriasis; vitamin D, folic acid, and protein are needed.

**Red skin around the cuticles** can be indicative of poor metabolism of essential fatty acids or of a connective tissue disorder such as lupus.

**Ridges** can appear in the nails either vertically or horizontally. Vertical ridges indicate poor general health, poor nutrient absorption, and/or iron deficiency; they may also indicate a kidney disorder. Horizontal ridges can occur as a result of severe stress, either psychological or physical, such as from infection and/or disease. A horizontal indentation in the nail (Beau's line) can occur as a result of a heart attack, major illness, or surgery. Ridges running up and down the nails also indicate a tendency to develop arthritis.

**Spooning** (upward-curling) or pitting nails can be caused by disorders such as anemia or problems with iron absorption.

**Thick nails** may indicate that the vascular system is weakening and the blood is not circulating properly. This may also be a sign of thyroid disease.

**Thick toenails** can be a result of fungal infection.

**Thinning nails** may signal lichen planus, an itchy skin disorder.

**Two white horizontal bands** that do not move as the nail grows are a sign of hypoalbuminemia, a protein deficiency in the blood.

**Unusually wide, square nails** can suggest a hormonal disorder.

**White lines** show possible heart disease, high fever, or arsenic poisoning.

**White lines across the nail** may indicate a liver disease.

If the **white moon area of the nail turns red,** it may indicate heart problems; if it turns slate blue, then it can indicate either heavy metal poisoning (such as silver poisoning) or lung trouble.

**White nails** indicate possible liver or kidney disorders and/or anemia.

**White nails with pink** near the tips are a sign of cirrhosis.

**Yellow nails or an elevation of the nail tips** can indicate internal disorders long before other symptoms appear. Some of these are problems with the lymphatic system, respiratory disorders, diabetes, and liver disorders.

## Nail Fungus (onychomycosis)

Infections of the fingernails and toenails by fungal organisms called dermatophytes can cause a white or yellow spot under the fingernail or toenail. As the fungus spreads, it may cause the nail to discolor and thicken and the edges to crumble or become ragged. This condition can be unsightly, embarrassing and even painful. If it infects between the toes and the skin of the feet, it's called tinea pedis or athlete's foot. The efficacy of the over the counter medications is highly questionable and the side effects are often more than interesting.

In the alternative world, the treatment for this is very simple: Weekly cold laser treatments to the nails along with daily soaks in Pao d Arco seems to work well. At home, in a bowl of warm water sprinkle the contents of two capsules of Pao d Arco. Soak the hands or feet for 15-20 minutes daily. If possible, soak twice a day, however, once a day will do.

Another proven treatment is to soak the hand or hands, foot or feet in a bowl or basin of water mixed with 2-3 teaspoons of oregano oil once or twice per day until resolved. Or mixing 1 drop of oregano oil, tea tree oil or grape seed extract in a teaspoon of olive oil or coconut oil and rubbing it on the skin or nail area. This same treatment can be used for athlete's foot.

## Nausea

Nausea, often called "feeling sick,"affects everyone at one time or another. Nausea can simply be an allergic reaction to food or an environmental condition. However, nausea can be a result of pregnancy, gastritis, a gallbladder condition, or an early warning sign of heart, GI or a kidney condition. Those generally come with other symptoms that would alert you to the cause.

Non specific nausea can be relieved in several ways.

Drink raspberry, peppermint or ginger tea.

Suck on a piece of peppermint candy.

Drink a tablespoon of Bragg's Apple Cider Vinegar with water or a juice.

Find the last crease of the arm before the palm of the hand. Find the spot two finger widths up the arm. Rub that spot on each wrist for 20 seconds. The nausea should be reduced almost immediately.

## Night Sweats (Nocternal Hyperhydrosis)

Night sweats or nocturnal hyperhydrosis can affect males and females alike. The condition can be very frustrating and very annoying. For women especially, night sweats are closely linked to decreased levels of estrogen.

A system detox and regular exercise will go a long way in reducing or eliminating night sweats. Be sure your diet contains protein, fiber, fruits, vegetables and grains. A multi-vitamin supplement along with extra vitamins C and D3 is always important. If over 25 years old, we strongly recommend enzyme and amino acid supplementation. Avoid alcohol, caffeine, tobacco, sugar and spicy foods.

Cell salt Calc.Iod. (Iodine of Lime) and Sage tea help reduce the night sweats.

## Osteoporosis

With age, some people's bones become brittle and fragile. Falls and accidents can be disastrous. It's estimated that over 40 million people are affected, 1 in 3 women and 1 in 5 men. For years it was thought that a deficiency of calcium was the cause of osteoporosis. However, recent studies have shown that certain drugs or a vitamin D deficiency can be the cause of the porous bones.

Osteoporosis drugs such as Actonel, Boniva or Fosamax are biphosphonate drugs. These are called antiresorptive medicines, which means they slow or stop the natural process of dissolving bones and laying down new bone. The result is increased bone density. This process is accomplished by killing off osteoclasts (cells that naturally eat away old bone cells) and promoting the production of osteoblasts (cells that lay down new bone). This leaves the victim with increased bone density but decreased bone strength. The bone can't naturally build new bone and adjust to the changing forces applied to it. The end result is thicker, weaker bones. Additionally, the side effects, as in many cases with drugs, are worse than the original problem. Typical side effects range from eye problems, liver damage and kidney failure to atrial fibrillation and esophageal cancer.

In the late 1800's a German anatomist and surgeon, Julius Wolff, put forth a theory which has now become a physiological law. It's known as Wolff's Law. To overly simplify it, it states: Any bone under stress will lay down calcium along the lines of stress." That means that if you put a bone under stress, as with exercising with weights, that bone will lay down calcium in the bone and make it stronger.

With that in mind, a mild exercise program to stop or even reverse osteoporosis would involve weights. We suggest light leg weights, arm weights and a vest with pockets to hold weights. The following are some suggested exercises – some can be combined to give a flowing motion.

- Walking with arm and leg weights – swing your arms as you walk fast enough to make it difficult to talk.
- Stand from a sitting position without using your arms and hands to push you up – repeat 10 times.
- Rise up on your toes then drop down to your heels – repeat 10 times.
- Rock back onto your heels and then back to your toes – repeat 10 times.
- Lunge forward and then back 10 times alternating the leading leg.
- Lunge to the right and then to the left 10 times.

- Do a half squat 10 times.
- Do 10 arm curls with each arm.
- Do 10 punches toward the ceiling with each arm.
- Do 10 step ups onto a stair or block leading with one leg and then the other.
- Jump up and down 10-20 times without the weights.

These can be combined to make a smooth, fluid motion. More reps can be added depending on your level.

Nutritional support is vital in the prevention and healing of osteoporosis. Just 15 to 20 minutes of sun each day can help maintain normal vitamin D levels. If this is not possible or practical, taking 5,000 to 10,000 units of vitamin D3 per day is a good option. It's important to have your vitamin D level checked by a qualified lab to determine your current level. Then you can determine the amount of supplementation to take. Taking animal based omega-3 fats and vitamin K (especially K2) are important in helping calcium to get absorbed into the bone.

Some studies have shown positive results by mixing1/8 to ¼ teaspoon of boron to one liter of water and drinking 1-2 liters each day. For years this was viewed as a miracle cure for arthritis. Boron capsules are also available. See the mineral section for more information.

## Ovarian cyst

An ovarian cyst is a very painful condition. According to the Mayo Clinic, ovarian cysts are fluid-filled sacs or pockets (like blisters) on or within the surface of an ovary. They can be quite small to quite large. Most agree that most cysts are harmless and cause little or no symptoms. The CDC has stated that most premenopausal women will have them one or more times in their lives. They are usually due to an imbalance between estrogen and progesterone with estrogen becoming abnormally dominant.

There are two common types of ovarian cysts – functional and pathological. The functional cyst is generally formed during ovulation because either the egg is not released or the follicle (sac) in which the egg is formed does not dissolve. These cysts generally don't last long and tend to go away on their own. On the other hand, pathological cysts grow in the ovaries and can be either harmless or cancerous.

Symptoms, if they occur, may vary significantly. They include, but not limited to:

> Pelvic pain, especially during the period
> Irregular periods
> Painful bowel movements
> Painful sexual intercourse
> Painfulness, fullness, or heaviness in the abdomen
> Tender breasts
> Nausea and/or vomiting
> Rectal or bladder pressure or heavy feeling
> Feeling a need to urinate
> Dizziness, rapid breathing or severe abdominal pain may be signs of a serious condition.

The standard medical approach is to either wait and see what happens, prescribe birth control pills, or perform surgery. If the mass is discovered to be cancerous, a hysterectomy, including the uterus and the ovaries, will be recommended.

Most successful natural treatments take time, in other words, they won't eliminate the cysts overnight. Give three to six weeks for any treatment to be effective. The goal is to restore balance and harmony to the system so that healing can take place. The following is what we have seen, singularly or in combination, that helped eliminate the cysts. These do not take the place of visiting with a holistic doctor to appraise your particular condition.

1. The Asyra will indicate which areas need addressing. The homeopathic drops will help balance the hormonal sys-

tem. In addition, avoid soy foods and BPA's in plastics. Both tend to increase estrogen levels. Avoid chemical additives as much as possible, i.e. in detergents, many foods, especially processed, and personal care products. Eat only organic meats and dairy. Avoid GMO's.

2. Herbs have been used for centuries to help balance the hormones. The following have been used to balance women's estrogen and progesterone levels: Milk thistle, black cohosh, chasteberry, dong quai, wild yam root, and red clover.

3. Detox the system, especially the liver. Drinking water with lemon, ionic foot baths, Epson salt baths, coffee colonics or enemas are a few safe ways to detoxify the system.

4. A good regiment of supplements specifically designed for you is necessary to maintain a strong immune system and balance organs and glands. Adding to a good foundation of supplements, evening primrose oil helps regulate hormonal imbalances and vitamin E and fish oil aid in healing.

5. Homeopathic remedies such as apis mellifica and bellis perennis help reduce inflammation and shrink cycts.

6. Apple cider vinegar helps shrink and dissolve ovarian cysts. Mix 1 to 2 tablespoons of vinegar with 1 tablespoon of black strap molasses and 8 ounces of warm water. Drink one or two glasses daily to help shrink the cyst.

## Parasites

Parasites are considered by many as the root cause of many diseases. Dr. Hulda Clark devoted most of her entire career researching the effects of parasites. In her books she describes the many varieties of parasites, their actions on the body and what can be done to eliminate them.

It is very easy to contract a parasite infection. Contacting an infected person, drinking contaminated water, improperly washed or undercooked food, and more commonly, touching pets are just a few ways of contracting parasites. It's estimated that billions of people worldwide are living with dangerous and harmful parasites within their bodies.

The symptoms may vary from individual to individual and from minor to severe. Some of the more commons symptoms include: Abdominal pain, gas, bloating, bad breath, grinding teeth at night, allergies, mood swings, loss of energy, skin conditions, food cravings, weight changes, sleeplessness, irritability, reddened eyes, creepy-crawly feeing in different parts of the body, including the brain, and many more. There are lab tests available to determine what kind of organism is causing the problems.

Our office offers the patient several ways to eliminate parasites. Dr. Clark describes in her books a simple apparatus that she calls a "**zapper.**" Instructions are given in her book **The Cure for All Diseases** with diagrams and parts lists. The instructions are to hold the two metal hand masses for 7 minutes and then rest for 20 minutes. Repeat that two more times. Make sure the hand masses don't touch. Evidence of dead parasites may appear in the stool by the next morning.

Dr. Clark often referred to a **frequency generator** for eliminating parasites. A great deal of research has gone into expanding her ideas for using a frequency generator. Most ailments, diseases, and parasites have been studied and specific frequencies assigned to either totally eliminate or assist in eliminating the condition. The patient simply holds a pair of hand masses for three minutes for each frequency. The healing frequencies generally come in sets for each condition. According to Dr. Clark, a condition can be reduced or completely eliminated by using the frequency generator.

Several herbal supplements have been reported to help rid the body of parasites. Unfortunately, not a great deal of research has been conducted to determine the effectiveness of each. Here's a list of some commonly used herbals:

1. **Garlic (Allium sativa)** – shown to have activity against As-

caris (roundworm), Giardia lamblia, Trypansoma, Plasmodium, and Leishmania.

2. **Goldenseal (Hydrastis Canadensis)** – historically used for infections of the mucous membranes in the body, i.e., respiratory tract infections, mucous drainage, etc. Goldenseal's active ingredient, Berberine, has shown to be effective against Entamoeba histolytica, Giardia lamblia, and Plasmodium.

3. **Pumpkin Seeds (Curcubita pepo)** – have traditionally been used to eliminate tapeworms and roundworms. Twenty five ounces of mashed seeds mixed with juice appears to provide the best results. A laxative is recommended 2-3 hours after drinking the juice to help cleanse the intestinal tract.

4. **Wormwood, Wormseed, and Grapefruit seed extract, oil of Oregano, cloves, thyme and tumeric** have been reported to produce positive results.

Again, we're not all made equally. Some of these remedies work for some but not for others. We recommend trying different combinations until the most effective one is found for the patient.

Diet is always important in the parasite cleansing process. The following ideas should help:

- Avoid coffee, alcohol, refined foods, artificial flavorings or colorings, refined or artificial sugar.
- Foods such as garlic, pineapple, and Papaya help clear parasites and improve digestion.
- Vitamins, minerals, enzymes, amino acids and probiotics are essential for good digestion, elimination, and cleansing parasites.

## Parkinson's Disease

Parkinson's Disease is a disease marked by uncontrollable tremors and jerking motions. It is progressive and very frustrating for those who suffer from it. It is classified as incurable, however, the body has the ability to heal itself of any disease, even supposedly incurable diseases. There are primary symptoms of Parkinson's and there are secondary.

Primary symptoms include:
Slowness in voluntary movement (Bradykinesia) – including standing up, walking, and sitting down. Delayed transmissions from the brain to the muscles cause this to happen. This is generally seen when initiating walking but can "freeze" a person while walking.
Tremors of the hands, fingers, forearms, foot, mouth, or chin occur generally while at rest.
Muscles become stiff or rigid and can produce muscle pain with movement.
An unsteady balance may occur due to the loss of reflexes that assist in posture. This can lead to falls.

Secondary symptoms include:
Anxiety, depression, isolation
Choking, coughing, or drooling
Constipation
Difficulty swallowing
Excessive salivation
Excessive sweating
Loss of bowel and/or bladder control
Loss of intellectual capacity
Scaling, dry skin on face or scalp
Slow response to questions
Small cramped handwriting
Soft, whispery voice

In working with someone with Parkinson's, patience is key. Changes come slowly and in small degrees. In order to heal itself, the body needs to eliminate toxins and address deficiencies. As with any "disease," we begin with an EAV evaluation and a thorough detox program. If there are any allergy problems, we will eliminate those with NAET. A calcium deficiency, along with others, has been shown to be responsible for many of the symptoms. We look closely at calcium and potassium deficiencies, as well as a malfunctioning Parathyroid gland. If a patient is deficient in potassium, we look to see if he/she has a dairy allergy. This can lead to a calcium deficiency. Along with a complete program of nutrients and supplements, we use a Parathyroid glandular supplement in correcting the condition.

Calcium is a sedative and relaxant. It should be taken through the day and evening. It helps reduce the shaking and helps with sleep at night. Bone Meal and Oyster Calcium are good non-allergenic sources of calcium.

B-complex vitamins are often deficient. I recommend the non-allergenic Bee Pollen as a source of potassium as well as Royal Jelly. Alfalfa, as a source of potassium, and Spirulina, as a source of calcium, are also recommended. Magnesium taken before going to bed is a very good muscle relaxant.

Although we do not prescribe drugs, nor do we advise any change in a prescription, a patient's medication can be evaluated using EAV. It can be determined if the medication is of any value to the patient and if so, the dosage and duration. Interaction with other drugs or supplements can also be evaluated. That information can then be given to the prescribing physician for his review. The determination to change any prescription medication lies with the patient and his/her prescribing doctor.

Several herbs or combination of herbs can help. Some of these are:

> Calms Forte – Helps relieve nervousness and insomnia.
> Cat Nip, Chamomile, Lobelia, Passion Flower, and Valarian Root are nerve relaxants and regenerators. Note: Don't use all at once.
> Gaba Plus – Helps stop nocturnal urination.
> Broad beans – Natural source of L-dopa – helps restore

dopamine in the brain. The lack of dopamine in the brain is the primary reason for the symptoms.

St. John's Wort – Helps alleviate depression and insomnia.

Acupuncture and massage help reduce the discomfort associated with muscle stiffness. In Parkinson's the muscles become very stiff and rigid causing an inflexibility of the joints. Exercise helps keep the joints flexible. Many Parkinson's patients balk at or refuse to exercise. Big mistake. Without exercise the joints become increasingly immobile and whole body mobility is greatly hampered.

## Premenstrual Syndrome (PMS)

Each month most women suffer from a condition known as premenstrual syndrome. It affects each person differently. For some the symptoms are severe while for others the symptoms are hardly noticeable. The symptoms may include:

- Anxiety
- Mood swings
- Irritability, even outbursts of anger
- Food cravings
- Headaches
- Loss of libido (sexual desire)
- Breast tenderness
- Bloating
- And more…….

The cause is generally accepted as an imbalance in the hormonal system. Without going into a long dissertation of the hormonal influences, suffice it to say that, like other systems in the body, balance equals good health and therefore the lack of symptoms. Some basic causes for this imbalance may be:

- Nutritional deficiencies

- Stress
- Extreme estrogen to progesterone ratio
- Improper carbohydrate and/or sodium metabolism

The medical approach for this condition, as with many others, is to suppress the symptoms. However, we've found that by balancing the system (re-establishing the body's equilibrium) the symptoms are reduced or eliminated. Here are some ways to approach PMS:

- In our office we stress the importance of an Asyra test to give us insight into a course of action, NAET protocols to eliminate allergies and boost hormonal glands, and thought field therapy to reduce or eliminate depression.
- Chasteberry (*Vitex agnus-castus)* is an herb that helps with breast pain or tenderness, edema, constipation, headache, irritability anger and depressed feelings.
- Dong quai (*Angelica sinensis)* along with black cohosh (*Cimicufuga racemosa)* helps with irritability, sleep disturbances, and depressed libido.
- We stress taking a multi vitamin and mineral daily but being especially vigilant before and during the period. Just before the period, extra chromium, calcium, magnesium and vitamin B6 (*pyridoxine)* could be a boost in relieving symptoms – chromium to stabilize the insulin and blood sugar levels, calcium and magnesium to help relax muscles and reduce cravings, and B6 to relieve depression and irritability. Extra vitamin E and essential fatty acids have also been shown to help.

## Prostate Enlargement (Benign Prostatic Hyperplasia [BPH])

The prostate gland is a small (walnut size) gland under the bladder in men. It wraps around the urethra (a small tube from the bladder through the penis to the outside). One of the duties of the prostate is to add a lubricating fluid to the seminal fluid which holds moves along sperm. For some unknown reason, possibly hormonal or bacterial, as a man ages the prostate enlarges. The condition is called benign prostatic hyperplasia (BPH). If it inflames, it's known as prostatitis. As it enlarges it clamps down on the urethra and restricts the flow of urine from the bladder. This can lead to frequent urination, a feeling of incomplete emptying, urine leakage, and urinary tract infections. The muscle reflex technique for prostate problems is performed by holding the index finger and the middle fingers apart and pointed downward at the pubic bone while the other arm is being tested (see the section on muscle testing). A weakness by doing that maneuver indicates that the prostate is involved.

Medical treatment for BPH includes drugs and surgery. However, there are alternatives. There are herbs that can reduce the size of an enlarged prostate and even prevent enlargement before it begins.

If the enlargement is caused by dihydrotestosterone, a combination of testosterone and an enzyme, Saw Palmetto extract is a very useful herb. Saw palmetto halts the production of dihydrotestosterone. This helps reduce the size of the prostate and reduces the frequency of urination and pain (very often after intercourse).

Zinc disables the enzyme that helps produce dihydrotestosterone. An alternative would be pumpkin seeds.

A morning drink of apple cider vinegar (2 teaspoons in 8 oz. of water, tea or juice) has been reported to help with symptoms of BPH including pain following intercourse.

Food allergies often cause an irritation to the urinary tract and can add to the problems associated with prostate enlargement. Elimination of the allergies with NAET is a large step forward in relieving prostate problems.

Studies have shown that lowering cholesterol levels help reduce BPH.

To reduce the symptoms, avoid caffeinated drinks, i.e. coffee, sodas, and chocolate. Also avoid alcohol and spicy foods.

Rosemary essential oil (2 drops in ½ tsp of carrier oil) rubbed beneath the testicles seems to help some men.

## Psoriasis

This irritating skin disease is characterized by itchy and/or painful patches of thick, red skin with silvery scales. Skin cells in these areas divide 1,000 times faster than normal. The result is a pileup of cells with an inflamed base capped by dead cells. These patches may appear on the elbows, knees, back, face, scalp, hands, and feet. Psoriasis is a chronic disease that may have periods of remission, but generally the condition is constant.

Symptoms may include:

- Dry, cracked skin prone to bleeding
- Itchy or sore skin
- Ridged or thickened nails

We have found that toxicities and allergiesare major factors in causing psoriasis. By eliminating those two factors, the skin will heal and the condition will be completely eliminated. Our approach is to do the following:

- EAV testing to locate deficiencies and toxicities.
- NAET testing and treatment to identify allergens and eliminate them.
- Nutritional therapy includes vitamins A and E, essential fatty acids including omega 3, 6, and 9, zinc and selenium.
- Applying a mixture of ½ cup coconut oil and 10 drops each of the essential oils lavender, melaleuca and frankincense
- See Eczema section for more therapy ideas.

## Raynaud's Phenomenon

Raynaud's Phenomenon (Raynaud's Disease) is characterized by a discoloration of the fingers and/or toes. It can also be seen in ears, nose and tongue. Typically seen in the fingers and toes, the normal coloration turns to white or blue. The digits are usually cold and painful. The disease is caused by spasming of arteries leading to cold hands and feet. Sometimes called an "idiopathic" disease (no known cause), it is generally accepted that stress and cold are contributing factors to its onset. Recently it's been thought that hyperactivity of the sympathetic nervous system contributes to the constriction of the arteries.

We begin our treatment of Raynaud's by doing an EAV test to determine any imbalances in the body. By eliminating imbalances we set up a better playing field to decrease the effects of the syndrome. A review of ALL symptoms experienced by the patient is accomplished to determine any trends that might affect the condition. In acute cases, ultrasound therapy in water is performed to decrease the immediate symptoms.

The following supplements have shown promise in relieving symptoms:

Arginine an amino acid that helps dilate arteries.
Ginko biloba has flavonoids (found in fruit and vegetables) and other compounds which thin the blood. A capsule of 40-60 mg per day is recommended.
Flavonoids, as mentioned above, are found in fruits and vegetables and help dilate arteries.
Fish oils have been shown to help with Raynaud's. Two to six softgels per day is recommended.

## Restless Legs Syndrome

Restless leg syndrome (RLS) affects approximately 10 percent of the population. In women the onset occurs commonly when they are in their 50s. The affliction generally occurs at night when rest is needed and desired but because of RLS, it's unattained. The victim is seized by an uncontrollable urge to move their legs. Their legs begin to twitch or jerk while at the same time they experience the sensation of something crawling or wiggling under their skin. They could experience pain, burning sensations, tingling and an uneasiness within their skin. All this occurs while lying still in bed. There has been a great deal of speculation concerning RLS, but to date, no known cause has been determined. The condition can lead to sleep deprivation, anxiety and depression.

An Asyra test is usually accomplished to begin to balance any imbalances within the body, including emotions. The patient is often told to get up and walk around at the first sign of an attack. Restricting coffee, tea, chocolate, sodas and any over the counter medications that contain caffeine might help. Whenever changing any medications, the patient is referred to their family physician or pharmacist for that determination. Nicotine and alcohol have a stimulating effect, so reducing or eliminating those sometimes helps. Other factors that seem to be helpful include: Taking a bath or getting a massage before bed; maintaining a regular bed time; yoga, meditation, visualization, or engage in a stress-less hobby.

Supplements that we recommend include:

Iron 200 mg (check iron levels)
5HTP 100-200 mg 20 minutes before retiring
Folic acid 35-60 mg/day (if familial)
Vitamin E 300-400 IU/day
Calcium1,000 mg/day
Potassium 300mg
Magnesium1,000 mg/day before bed
Zinc 100 mg/day

## Ringworm (Dermatophytosis)

Ringworm is a common, especially among children, fungal infection that is non-life threatening. It can affect the skin, nails and scalp. On the skin it appears as circular, reddish patches. As the patches grow larger the borders will raise slightly and the centers will become clear. They begin to look like a ring.

The most common symptoms are:

1. *Tinea capitis (scalp):* Begins as a small lump and grows to a circular pattern.
2. *Tinea corporis (body)*: Appears as flat, round and scaly spots on the skin.
3. *Tinea cruris (groin)*: Jock itch. Appears as an itchy, reddish rash in the groin area.
4. *Tinea faciei (face):* Appears as red scaly patches on the skin.
5. *Tinea manus (hand):* Usually affects the palms and sometimes between the fingers.
6. *Tinea pedis (feet):* Appears as scaling between the toes and occasionally as a thickening and scaling on the heels and soles.
7. *Tinea unguim (nails):* Fingernails/toenails can become yellow, thick and crumbly.

Natural treatments for ringworm include:
*Coconut oil:* Apply to the affected area, especially at night.
*Tea Tree Oil:* Soak cotton ball in TTO and apply three times daily to the affected area.
*Lavender oil and Jojoba oil:* Drop one drop of the essential oil of Lavender into a teaspoon of Jojoba oil. Mix and apply with a cotton ball to the affected area.
*Aloe vera:* Apply the gel from the plant itself or from a container of pure Aloe vera to the skin and leave it on overnight.
*Apple cider vinegar: Soak a cotton ball in pure ACV.* Apply pure

ACV (preferably Bragg's) 3-5 times daily to the affected area.

The above treatments can be used separately or in combination. In each case, results should be seen within 5-6 days.

## Rosacea

Rosacea is a chronic condition characterized by redness (erythema) of the cheeks, nose, and forehead. This is a typically harmless condition unless it affects the eyes (ocular rosacea). This generally affects people between the ages of 30 – 60, fair-skinned and more often women. A red, bulbous nose (rhinophyma) may also result. In some cases, a semi-permanent redness (telangiectasia) caused by dilation of superficial blood vessels may cause a person to seek help.

Treatment: Topical steroids can aggravate the condition. Therefore, a more natural approach is recommended. Cold laser therapy helps reduce the flushing and the appearance of blood vessels. Colonics help eliminate toxins from the colon and thereby improve skin conditions. Baking soda baths also improve skin conditions by drawing toxins through the pores of the skin. Digestive enzymes with each meal have been shown to reduce indigestion and rosacea.

Other treatments include:

- Chrysanthellum Indicum Cream – Some of its compounds help strengthen
capillaries. One study showed improvement in 12 weeks.
- Green Tea Cream –One small study showed improvement in 4 weeks.
- Niacinamide Cream
- Licorice – Improvements may be seen in 4-8 weeks.
- Eliminate food allergies
- Apple Cider Vinegar – Taken orally helps balance bacteria in the intestine.

## Seizures

Seizures are generally symptoms of a problem in the brain. Any sudden malfunction in the brain that causes a person (adult or child) to convulse, collapse or experience a temporary change in brain function with or without a change in consciousness is termed a seizure.

There are two groups of seizures: Generalized seizures are those that display abnormal activity in both sides of the brain. Focal or partial seizures are limited to abnormal activity in one side of the brain. When seizures are recurring the condition is called epilepsy. When this occurs, they are categorized into four types:

Grand mal: major episodes with loss of consciousness.
Petit mal: mild episodes with no loss of consciousness
Psychomotory: characterized by different types of movement
Autonomic: abnormal symptoms including rapid heartbeat, high blood pressure, flushing or pale appearance, abdominal pain, nausea, sweating

Much can be done to help reduce or eliminate seizures. They are listed below in no specific order.

- Do a complete, <u>full-body evaluation</u>. We use the Asyra testing for the initial scan.
- <u>Eliminate allergies</u>. We use NAET procedures.
- Make <u>dietary changes</u>. We suggest the Ketogenic diet (under the care of a doctor familiar with the diet). The high fat, low carbohydrate diet has been shown to be effective in reducing the frequency of seizures.
- Do a <u>bowel detox</u>. We suggest using enemas or hydrocolonic therapy.
- <u>Rest and reduce stress</u>. Get more sleep. Take walks or do yoga or listen to soothing music or use biofeedback.

- <u>Avoid anything with</u>: GMO's, MSG, artificial sugars, i.e. aspartame, anything hydrolyzed, anything that says "natural flavors," yeast extracts.
- <u>Avoid stimulating supplements and foods</u>, such as coffee, colas, caffeinated teas, ephedra, ginkgo, tyrosine, etc.
- Adults should <u>take a multi vitamin and mineral</u>, multi amino acid, multi enzyme additional vitamin B6 and magnesium. Children should take proportionately less.
- The <u>essential oil Frankincense</u> helps normalize and stimulate normal brain activity. Each night apply one drop to the bottom of each big toe and at the base of the neck.
- <u>Essential oils to avoid</u> (alphabetically): Eucalyptus, Fennel, Hyssop, Pennyroyal, Rosemary, Sage, Savin, Tansy, Thuja, Trupentine and wormwood.

## Shingles (Herpes Zoster)

Shingles is a painful activation, or reactivation, of a varicella zoster virus (also known as a herpes zoster virus). This is the same virus that causes chicken pox. Therefore, it's believed that once you've had chicken pox the virus lies dormant in a single or group of sensory nerve roots. It can be reactivated months or even years later. Shingles usually strikes people between the ages of 60 and 80 with weakened immune systems. A physical or emotional stress can be the triggering factor to set shingles in motion. Symptoms include: Fever, chills, headache, a red band may develop at the site of the future rash. Some have reported that three to four days prior to the blisters appearing, chills, fever, malaise, and gastrointestinal symptoms have appeared. Finally, very painful patches or groups of blisters appear generally on one side of the body. The skin becomes reddened for three to five days. After that the blisters dry out and scab over. Generally, the blisters will be gone within two weeks. However, during the blister phase, they are infectious for up to a week. The very severe pain from shingles, called postherpetic neuralgia, may persist for months or years.

Medically, there is no specific cure for shingles, however, anti-viral and anti-inflammatory drugs may be tried to shorten the infection and reduce the risk of complications.

Our recommendation is to first perform an Asyra test to discover what markers might be present that might lead to or perpetuate shingles. If there are indicators of a viral infection, and/or if there is an accepted medical diagnosis by an MD, (remember, electronic equipment cannot legally diagnose or indicate a diagnosis), then the patient is given a NAET treatment. In this treatment, the patient is treated for viruses, neurotransmitters, the nervous system and shingles itself. Isode therapy is also added to the treatment.

Some of the following might be recommended depending on the individual case:

**Olive Leaf Extract** – Two 250 mg capsules, 4 times per day (breakfast, lunch, dinner, bedtime) for one week or until symptoms disappear. OLE has strong anti-viral properties.
**Garlic** – 2 capsules twice a day for one week for more anti-viral protection.
**Lysine** – 1,000 mg three times per day.
**Vitamin C** – 500 to 1,000 mg three to five times per day.
Topically: **Capsaicin (or Capsicum) cream, Apple Cider Vinegar, Tea Tree Oil,** or **Hydrogen Peroxide** can be applied to the skin for pain relief and to expedite recovery.

## Sinus Conditions

Sinus congestion or chronic drainage is usually the direct result of inflammation. That inflammation of the sinus cavities (sinusitis) is caused by allergies, certain drugs or a viral or bacterial infection. The swelling of the membranes leads to congestion and irritation and then to inflammation of the mucus membranes which then leads to symptoms. The symptoms may include stuffy nose or runny nose. If the minor symptoms persist it can lead to chronic sinusitis or nasal polyps.

We have found that, in most cases, by eliminating the patient's allergies, the sinus condition resolves. We also check for Pantothenic acid (vitamin B5) deficiency, as well as sodium and potassium deficiencies. Proper balance of those nutrients will clear many sinus conditions that are not allergy related. When we treat the allergies, we also treat (boost) the adrenal system. We have found that most sinus conditions are accompanied by weak adrenals.

Other protocols that we suggest that patients try include:

- Drink bayberry tea or take capsules in the evening.
- Drink blackberry tea or take blackberry capsules.
- Drink 2-3 cups of sage tea daily until the condition is resolved.
- Essential oils help many patients with chronic sinus conditions. Simply put 1 or 2 drops of an essential oil in a diffuser, inhaler or in a cup of hot water and breathe the steam deeply. The most recommended is 2-4 drops of peppermint alone or 2-4 drops of peppermint plus 2 drops each of lemon, lavender and cinnamon. Oregano can be added to make it stronger. Other essential oils that can be tried include clove, ginger and Melaleuca.

## Skin Tags (Acrochordon)

Skin tags are harmless growths of skin that can appear anywhere on the body. Most commonly they appear on the neck or in the arm pits. They can also appear on the eyelids, upper chest, under the breasts, buttock folds, and groin folds. They generally appear in areas that are rubbed frequently, either intentionally or unintentionally by skin (folds) or clothes. They usually appear smooth or slightly wrinkled and irregular. They appear flesh colored or slightly brown and hang from the skin by a small stalk.

Skin tags can occur to anyone at any stage of their life. They occur more often in adulthood and tend to increase until around 60 years old. They are thought to occur because of genetics, hormones, weight, metabolism, or toxicity. The truth is, no one really knows for sure. Some doctors believe that skin tags are a sign of a sugar metabolism problem, i.e., hyperglycemia or hypoglycemia. Others believe that tags are an outward manifestation of internal toxins. By changing the diet, one can manage the sugar problem. By detoxifying the system with a liver cleanse, kidney cleanse and a colon cleanse very often skin tags will disappear.

There are three non-surgical ways that have helped people remove skin tags at home.

1. The tags can be removed by cutting them off with sterilized nail scissors or clippers. The ensuing wound should be cleaned completely to avoid infection. (Skin tags on the legs or under the arms are often removed while shaving.)
2. The blood supply to the tags can be stopped by tying dental floss or thread around the base of the tag. Over the course of hours or days the blood supply should be cut off and the tag will die or fall off.
3. Another way of removing a skin tag is to freeze it off much like most MD's do. There are quite a few products at the local drug store that do exactly the same thing at much less expense. It may take a little longer than in a doctor's office but the results are the same.

## Skin Bumps or Growths

There are a few common lumps or bumps on the skin that cause concern. The three most common are epidermal inclusion cysts, sebaceous cysts, and lipomas.

**Epidermal inclusion cysts** are similar to sebaceous cysts except that the contents are keratin. They appear as flesh-colored, dome-shaped nodules that feel firm but not hard. They are painless unless pressed onto an underlying nerve or sensitive area. When the pore is found the contents can be expressed. The contents will present as a whitish, cheesy, foul-smelling keratinous pasty fluid.

**Sebaceous cysts** are similar except that the fluid expressed is generally clearer and of a different texture. These are sometimes referred to as a "blackhead" in that the sebaceous pore will plug with dirt or other material and appear black. Therefore, the initially expressed fluid will generally have a dark spot at the beginning.

A **lipoma** is a fatty tissue that is usually deeper and feels less malleable. Any of these can appear anywhere on the body but don't present a problem unless they are near a nerve or sensitive structure. Lipomas can be surgically removed safely. Epidermal cysts and sebaceous cysts can be safely treated at home.

See also Keratosis pilaris (Chicken Skin)

## Skin Cancer or Lesions

It's always advisable to see a dermatologist or natural healthcare provider when in doubt about a skin condition. Special attention should be paid if there are skin changes that do not heal promptly or properly. When a longstanding pigmented patch suddenly changes in appearance, color or size, an analysis should be made. However, most skin cancers are among the least dangerous of all cancers. See the section on Cancer and the appendix on successful cancer treatments.

Some have found that equal amounts of essential oils Frankincense, Tea Tree, and Raspberry seed mixed with a carrier oil (coconut or olive) and rubbed on the skin three times daily seems to eliminate the condition.

## Sleep Apnea

See Sinus Conditions

## Sleeplessness

See Insomnia

## Snoring

It's been estimated that 45% of all adults (male and female) snore at least occasionally. This can cause problems with restful sleep and even with good marriages. Just as seriously, it's estimated that 75% of those who snore have obstructive sleep apnea (stopping breathing for short periods). Sleep apnea increases the risk of developing heart disease.

There are several natural solutions to snoring that we suggest. As with most things, not every one of these works with everyone. Experiment until the right combination is found.

- Peppermint oil – rub (with finger or Q tip) a few drops of peppermint oil onto the lower portions of both sides of the nose. Vicks mentholatum can also be used as a substitute for peppermint oil. Peppermint oil can also be taken as a steam inhalation or as a gargle using one drop in a glass of water.
- A homemade saline solution can be made by adding ¼ tsp of sea salt to ½ cup of distilled water. This solution can be sprayed into each nostril or two drops with a dropper into each nostril before bedtime. Don't keep the solution over 5 days.
- Olive oil (two drops into each nostril) at bedtime is said to lubricate the tissues of the nasal passages and reduce friction and thereby reduce snoring.
- Inhaling Eucalyptus oil helps liquefy mucus and reduce inflammation in the nasal passages. Simply add 2 drops of eucalyptus oil to hot water and inhale the steam through the nose and mouth. The same procedure can be used for mint tea.

- Essential oil blends can stop snoring and give a restful night of sleep. First begin by adding 5 drops of lavender oil and 5 drops of rose oil into a carrier oil (olive oil or coconut oil). Mix well and either massage this mixture into the chest before bedtime or, without the carrier oil, inhale the vaporized essential oils from a vaporizer. If that combination isn't as effective as desired, other essential oils can be added in any combination. Suggested oils are: Basil, cary sage, cinnamon bark, clove bud, eucalyptus and myrtle.

Suggestions that seem to help in most cases:

- Eliminate allergies by using NAET procedures.
- Sanitize the bedroom including the bed – dust for dust mites, vacuum the bed and wash the sheets and pillow cases, clean the blankets, keep pets out of the bedroom, change the pillows
- Try sleeping on the side rather than on the back or raise the head of the bed slightly.
- Lose weight if overweight. This doesn't apply to everyone – even thin people snore at times.
- Practice good sleeping habits, i.e., sleeping when over tired (pushed to the limit), can lead to snoring.
- Avoid alcohol and smoking.
- Exercise regularly.
- Drink plenty of water – stay hydrated.

## Splinters

When working with wood or bark dust, often a pesky splinter creeps into your hand. If you can't get it out with tweezers or it's too small to see, I often recommend two things. Wet a small piece of white bread and place it over the splinter. Wrap a band-aid over it and leave it over night. As the bread dries, the splinter will draw up into the bread. A second method is to tape a piece of banana peel to the spot. The digestive enzymes seep into the skin and draws out the splinter. After an hour, remove and rinse with soapy water. The vitamins B6 and C and the polysaccharides in the peel will accelerate the healing process.

## Sprains and Strains

Very often the terms strain and sprain are used interchangeably. However, there is a significant difference. A sprain is an over stretching or overexertion of a ligament. Ligaments attach bones together around a joint. They give stability to a joint. A strain is an overstretching of a muscle or tendon. The tendons of the muscles attach to bones and give flexibility and strength to joint. An injury to each one is classified by the severity of the injury. One form of classification that is shared by both is by the severity of the symptoms, i.e., acute, sub-acute, and chronic. Simply put, acute is a recent painful condition whereas sub-acute is less recent or less painful, and chronic reflects a long standing condition.

A **mild sprain**(grade 1) is characterized by tenderness over the affected ligament, mild swelling, and negligible joint instability.

A **moderate sprain**(grade 2) involves a partial laceration of the ligament and is characterized by the same indications as a mild sprain plus a lack of normal ligamentous resistance on digital pressure and increased joint movement on x-ray studies or palpation.

A **severe sprain**(grade 3) involves a complete laceration of the affected ligament and is characterized by all the above plus a marked excess of joint motion indicating a definite separation of the bony structures on motion or tension.

Strains, overstretching of muscles or tendons, are generally classified as acute or chronic. **Acute strains** are caused by over stretching, excessive muscle contraction, or a direct blow to the affected area. **Chronic strains** are the result of prolonged or excessive overuse of muscles or tendons. Chronic strains, if left untreated, my lead to myofascitis or myofibrositis.

A sprain usually elicits pain on movement of an affected joint even without muscular effort. A strain, on the other hand, elicits pain on muscular effort even without joint movement. As with sprains, the mild, moderate, and severe classifications apply. Pain, muscle spasm, muscle weakness, swelling, inflammation, and cramping are typical indications. A mild strain will demonstrate a mild version of the above symptoms. With a moderate strain, some muscle function will be lost due to overstretched and slightly torn muscles. In severe strains, the affected muscle or tendon is partially or completely torn or ruptured very often incapacitating the individual.

Treatment is rather simple for mild or moderate cases – RICE – Rest, Ice, Compress, and Elevate. Severe strains/sprains should be x-rayed and then attended to by a sports doctor. Mild and moderate strains/sprains should follow the RICE principle for the first 24-48 hours. After that, alternating hot/cold packs for five minutes each (start and end with hot), splinting the area with a brace or elastic wrap, and mild range of motion exercises will help expedite recovery. We have found that ultrasound therapy will hasten recovery and minimize pain.

## Spider Veins

Arteries carry blood from the heart to the body and veins transport blood from the body to the heart. Veins that have become swollen, raised, and snakelike are called spider veins. Blood can pool or even flow backwards if one or more of the one-way valves in the superficial veins don't function properly. The blood stretches the vein and often nearby veins. When other nearby veins are affected, their valves can also malfunction. As the blood pools it stretches the veins and they become kinked and swollen as the blood stagnates. The veins can then be seen on the surface as purple or dark blue or even cranberry in color. Spider veins are most commonly seen in the lower extremities. If several veins are affected, nutrients and oxygen can be prevented from reaching the local area and the removal of waste products is severely restricted. The skin around the affected area may become thin, hardened, sunken, discolored or prone to ulcers.

Some possible symptoms may include: visibly displeasing, a burning, itching, or throbbing feeling, an inflamed feeling, swollen ankles and feet. The symptoms are generally worse during the day or after prolonged standing or sitting with the knees tightly flexed. Spider veins can also cause blood clots, inflammation in the veins, and bleeding if the vein is bumped or cut.

Spider veins are familial and most likely to occur in women more often than men. Some factors that may contribute to spider veins include: lack of exercise, overweight, prolonged standing or sitting, premenstrual or menopausal hormones, pregnancy, birth control pills, excessive lifting, high heels, tight clothing, smoking, muscular atrophy, poor circulation, prolonged bed rest, and chronic constipation.

Several remedies have been found to be effective for reducing spider veins. The most successful we've found is **Horse Chestnut**. It reduces most symptoms while increasing circulation, decreasing inflammation and strengthening the capillaries and veins. We recommend 500 mg per day. Horse Chestnut cream can be topically applied to the affected areas. If taken orally and applied topically, healing time can be reduced significantly.

**Apple Cider Vinegar** can reduce the appearance of spider veins by increasing circulation to the area. Saturate a cloth with ACV and apply it as a compress directly to the spider veins for 15 to 20 minutes. If this is done once or twice per day for at least a month, the spider veins should no longer be seen.

Other herbs and supplements that have been shown to be effective in diminishing spider veins include:

> **Witch hazel** - applied directly a few times per day
> **Ginkgo Biloba** – 40 mg three times a day
> **Grape seed extract** – 100 mg, 3 times a day
> **Vitamin C** – 2,000 – 3,000 mg per day
> **Bilberry extract** – 20 – 40 mg, 3 times a day

**Hawthorn extract** – 200 mg, 3 times a day

The essential oils Helichrysum, Cypress, and Tansy have been shown to dissolve coagulated blood and strengthen the capillary walls.

**Exercise** (walk, run, ride a bike) causes leg muscles to contract and act like a venous pump to push blood back to the heart.

**A high fiber diet** decreases the risk of getting spider veins or varicose veins. The recommended about of fiber each day (by diet or supplements) is 35-50 grams.

## Stomach ache– See Gastritis

Stomach ache or abdominal pain is a common symptom for a variety of disorders. The pain may result from problems in the GI tract, glands, organs, digestive system, muscular system, etc. In other words, it may come from anywhere. However, if the pain is severe and persistent, it is likely to require medical assistance. If the pain is accompanied by nausea, vomiting, abdominal distention, fever and signs of shock (rapid heartbeat, low blood pressure, irregular breathing), the most common cause is acute appendicitis. Immediate medical attention should be sought. However, if there is pain without the accompanying conditions listed above, it is most likely benign. The most common causes are trauma, food poisoning, allergies, insufficient food or gastric hydrochloric acid, or an over abundance of food.

A common remedy is to add one teaspoon of cinnamon powder to two tablespoons of honey and ingest slowly.

Another approach that helps in most cases is to suck on a piece of peppermint candy.

Finally, if the above two are not convenient, measure two finger widths above first wrinkle in wrist closest to the palm. With two fingers of the opposite hand, lightly rub that spot in a clockwise motion.

## Stye

A stye is a bacterial infection around the eye. It usually manifests as a swollen and often painful bump. Place a warm compress over the eye for 5-10 minutes. Mix 2-3 drops of Lavender, Melaleuca and Lemon oils into one ounce of virgin coconut oil. Rub a small amount over the stye and let it sit for a couple of minutes. Gently press a warm wash cloth to the eye until it cools. Repeat two or three times daily until gone.

## Sugar Cravings

In today's society, sweet-tasting foods have not only become one of life's simple pleasures, but have also become an endorsement for love and friendship. Sugar has the ability to increase the levels of serotonin and endorphins thus leading to energy and improved mood.

The consumption of sugar causes insulin to be released. Insulin then binds to amino acids and goes right to the muscles. This leaves the amino acid tryptophan a clear path to the brain where it is used in the production of serotonin. Studies have shown that increased levels of sugar consumption along with depleted levels of tryptophan are present in overweight individuals. It's estimated that the average American consumes 150 pounds of sugar each year.

There are several "causes" for sugar cravings. Psychological causes include boredom, stress, life problems and low self esteem. Some people get comfort or a feeling of control by eating sweets. Unfortunately the cycle of peaks and valleys (sugar highs and lows) begins by consuming sugar to feel better.

There are several physical causes of sugar cravings. Here are just a few:

**Hormones:**
**Serotonin:** This hormone is released into the body when

sweets are ingested. It causes a temporary burst of energy and a feel good feeling. These feelings don't last long and they're usually followed by a sugar low and an increased craving for sugar.

**Endorphins:** Sugar increases the levels of endorphins in the body, thereby producing a pain relieving quality. That becomes addictive much like alcohol. So when in pain, some reach for the bottle while others reach for the sweets.

**Adrenaline:** Stress takes its toll on the body. To keep going, the body produces adrenaline. However, insulin is an antagonist to adrenaline. Therefore, by ingesting sugar, insulin is produced and adrenaline is reduced. Continued behavior such as this leads to adrenal fatigue or adrenal exhaustion.

**Allergies:** Allergies cause a great deal of stress in the body. A reaction of the immune system towards a suspected allergen produces immunoglobulin type E (IgE) antibodies. These IgE antibodies react with allergens to release histamines. The immune system will then immediately release adrenaline and many other substances to counteract the allergens. As adrenaline is consumed, the body becomes tired. Fatigue from the body fighting the allergies, often causes one to reach for a sweet for an energy boost.

**Digestive Problems:** An imbalance in the beneficial bacteria of the intestinal tract can lead to yeast and fungal overgrowth. This overgrowth has a high craving for sugar. Once again the digestive tract is involved in a multitude of reactions that affect how we feel.

There is a condition known as pica which triggers the cravings. This is often caused by pregnancy, malnutrition, and eating a diet loaded with processed foods. These cravings have been linked to a deficiency of the trace minerals chromium and vanadium. Both are essential in normal glucose metabolism and normalizing blood sugar.

Eliminating the allergies by using the NAET procedures and

then testing and treating with the Asyra, the craving for sugar is virtually eliminated. The test will also help determine areas of toxicities and deficiencies. Retesting will determine critical areas that need to be addressed. An organic, non GMO nutritional program low in sugar and having adequate supplementation will help eliminate deficiencies. Detoxing the body by way of colonic hydration, saunas, baking soda baths and ionic foot baths are safe and effective methods.Stress and boredom can be relieved with meditation, exercise, prayer and a hobby that provides self satisfaction and a sense of accomplishment.

## Sunburn

UVB (ultraviolet) rays, when they strike the skin, converts cholesterol to vitamin D3. But too much exposure can lead to an inflammatory response in your skin. When this happens, the skin will become red and feel hot to the touch even by clothes. If prolonged, the skin can blister with liquid filled boils, cause peeling or flaking of the skin and eventually dryness and wrinkling. First and second degree sunburns are usually temporary and manageable at home. However, third-degree sunburns with blisters and/or fever and chills require immediate medical attention.

The most successful treatment we have found is by lightly rubbing raw aloe vera gel onto the surface of the skin. It will accelerate the healing process. The gel can be applied 5-6 times daily without adverse side effects.

Other remedies that our patients have used include:

Bragg's Apple Cider Vinegar (ACV) on the skin either by dabbing or by adding ½ cup to bath water and soaking in a tub.

Coconut oil rubbed over the skin gives relief and promotes healing.

Coriander essential oil dabbed onto the skin gives relief and promotes healing.

Green tea, from soaking two bags in water, either dabbed on the skin or use the bags as a cold compress.

## Sweating – Hands, feet, body (Hyperhidrosis)

A condition characterized by abnormal sweating of the hands or feet or under the arms, in fact, anywhere, is called hyperhidrosis. Primary or focal hyperhidrosis refers to localized sweating (palms, soles, underarms). Secondary hyperhidrosis involves the whole body and may be caused by diabetes mellitus, gout, menopause, tumors, mercury poisoning or disorders of the thyroid or pituitary glands.

Some signs and symptoms of hyperhidrosis include:

- Sweaty palms and/or soles of the feet
- Foot odor
- Cracking and scaling of the skin
- Visible discoloration of the skin in the affected area

An Asyra test to determine deficiencies and/or toxicities is always advisable to expedite finding the cause. This may take some time, so in the meantime, the following are some suggestions that have worked for our patients.

- Coconut oil – mix 2 tsp. of camphor in a bowl of coconut oil and apply to the trouble area.
- Tea Tree Oil – apply a thin layer of the TTO to the affected areas. TTO is a natural astringent.
- Natural vinegar (2 tsp) plus 1 tsp of Bragg's Apple Cider Vinegar and drink three times per day to stop the sweating. This mixture can be added to apple juice or grape juice to soften the taste. Take this mixture on an empty stomach – at least one half hour before or after a meal.
- Sage tea (one cup daily) reduces the activities of the sweat

glands especially under the arms.

- Steep some strong tea in boiling water. When cooled, immerse the hands in this solution for 3-5 minutes.
- Homeopathic medications include:
  Silicea for sweaty feet
  Acidum hydrofluoricum for sweaty palms
  Calcarea for sweating due to obesity
  Botulinum for sweating under the arms

## Tachycardia (Rapid Heartbeat)

There are many reasons for a benign rapid heartbeat (more than 100 times a minute). Exertion, excitement, menstruation, pregnancy, menopause, hyperthyroidism, heart failure, hypoglycemia, anemias and many drugs can cause a rapid increase in heartbeat. Overindugence in coffee or alcohol can also cause an increase. Ingesting, inhaling or touching something that causes an allergic reaction can rapidly increase the heartbeat. Eliminating allergies via the Asyra or NAET often resolves the problem.

Symptoms:rapid heartbeat (100 plus times a minute), possible nausea, weakness, pallor, fainting, even shock.

Treatment: One of the best ways to reduce the frequency of episodes of tachycardia or eliminate tachycardia completely is to take coconut oil. One doctor noted that he recommends 4 tsp. of coconut oil a day to virtually eliminate his patients' tachycardia. To stop an attack, several ways have worked:

1. Lie down with the feet elevated.
2. Bending forward as far as possible from the waist.
3. Placing the fingers over the eyeballs and applying pressure.
4. Inducing vomiting.

# Thrush (Oral Thrush, Oral Candidiasis)

Thrush is a yeast infection of the mucous membranes of the mouth and tongue and is often very painful. The affected mucosal membrane may appear to be coated with a white layer or may be red and slightly raised. When scraped, a mild bleeding may occur. Small amounts of fungus in our mouths are generally kept in check by our immune system. However, certain medications such as antibiotics and a weakened immune system can allow the fungus to infect the membranes.

If antibiotics are used for any length of time, a good probiotic should be used to replace the good bacteria that have been eliminated by the antibiotics. A good self-diagnosis test for candida is called the "spit test." The test goes like this: Rinse your mouth out the first thing in the morning and then spit a large glob into a glass of clear water. If candida is present there will be strings descending from the saliva floating on the surface, or there will be cloudy specks in the water, or there will be disgusting looking saliva on the bottom of the glass. Any or all three are indicative of candida. If you don't have candida, the saliva will remain floating on the top and the water will be clear.

Several home remedies have shown to be successful.

1. Swishing the mouth with baking soda and water (one teaspoon of baking soda to eight ounces of water or one half teaspoon of salt to one cup of water) and then spitting it out. Don't swallow.
2. Brushing the teeth and mouth with baking soda, rinsing and then holding a cap full of hydrogen peroxide in the mouth for 5 minutes. Spit it out and don't swallow. Brush thrice daily.
3. Frequently change your tooth brush or soak it in hydrogen peroxide.
4. The most effective remedy is to mix Bragg's Apple Cider Vinegar, warm water and salt. Swish this mixture, gargle and spit out.

Onions help heal the white layer while garlic helps eliminate the fungus.

To increase the amount of healthy bacteria in the mouth, swish the mouth with fresh yogurt and drink some water afterwards.

## Tinea Versicolor (pityriasis versicolor)

*Pityrosporum ovale* (a fungus) is a type of yeast that is found commonly on human skin. When it gets out of control it can cause discoloration of skin. Patches of altered pigmentation, whether lighter (hypopigmentation) or darker (hyperpigmentation), can occur. These spots most often occur on the chest, back, upper arms and shoulders and can progress to the neck. They are more embarrassing than anything else.

Medically the condition is attacked by using chemicals, of course. However, there are some safe, natural and effective ways to eliminate the condition. The following are some suggestions that can be used singularly or in combination. Try a small area first to determine if there are any allergic reactions.

1.  Aloe vera can be applied to the areas 2-3 times daily.
2.  Yogurt can be applied to the areas, left on for ½ hour and then washed off.
3.  Apple Cider Vinegar – 1 tsp. in a cup of water or coconut oil and applied.
4.  Selenium sulfide (anti-dandruff shampoo) can be applied to the skin and left on for 10-15 minutes and then wash off. You should see results in 12-14 days.

## Tinnitus

Tinnitus can be annoying and even maddening. It's characterized by distracting sounds in the ears such as ringing, hissing, buzzing or whistling. It can be intermittent or it can be constant.

Possible causes include: TMJ disorders, nerve damage, inner ear damage, high cholesterol and allergies. There is no medical cure for tinnitus, however, there are several holistic ways to help reduce or eliminate the condition.

An Asyra test can help give direction as to which course to pursue. If allergies seem to be a problem, NAET treatments are prescribed in our office. Very often clearing the allergies, eliminating deficiencies and toxicities will resolve the problem.

If more is necessary, there are other remedies that seem to help.

- Ginko biloba increases blood flow to the head, neck and brain while it reduces inflammation.
- CoQ10 also increases blood flow. This taken (1 mg/pound of body weight) along with Ginko is especially effective.
- Garlic helps reduce inflammation and increase circulation.

Things to avoid that aggravate tinnitus include smoking, use of alcohol, caffeine, aspirin, and loud noises.

Sometimes excess ear wax (cerumen) builds up in the ear canal causing hearing loss and tinnitus. Ear irrigation is recommended to flush out the unwanted wax. Q tips and doctors who want to put a wire probe into the ear should be avoided. Flushing the ears with warm water is the safest and most effective procedure.

A technique that has not been used in our office but has been strongly recommended is called the finger drumming technique. Place the palms of the hands over the ears with the middle fingers approaching each other behind the head and just above the base of the skull. With the index fingers atop of the middle fingers, snap them onto the skull. This will make a loud drumming sound. Repeat this 40-50 times. This technique can be repeated several times during the day. Some have told us that they have received immediate relief.

## TMJ (Temporomandibular Joint Syndrome)

It is common to see patients with TMJ problems. Complaints of clicking and popping in the jaw to joint pain to difficulty opening the mouth are quite common. Some have even noted that their jaws "lock" open. One young lady complained that her husband refused to take her out to eat because of the loud popping her jaw made when she ate. The medical/dental world is quick to suggest a mouth guard or surgery. However, we've found that a simple TMJ adjustment along with some home exercises can eliminate the condition most of the time. Not all chiropractors perform TMJ adjustments. So simply calling around to find one who is proficient in this procedure is recommended.

The TMJ is a bony junction between the skull and the jaw. Between the two is a complex disc. Assisting in the movement are four muscles. The temporalis and masseter muscles are superficial muscles that assist in closing the jaw. The two pterygoid muscles lie deep in the jaw. Working together they provide smooth opening and closing of the jaw. If for some reason, such as trauma, being held open for long periods of time or biting into a hard object, the muscles can get strained and cause an asymmetry of movement. Dysfunction then occurs.

The exercises to help balance the muscles are very simple. First, warm up the muscles and increase flexibility by jutting the jaw in and out a few times. Then move the jaw left and right a few times. If the TMJ pops or grinds while doing these exercises, press on the TMJ (just below the zygomatic arch or bone you feel in front of the ear).

The first rehabilitative exercise is to put your thumb or the back of your hand underneath the center of your chin. Slowly open your mouth while applying a steady light pressure upward with your hand against the opening jaw. Hold this for 3-5 seconds then close your mouth slowly. Repeat this exercise 5-6 times.

The second exercise starts with an open mouth. Place your thumb or palm under the center of the chin. Place the middle two fingers at the TMJ (below the bony arch). As you close your mouth slowly, push in with your fingers while pulling your thumb or palm toward your fingers. Repeat this 5-6 times on both sides.

When finished with those exercises, close your mouth and place your tongue on the roof of your mouth just behind the front teeth. With the teeth closed, run the tip of the tongue back until you feel the soft tissue called the soft palate. Now with the tongue in that position, slowly open your mouth. Stop if it begins to hurt, your jaw starts to pop, or you feel the tongue move away from the soft palate. Repeat this just once or twice.

## Toe Nail Fungus

See Nail Fungus

Infections of the fingernails and toenails by fungal organisms called dermatophytes can cause a white or yellow spot under the fingernail or toenail. As the fungus spreads, it may cause the nail to discolor and thicken and the edges to crumble. This condition can be unsightly, embarrassing and even painful.

The treatment for this is very simple: Weekly cold laser treatments to the nails along with daily soaks in Pao d Arco. At home, in a bowl of warm water sprinkle the contents of two capsules of Pao d Arco. Soak the hands for 15-20 minutes daily. If possible, soak twice a day, however, once a day will do.

Another proven treatment is to soak the foot or feet in a bowl or basin of water with 2-3 teaspoons of oregano oil in it. Or mixing 1 drop of oregano oil in a teaspoon of olive oil or coconut oil and rubbing it on the skin or nail area. This same treatment can be used for athlete's foot.

## Tongue Analysis

The tongue accurately reflects the state of the digestive system. A quick look at the tongue can save a battery of tests to determine what part of the digestive tract is in distress.

The following correspondences exist in the relationship of the tongue and the digestive tract:

The tip area reflects the rectum and the descending colon.

The peripheral area reflects the large intestine.

The middle region corresponds to the small intestine.

The back edge region relates to the liver, gallbladder, duodenum, and pancreas.

The near back region corresponds to the stomach.

The back region ('the root of the tongue') reflects the esophagus.

The underside of the tongue reflects the quality of blood and lymph circulation in each corresponding area.

The structure of the tongue can reflect an individual's basic constitution.

**Width:**

A wide tongue reflects an overall balanced physical and psychological disposition.

A narrow tongue reflects a lack of physical adaptability with pronounced strengths and weaknesses. Mentally, thinking may be sharp but tend toward seeing a narrow view.

A very wide tongue reflects a generally loose and expanded physical condition and a tendency toward more psychological concerns.

**Tip:**

A rounded tip reflects a flexible yet firm physical and mental condition.

A pointed tip reflects a tight, perhaps even rigid physical condition and an aggressive or even offensive mentality.

A very wide tip reflects an overall weakness of the physical body and a flaccid or even "spaced out" mental condition.

A divided tip reflects a tendency toward physical and mental imbalances with the possibility of sharp fluctuations in thinking and mood.

**Thickness:**
A flat tongue reflects a balanced condition and the ability to flexibly adapt to circumstances.
A thin tongue reflects a more mental orientation, with a tendency to be more gentle and easy going.
A thick tongue reflects a more physical orientation, with the tendency to be assertive or even aggressive.

**Color:**
Dark red: indicates inflammation; lesions or ulceration; and sometimes a degeneration of the related organ.
White: indicates stagnation of blood; fat and mucus deposits; or a weakness in the blood leading to such conditions as anemia.
Yellow: indicates a disorder of the liver and gallbladder, resulting in an excess secretion of bile; deposits of animal fats, especially in the middle organs of the body; and possible inflammation.
Blue or Purple: indicates stagnation of blood circulation and a serious weakening of the part of the digestive system that corresponds to the area of the tongue where the color appears.
Under the tongue, Blue or Green in excess reflect disorders in the blood vessels and in blood quality and circulation.
Under the tongue, Purple in excess reflects disorders of the lymphatic and circulatory system. It indicates a weakening of the immune ability and of the blood vessels.

**Indicators:**
**Body Shape:** Indicates blood and immune health. It reflects a full or empty condition; full equates to excessive or inflammatory condition, empty equals a deficiency, weakness, or paleness.

**Blisters**: Show inflammation affecting the organs according to the organ location on the tongue.
Apis Mellifica – blisters that sting and burn.
Arsenicum album – burning that is better from heat; includes restlessness.

Lycopodium – digestive issues with all symptoms worse from 4 to 8 pm.

Nitric acid – splinter-like pains.

Blisters under the tongue: With a dark purple color may indicate a serious condition, tumor or cancer growing somewhere in the body.

Blisters on the sides of the tongue: Show signs of stomach mucus and congestion.

Carbo animalis – burning with thick mucus coating and indigestion.

Spongia tosta – burning with pancreas problems, indigestion, and respiratory problems.

**Burning tongue:** A burning sensation may indicate stomach dysfunction, fungus problems, or a vitamin B12 deficiency.

Cantharis – burning, cutting and smarting pains; better from warm applications.

Causticum – Burning, rawness, and soreness; better from cold drinks; possible local paralysis.

Urtica urens –ill effects of burns; first degree burns, worse from application of water.

Cancer of the tongue: Generally seen on the side of the tongue and not painful in the beginning. Warts or cysts on the tongue may turn malignant.

Kali cyanatum – cancer of the tongue with hardened edges.

Conium maculatum – growths without pain and can have dizziness.

Hydrastis – severe cancer exhaustion; bitter, peppery taste in mouth.

Thuja – growths where the person expresses disgust.

Silicea – for cysts with people that usually feel cold.

Cankers on the tongue: painful sores from digestive problems relieved with 2,000 to 6,000 mg. of Lysine per day.

Borax (#1) – cankers when sensitive to sudden noises and downward motion, i.e., a descending elevator; thrush may be present.

Arsenicum album – when sore are burning and the person is restless.

Mercurius vivus – when there is lymphatic disturbances and glandular swelling.

## Tremors in the Hands

Involuntary hand tremors or shaking can occur at any age but are more common in older people. Static tremors occur while the hand is at rest. Kinetic tremors occur when the hand is in use but go away when it's at rest. Postural tremors occur when a hand is held in one position for a long time. There are many reasons for hand tremors. Listed below are just a few:

Nerve irritation or compression
Muscle contraction
Caffeine or alcohol
Fatigue or stress
Medications
Low blood sugar
Parkinson's disease

If after a thorough history and examination, blood tests may be requested to rule out some conditions and give a general picture of the patient's health. We usually do an Asyra test to determine if there are any harmonic resonance issues. If so, those will be addressed homeopathically or by NAET treatments. Musculoskeletal conditions are treated with chiropractic adjustments or referred to a massage therapist or acupuncture therapist. Magnesium helps relax muscles.

By reducing alcohol and/or caffeine consumption or eliminating both entirely, the body is stressed to a lesser extent and tremors often disappear. In like manner, emotional stress or anxiety can cause tremors. By using relaxation techniques, TFT and exercise, the effects can be minimized. Low blood sugar can cause hand tremors with or without the person being hypoglycemic. A small protein snack should eliminate the problem. Certain medicines or combination of medicines can cause hand tremors. Although most MD's are reluctant to take you off medications (drugs) but would rather change the drugs, some holistic MD's find that the patient benefits more by being off certain meds rather than switching them.

## Trigger finger/thumb

Trigger finger, also known as stenosing tenosynovitis, is caused by a narrowing of the sheath that surrounds the tendon in the affected finger/thumb. People who require repetitive gripping in their work or hobbies (i.e. gripping bicycle handle bars), are more susceptible. It's more common in women than in men. A proven cure, although it might take as long a six months, is Vitamin B6 (pyridoxal-5-phosphate (P5P), 100 mg taken three times daily. One M.D. that I highly respect stated that in his 36 years of practice, this has worked every time.

To naturally lubricate our joints, hyaluronic acid (HA) is required. As we get older, our natural production of HA starts to decrease. HA is a water-gelling molecule contained in the synovial fluid surrounding our joints, cartilage and skin tissues. Synovial fluid functions as a lubricant, nutrient carrier and shock absorber for our bones and joints. By taking quality supplements that contain HA, collagen and chondroitin sulfate will help maintain joints and synovial fluid. Vitamin C also helps in the production of synovial fluid.

Ultrasound therapy has been used in our office for several years to help joint mobility and reduce discomfort. Along with the above therapies, ultrasound can expedite healing.

## Triglycerides – High

Many people talk about triglycerides but few really understand what they are. Triglycerides are an essential type of fat found in the body. They are necessary to provide the body with energy. Sometimes the levels can get too high. When they do, the body begins to store them as fat. This increases the risk of heart disease including heart attack and stroke. Generally the reference ranges (units of measurement are in milligrams per deciliter [mg/dL]). Normal is less than 150. Borderline high is 150-199. High is 200-499. Extremely high is anything above 500. These numbers can vary a little bit between labs. Metabolic syndrome can be associated with high triglyceride levels. Metabolic syndrome is a combination of medical disorders including too much fat around the waist (40 inches or more for men and 35 inches or more for women), high blood sugar, high blood pressure, high cholesterol and triglyceride levels. This increases the possibility of having heart disease and diabetes.

There are several things that can cause elevated triglycerides level:

- Medication such as hormone replacement therapy, steroids, diuretics, birth control pills, beta-blockers, Tamoxifen
- A diet of too much sugar, carbohydrates and alcohol
- A thyroid condition, especially hypothyroidism
- Conditions such as diabetes, obesity, kidney disease, liver disease

Without relying on chemicals with side effects, there are some proven ways to lower triglyceride levels.

- We recommend having an Asyra test performed and eliminate the allergies with NAET procedures.
- Losing 5-10 percent of body weight can reduce triglyceride

levels by 20%.

- Reduce or eliminate sodas and added sugar. Totally eliminate artificial sweeteners. Carbohydrate foods cause elevated blood sugar levels as well as elevated cholesterol and triglyceride levels.
- Increase fiber intake. Eat more organic, non-GMO fruits, vegetables and grains. Psyllium fiber supplements are a good way of decreasing triglycerides, especially when a good diet is not possible.
- By exercising 30-45 minutes per day, triglycerides begin to drop and HDL's (good) cholesterol increases. "Exercise" could be simply walking 30-45 minutes a day for 3-5 days per week.
- Omega 3 fatty acids help lower triglycerides. It's difficult to get a good amount in the diet, therefore, supplements are the best alternative. It's best to get a supplement that contains omega 3, 6 and 9. Be sure that the amounts of omega 3 plus DHA equal 1000 mg.

## Ulcerative Colitis

See Colitis

## Ulcers (Stomach ulcers, peptic or gastric ulcers)

Stomach ulcers are open sores in the lining of the stomach. They are often extremely painful due to the amount of acid in the stomach. Too often they are caused by prescription or non-prescription drugs such as pain killers, aspirin, and anti-inflammatory drugs. Most often they are treated by more drugs.

However, as in most things, we have been provided with alternatives to man-made "cures." One of the most effective is **deglycyrrhizinated licorice (DGL)**. When the sweet part (glycyrrhizin) of this natural plant source has been removed, studies have shown that it works as well as prescription medications in treating peptic and duodenal ulcers. Apparently it helps the stomach and intestines produce more protective mucus. It should be taken between meals and best at two 380 mg tablets three times per day until the ulcers have healed.

**Garlic,** among the many other health benefits, helps keep the levels of *Helicobacter pylori (H. pylori)* low. The H. pylori bacteria is known to be a causative factor in many ulcers.

**Cabbage juice** taken daily has been shown effective in preventing ulcers. It helps maintain a good balance of bacteria in the bowels. Acid fermented foods such as homemade sauerkraut and pickled vegetables can provide what's needed. Add yogurt and buttermilk to the diet to make it even more effective.

Two tablespoons of local, natural, unprocessed **honey** has been shown to be effective in killing harmful bacteria that contributes to the formation of ulcers.

## Urinary Tract Infection (UTI)

Urinary tract infections (UTIs) are painful, aggravating and frustrating bacterial infections. They are caused by the E. Coli bacteria that adhere to the bladder and urinary tract. Cranberry (Vaccinium macrocarpon) actually helps prevent bacterial adhesion. UTIs attack mostly younger, sexually active women, however, UTIs can attack anyone. Once you have had an attack, you are more prone to get another one. Therefore, prevention is the key. Some of the most common symptoms are: burning with urination (dysuria), frequency of urination, shorter duration of urination, a frequent urge to urinate. Other possible signs might include: foul smelling urine, cloudy urine and blood in the urine.

A quick dip-stick test can determine the pH of the urine and if there's any blood present. The more acidic the reading, usually the more severe the symptoms. A quick EAV scan of the urinary system, kidneys and bladdercan help find any imbalances that might affect the condition.

Some proven remedies for helping eliminate UTI's and their symptoms:

- A very effective treatment is 1 teaspoon of D-mannose for adults, ½ to 1 teaspoon for children (depending on their age and size). Dissolved in a glass of water. Repeat this every 2-3 hours until symptom free. Continue for two days after symptoms have disappeared. For prevention of post-intercourse UTI's, take one tablespoon of D-mannose before and the same immediately after intercourse.
- At the first sign of a UTI, drink large amounts of water — purified, alkaline water is best.
- One teaspoon of baking soda in a full glass of water helps ease the burning sensation. Don't use when taking cranberry juice — they will cancel each other out. Offset their use and use baking soda sparingly.
- Drink two 8 oz. glasses of 100% unsweetened cranberry juice daily until the infection disappears. Blueberry juice can be substituted for cranberry juice. Drink this periodically as a preventative. Cranberry extract capsules can be taken as an alternative.
- Pao d'arco tea taken three times a day will enhance other remedies.
- Daily drinking half a cup of fresh squeezed lemon juice first thing in the morning helps eliminate the infection quickly.
- Parsley tea made by adding a pinch of parsley to a cup of boiling water, steeping for a few minutes and then filtering it off, normally relieves the pain within 20 minutes. Do not use if pregnant as this can induce labor.
- Half a teaspoon of a tincture made from Echinacea and Oregon grape root or goldenseal every hour helps fight acute cases.
- A cap of apple cider vinegar to half a glass of water four times daily helps kill the bacteria.

- Equal parts of Juniper berries, Licorice root, Uva ursi leaves, Couch grass root, and Marshmallow root combined into one compound and taken as a tea or in capsules has shown to be very effective in relieving UTI's.

Cell salts number 4 (Ferr. Phos.) and number 10 (Nat. Phos.) are acid neutralizers. Four small tablets of each dissolved under the tongue six to eight times a day helps reduce the acid in the system. Specific frequencies for UTI, bacteria, and especially E.coli, used with the frequency generator help to hasten recovery.

If symptoms persist after two or three days, an antibiotic can be used to relieve the pain. Be sure to use a probiotic for a short time after using an antibiotic. A qualified naturopathic doctor can best guide in the use of antibiotics.

For immediate pain relief for some, a medicine called phena-zopyridine (brand names AZO Standard and Cystex) are sold OTC at pharmacies. Be aware that the urine will become bright amber/orange while taking. Use no more than for two days.

For more information, see Bladder Infection.

## Valley Fever (Coccidioidomycosis)

This condition is found primarily in the southwestern United States, especially Arizona and southern California. It is also known as desert fever, San Joaquin Valley fever, and desert rheumatism. It is most often seen between June and November. Symptoms may include: Fatigue, headache, cough, chest pain, joint pain, fever, rash and muscle pain. The cause is by inhalation of fungal particles (Coccidioides immitis or Coccidioides posadasii) found in the dirt.

The best treatment for Valley Fever is prevention. By keeping the immune system strong, the chances of contracting or demonstrating symptoms of Valley Fever are minimal. Less than 40% of those infected show symptoms. If symptoms occur, increase supplements to stimulate the immune system and add one or two cloves of raw garlic to the diet each day. Garlic has antibiotic and antifungal properties.

## Varicose Veins

Varicose veins are unsightly and often embarrassing. They can be stripped, compressed with support hose, or simply hidden. The name "varicose" comes from the term "varix" in Latin. It means twisted. As the name implies, the affected veins are usually enlarged, twisted and purple in color. Our veins and arteries have one way valves that assure the blood flows in one direction – veins to the heart and arteries away from the heart.

There are some natural treatments for varicose veins, but like all conditions, no one thing is going to work for everyone. We suggest the following:

Horse chestnut (*Aesculus hippocastanum*) is the most widely used alternative treatment for varicose veins. Studies have shown a significant reduction in pain and swelling with the use of Horse chestnut. Because there is a poison (esculin) in the chestnut, capsules from the seeds are suggested as the best way to take this herb. The recommended dose is 300 mg of horse chestnut seed extract twice per day.

Oligomeric proanthocyanidin complexes (OPCs) are very strong antioxidants found in grape seed extract and pine bark extract. Both of these extracts appear to strengthen the connective tissue structure of the blood vessels and reduce inflammation. However, these should not be taken when taking any medication that suppresses the immune system. Because of the effects on the immune system, people with rheumatoid arthritis, multiple sclerosis and Crohn's disease should avoid this herb. Children and women who are pregnant or nursing should avoid these herbs. Recommended dosage if taken by capsule is 50-100 mg three times a day for pine bark extract and 50 mg three times per day for grape seed extract. It is strongly recommended that a medical herbalist be consulted before taking either of these two extracts.

Genetics, prolonged standing, especially on a hard surface or concrete floor, prolonged sitting, being overweight and aging all contribute to the enlargement of the veins.

Grape seed oil (3 tsp) mixed with 3 tsp of coconut or jojoba oil and 8 drops of an essential oil can be gently massaged over the affected veins to give relief. Massage strokes should be from the feet toward the heart.

Any combination of the following essential oils can be used as a compress or as a massage lotion. They include three drops each of: chamomile, carrot seed, lavender, cypress, lemon, geranium, grapefruit, juniper berry, orange, rosemary. Three or four at a time can be used mixed with water or coconut oil.

Mixing apple cider vinegar with a massage oil or skin lotion and gently massaging the area toward the heart has helped many people. Also soaking a cloth or gauze in ACV and placing it on the affected area(s) for 20-30 minutes is reported to gain relief.

Avoid sitting or standing for prolonged periods of time. Avoid sitting with legs crossed or wearing high heel shoes. Avoid wearing clothes that are tight around the legs and groin areas. Other helpful suggestions: lose weight, stop smoking, avoid alcohol, exercise regularly and eat a balanced diet.

## Vertigo (Motion sickness, Benign Positional Vertigo BPV)

Vertigo is often described as a loss of balance or an uncomfortable sensation of rotating or swaying. The symptoms are often accompanied by nausea and are increased or induced by looking up or rapidly rotating the head. Simply rolling over in bed can bring on a bout of vertigo. A temporary form of vertigo is known as motion sickness. Symptoms generally subside when motion is stopped. However, the sensation may last for hours. Another form of vertigo is known as Benign Positional Vertigo (BPV). Some believe this is due to small crystals of calcium accumulation in the inner ear, although, others disagree. Other possible causes include: subluxation of the cervical vertebra causing nerve impingement and/or reduced oxygen flow to the brain, middle ear infections, shingles, ear canal inflammation, obstruction of the eustachian tube (from the back of the mouth to the ear), inflamed nerve or a tumor, high blood pressure and certain medications.

The treatment, as with most treatments, varies from individual to individual. Begin by making sure allergies and toxins are eliminated and deficiencies have been addressed or eliminated. Avoid aspartame, alcohol, caffeine, chocolates, drugs, fried foods, and nicotine as much as possible, reduce stress and get adequate sleep. Ask your chiropractor to correct any cervical misalignments, especially upper cervical. Acupuncture and Naturopathy have also been helpful in alleviating vertigo.

The test for BPV is called the Dix-Hallpike test. Simply lie on the back with eyes open. Turn the head to one side. If no dizziness or nystagmus (involuntary rapid medial/lateral movements of the eye), the side is not affected. If by turning to the other side the dizziness and nystagmus is induced, that is the affected side.

The treatment(Epley Maneuver) is as follows: Sit on a table and lean the head back approximately 45 degrees. Turn the head 45 degrees to the affected side and extend slightly. Lie down rapidly on the affected side with the head maintaining a 45 degree rotation and extension. Hold this position for 20 seconds to two minutes (variations differ with therapists). Turn head 45 degrees further to the affected side with neck extended slightly for another 20 seconds or more. Roll to the unaffected side with the face turned to the unaffected side 45 degrees. Hold for 20 seconds or more then turn another 45 degrees, now facing toward the floor. Hold this position for another 20 seconds or more. Bend the knees and move the feet off the table toward the floor. Sit up holding the head down for 2-5 minutes. This will move the crystals to a neutral position and the vertigo should subside. This maneuver may be performed again at a later date depending on the severity of the condition. Many times one treatment is sufficient.

Some useful home remedies may include:

Vitamins: Be sure to maintain a good, foundational multi-vitamin and mineral supplement. Add to that a vitamin B complex, vitamin B3, vitamin B6, vitamin C plus bioflavonoids and rutin, vitamin E, calcium, choline, and adrenal glandulars.

Flower Essences: Scleranthus and Rescue Remedy.

Herbs: Ginko Biloba and Ginger. Participants (47%) in a three month study of vertigo showed complete recovery using Ginko in the amount of 120 mg to 160 mg per day.

During an attack, remain calm and still. Avoid any rapid body movements.

## Vitamin D toxicity

Lately the medical world has become obsessed with the benefits of vitamin D3. For many, many years the AMA and big pharma have warned the public that vitamin D was harmful and even deadly. The RDA for vitamin D was 400 IU per day. Anything over 400 was considered deadly because it is fat soluble and believed to accumulate in the body. Now 6,000 – 10,000 IU per day is common. Even with all the warnings from biochemists, vitamin D2 was added to commercial milk.

When vitamin D's storage form, 25(OH)D or calcidiol, becomes too high, adverse systemic effects begin to occur. Although toxicity levels may vary from individual to individual, the established toxicity threshold level is 200-250 ng/mL (500-750 nmol/L). Published cases of toxicity have generally been above 40,000 IU (1000 mcg) per day. Even cases in excess of 200,000 IU per day, the patients survived.

Signs of vitamin D toxicity are high urine and blood calcium (hypercalcemia).

Symptoms of vitamin D overdose or toxicity include:

- Abdominal cramps

- Nausea
- Vomiting
- Poor appetite
- Consitpaiton (possibly alternating with diarrhea)
- Weakness
- Weight loss
- Tingling sensations in the mouth
- Confusion
- Heart rhythm abnormalities

## Warts

Warts are benign skin growths that may resemble a blister or a cauliflower. Warts are caused by a viral infection. The human papillomavirus (HPV) is highly contagious and can enter the skin through any opening such as a cut or scratch from scratching, shaving, or biting nails. Warts are spread by contact and they can grow on any part of the body. They can be skin colored and rough or dark brown or gray and flat and smooth. There are over 10 varieties of warts, most of which are harmless. They may disappear after a few months or linger for years.

The following list includes six of the most common warts:

- Common wart (*Verruca vulgaris*), raised with rough surface, can grow anywhere but most commonly on the hands.
- Flat wart (*Verruca plana*), smooth, flat, flesh colored wart most commonly on the face, neck, hands, wrists and knees.
- Plantar wart (*Verruca plantaris*), hard, often painful, lump on the bottom of the feet sometimes with black specks in the center.
- Genital wart (venereal wart, *Condyloma acuminatum, Verruca acuminate*), found on the genitalia.
- Filiform or digitate wart, a finger-like wart most commonly

found on the face near the eyelids and lips.
- Periungual wart, a cauliflower-like cluster of warts most commonly around the nails.

Conventional treatment meets with varying degrees of success. The treatments include freezing, burning, injecting, shaving, electrocution, poison, or surgically removing (digging them out). However, in over 60% of the time, the warts will go away by themselves. As with any condition, locating and correcting the cause rather than attacking the symptom is the best means of permanent relief.

In a study reported in the October 2009 issue of the Archives of Pediatrics and Adolescent Medicine, patients wore duct tape over their warts for six days and not on the seventh. In the evening, they removed their tape and soaked the affected area in water. An emery board or pumice stone was used to scrape the area. The next morning, the duct tape was reapplied. This procedure continued for two months or until the wart disappeared. Apparently there is a chemical in the adhesive that irritates the wart and causes the immune system to react and attack the growths. We have found this to be the most effective method to permanently eliminate the wart.

Homeopathic remedies include Antimonium crudum (Ant-c.), Nitricum acidum (Nit-ac.), and Thuja occidentalis (Thuj.).

Some have reported success by using ground up vitamin C or garlic made into a paste and placed on the wart daily. The wart is known to fall off within a week.

There are many other remedies including covering the wart with a cotton ball soaked in vinegar, birch bark, a banana peel, a lemon peel, papaya, a raw potato, vitamin E oil, aloe vera and more.

I highly suggest taking a capsule or two each day of olive leaf extract as a preventive from viruses.

## Water retention

Sometimes fluid will leak from the blood into body tissues. There is a series of tubes called the lymphatic system that drains this fluid from the tissues back into the bloodstream. Edema or fluid retention occurs when this fluid isn't completely removed from the tissues. Localized edema occurs in specific parts of the body as opposed to generalized swelling that occurs all over the body. There are many causes of water or fluid retention, most of which are minor. However, if the swelling persists after trying some home remedies, a natural, holistic doctor should be consulted to rule out heart, kidney or liver disease.

Some symptoms include:
Swelling of affected parts, especially the feet, ankles and hands
Constant ache in a particular area
Stiff joints
Rapid weight gain or unexplained weight fluctuations
Pitting edema – skin holds the indentation after being pushed – check the heart
Non-pitting edema – indent bounces back

Some causes may include: Medications, stress, standing for long periods, hot weather, dietary deficiency (protein or vitamin B1), burns, menstrual cycle, pregnancy, oral contraceptives.

Some conditions cause fluid retention: Allergic reactions, thyroid conditions, arthritis, liver, lung, heart and kidney diseases.

We recommend that our patients:
Address allergy issues
Take supplements – B complex, vitamin B6, vitamin B5, multi vitamin & mineral
Take minerals –calcium, magnesium, manganese, evening primrose oil
Take herbs – dandelion leaf, corn silk, horsetail, parsley, nettle
Drink plenty of water

414

Reduce or eliminate coffee, alcohol and tea

Drink cranberry juice (mild diuretic)

Exercise

Drink apple cider vinegar – 1-2 teaspoons in water each day

Epsom salt baths – 2 cups in bathtub, soak 15 minutes, 3 times per week

## Yeast infection

See Candidiasis

# Appendix 1
## SUCCESSFUL CANCER THERAPIES

Cancer is the fastest growing killer in America. Millions of people die each year of cancer or cancer related illnesses. All this after billions of dollars have been spent on cancer research. In 1971, President Nixon declared war on cancer. At that time the cancer survival rate was 3%. After years of research and billions of dollars, the cure rate at this time is very slightly over 3%. It's been said that the cost for cancer treatment from initial diagnosis to termination is approximately $375,000. It's no wonder the cancer machine is the second largest industry in America.

Even though the "Machine" has been busy researching and giving us tidbits of hope, they continue to rely on radiation and chemotherapy, neither have been proven completely effective for the various forms of cancer. In fact, both cause more damage than good. At the same time, doctors and researchers around the world have been busy studying and implementing ways to beat cancer. Many of these doctors and scientists have been ridiculed and humiliated by the AMA, FDA and Big Pharma when their research and trials have proven various cures for cancer work. The "Machine" cannot afford to endorse anyone who has developed a cure for cancer.

The following is a list of treatments and their protocols. In researching successful treatment programs, I included only those programs that had a very high success rate, large numbers of those treated, and procedures that could be employed at home or by any holistic doctor. I did not include successful cancer clinics in Germany and Austria whose treatment programs last only 2-3 weeks and cost less than a used car. Also not included are several successful holistic cancer clinics in the U.S. There are other successful cancer protocols not listed due to specialized procedures or costs. There is more to most of these protocols but listed are just the primary factors of the protocol.

With any cancer treatment program, to be successful the person needs to look carefully at diet and detoxification. For many years and in many ways we accumulate toxins and store them in our bodies. Those toxins interfere with our body's defense system and metabolism. Begin your approach to cancer with detoxification, especially of the liver and colon. Coffee enemas or colonics followed by a yogurt enema or colonic is a good way to start. The next step is to eliminate the body's deficiencies.

Disclaimer: These treatments are presented in no particular order. One therapy or combination may work for one person and something else might work for another. These are presented for your reference and not as a substitute for good care but as a complement. Once again, the following procedures and protocols are not meant to diagnose or treat any condition.

## Essiac Tea

Developed in 1922 by nurse Rene Caisse, Essiac tea was originally a combination of 8 herbs. Later Ms. Caisse reduced her formula to four therapeutic components. These herbs are sheep sorrel (*Rumex acetosella*), burdock root (*Arctium lappa*), slippery elm inner bark (*Ulmus fulva*), and Turke rhubarb root (*Rheum palmatum*). Ms. Caisse refused to have extensive research done on her tea to make it Canada's official cancer drug. Had she agreed to the research, she would not have been able to use it while the testing was being performed. Instead she used her formula, free of charge, to save hundreds, if not thousands, of lives that would have been lost.

Essiac tea is not recommended for pregnant or lactating women. By taking too much, reports of temporary dizziness, headache, and/or nausea have been reported.

The recommended dose is usually two ounces, twice a day, combined with an equal amount of purified or distilled hot water. Sip the tea mixture slowly on an empty stomach. Take about four minutes to sip the entire cup. The best time to take the tea is an hour before breakfast and again in the evening, two hours after the last meal. If the cancer is severe, a third two-ounce dose may be added for a twelve-week period. If taken for prevention, one ounce per day or one ounce per week appears to be sufficient. However, no one knows for sure how effective this is.

While doing his research, one doctor in Florida noted that by placing a drop of Essiac tea on top of cancer cells on the skin dissolved the cells. Other benefits of Essiac tea include strengthening the immune system, reducing inflammation, helps detoxify the body and reduce intestinal problems. Before taking Essiac tea, a holistic healthcare provider or your pharmacist should be consulted if you are diabetic, had a cholecystectomy (gallbladder removal), have osteoporosis, taking cardiac glycosides, pregnant, under 12 years of age or have a kidney condition.

## Noni Therapy

Noni (*Morinda* citrifolia) is an extract of a tropical fruit. It is known to have anti-inflammatory properties. It has been used for a variety of health problems. However, when used in conjuction with other natural cancer fighters, its effectiveness is greatly increased. Doctors have used Noni for the treatment of hypertension, hypoglycemia, Type II diabetes, fibromyalgia, cancer, inflammatory arthritis, systemic lupus erythematosus, and most other connective tissue diseases. It has been shown to be effective for headaches when used in conjunction with feverfew.

Noni acts as an adaptogen to rebalance malfunctioning systems and bring them back to normal. It effectively targets cancer cells by stimulating the production and activity of white blood cells.

Most doctors recommend only two sources of Noni: Pacific Island Imports of Torrence, CA (www.pacificislandimports.com) and American Nuriceuticals, Inc. of Sarasota, FL (www.888vitality.com).

## Brandt/Kehr Grape Cure (Concord)

In 1928, Dr. Johanna Brandt, a South African naturopath, published a book reporting her success in dealing with cancer. She noted that grapes contain high amounts of antioxidants, including: beta carotene, ellagic acid, catechin, lycopene, quercetin, and selenium. The grape seeds contain laetrile, a proven cancer fighter.

Based on the Trojan horse principle, a 12 hour fast (8 p.m. to 8 a.m.) starves the cells, especially cancer cells, of sugar. It is a known fact that cancer loves sugar. During this time, drink only ionized or alkaline water. For the next 12 hours, eat and/or drink only organic, non-GMO concord grapes, including the seeds. The starving cancer cells gobble up the grapes for the sugar and also ingest high amounts of antioxidants. This, in effect, kills the cancer cells and spares the healthy cells. Eat ½ gallon to 1 gallon of grape mush (from a food processor) or drink grape juice divided into equal portions every hour for the next 12 hours. Drink at least one gallon of water every day to flush out the toxins.

Take the following supplements along with those regularly taken:

> Grape Seed Extract – in most OPC's and Resveratol
> Quercetin
> Vit. C – 12-15 grams per day, spread throughout the day.
> Cayenne Pepper
> Niacin – 1 gram spread throughout the day

Warning: Don't use Cesium Chloride with this treatment. It's best not to use other alternative treatments along with this one in that it may interfere with the Trojan horse effect.

Do this on a six week cycle: 1$^{st}$ 5 weeks – eat nothing but grapes.

6$^{th}$ week – eat only raw fruits and vegetables.

Repeat this procedure as necessary.

## Budwig Diet

Dr. Johanna Budwig, a German biochemist, found that the blood of seriously ill cancer patients was deficient in certain important essential ingredients, including phosphatides and lipoproteins, whereas the blood of a healthy person always contained sufficient quantities of these ingredients. She found that by replacing these ingredients the cancerous tumors began to shrink. The two essential fatty acids that she used were alpha-linolenic acid (ALA) an omega-3 fatty acid and linoleic acid (LA), an omega-6 fatty acid. The ideal ratio is around 1:2. Omega-3 fatty acids are highest in ocean fish (salmon, tuna, mackerel) and some nuts/seeds (flax/linseed and walnuts). Omega-6 fatty acids are highest in some vegetables and nuts (corn, safflower, cottonseed, peanuts, and soybeans). Dr. Budwig's therapy is based on cell oxygenation. Essential fatty acids combined with sulfur-rich proteins (as in cottage cheese and yogurt) increases oxygenation of the body.

Sources of sulfur-rich proteins are nuts, onions, chives, garlic, and especially cottage cheese and yogurt. The flaxseed oil should be virgin, cold-pressed, organic, liquid, refrigerated, and unrefined.

The following blend should be a part of a cancer patient's daily diet. Mix one cup of organic cottage cheese with two to three tablespoons of flaxseed oil. Mix thoroughly and let sit for several minutes. This will convert the oil-soluble omega-3 into water-soluble omega-3 and helps bind to the proteins. Stay away from sugar, animal fats, salad oils, and hydrogenated oils.

Use Bill Henderson's book, Cancer-Free, for the Budwig Diet protocol.

For more information: www.beating-cancer-gently.com.

**Cellect-Budwig Protocol**

The Cellect-Budwig protocol is actually five cancer treatments in one. Cellect is a multi-vitamin, mineral, amino acid supplement with some anti-cancer ingredients added.

Cellect Powder – Quickly increase up to 4 scoops/day.

Advanced cases can go as high as 6-8 servings per day.

If you become constipated, take 2-3 cod liver capsules.

Psyllium husk and fresh vegetable juice helps.

Mix with concord grape juice.

www.cellect.org.

Use the Budwig Diet – see above.

Don't take Cellect and the Budwig diet within 1 ½ hours of each other.

Take Cod Liver Oil with Cellect and Flax Oil with Budwig.

Vitamin B17

It's best to eat the seeds rather than take the pills.

Start slowly and build to 30 seeds/day.

Take on an empty stomach and throughout the day between meals.

Organic Juicing

Daily drink 1 oz. of fresh vegetable juice for every 4 pounds of body weight.

Sunshine (Vitamin D)

Get 30 minutes/day of sunshine or take Vitamin D3 (5,000 - 10,000) IU.

**Gerson Therapy**

The Gerson therapy is based on cleansing the system with cof-fee enemas or colonics and then restoring the immune system with proper nutrition.By eating well and taking colonics or enemas, the body can detoxify by eliminating wastes, improve the body's defenses by reactivating the immune system, and regenerate the liver.

The diet consists of drinking a glass of organic apple, carrot and green leaf juices (fruits and veggies) each hour for 13 hours and eating three plant-based meals per day. These can be made up as salads, cooked or baked vegetables, soups and juices. Fresh fruit and vegetables can be used as snacks throughout the day. Eat only salt-free, fat-free, organic, non-GMO vegetarian food.

Take Pancreatic Enzymes (especially Trypsin and Chymotrypsin).

Eat no meat protein.

Don't eat any processed foods.

www.gerson.org

## Dr. Kelly's Enzyme/Metabolic Therapy (Trophoblast Theory)

The trophoblast theory is not new to the successful treatment of cancer. It was first proposed by Scottish embryologist John Beard in 1905. He showed that trophoblasts (infiltrative components that form the placenta) produce human chorionic gonadotropin (HCG) in the same manner as cancer cells. After a great deal of research and observation, he theorized that at a certain point, pancreatic enzymes transformed the malignant cells to benign cells. With the advent of Madam Curie's work with radiation for treating cancer, Beard's work was dismissed.

In the 1960's, William Kelly, DDS revived Beard's trophoblastic theory. Despite considerable success in treating cancer patients, mainstream medicine was bitterly opposed to Kelly and his work. He was convicted of practicing medicine without a license in 1970 and lost his dental license in 1976.

In 1981, as a medical student, Nicholas Gonzalez reviewed 1300 patients treated by Dr. Kelly. He was so impressed with the results that he incorporated the trophoblastic theory into his own oncology practice in New York City.

Some of his protocol follows:

Eliminate pasteurized milk, peanuts, white flour and sugar, chlorinated water and all processed foods.

Restrict protein.

Eat 70-80% raw foods.

Emphesize whole grains, fruits, vegetables, raw juices and sprouts.

Take Pancreatic Enzymes.

Begin with coffee enemas or colonics.

See Dr. Kelly's book: Cancer: Curing the Incurable Without Surgery, Chemotherapy or Radiation. www.dr-gonzalez.com

See Dr. Kelly's Enzymatic/Metabolic Therapy below for more information and a protocol for cancer elimination.

## Vitamin B17 (Nitrilosides, Laetrile)

Nitrilosides are found in the seeds of apricots, peaches, apples, millet, bean sprouts, buckwheat, and other fruits and nuts, including bitter almonds. Each molecule of B17 contains one unit of hydrogen cyanide, one unit of benzaldehyde and two of glucose bound tightly together. The cyanide can only become dangerous if is unlocked by an enzyme called beta-glucosidase. This can happen in minute quantities all over the body but in huge quantities in cancer cells. This cyanide is harmless to the body but deadly to cancer cells. The combination of cyanide and benzaldehyde together are 100 times more effective than either one separately. The enzyme, rhodanese, is always present in larger quantities than beta-glucosidase in healthy tissues. It has the ability to break down both cyanide and benzaldehyde into thiocyanate and salicylate, both harmless to healthy cells. However, malignant cancer cells have no rhodanese, leaving them at the mercy of the two deadly cancer poisons. This is called selective toxicity. Trypsin, acting as a co-enzyme to B17, provides hydrogen cyanide, a harmless molecule, to digest the protective coating of cancer cells.

The most effective treatment of cancer with B17 has been six grams, intravenous once a day, usually for three weeks. Zinc is the transport mechanism for B17 and should be added to this procedure. Pancreatic enzymes are also important to make this procedure effective. It's difficult to find a doctor to perform this procedure, but there are some who understand and believe in its effectiveness.

As a preventative, 50 mg of B17 per day should be taken.

For information about B17, look at: www.oasisofhope.com.

To purchase B17 tablets:

Medicina Alternativa: www.tjsupply.com.Or

CytoPharma: www.cytopharma.com.

**Intravenous Vitamin C**

Hyaluronidase is an enzyme secreted from cancer cells that helps the cells eat away at collagen and break out into the rest of the body. Vitamin C along with increased consumption of the amino acids L-Lysine and L-Proline and EGCG (a polyphenol catechin found in Green Tea) prevents hyaluonidase from dissolving collagen. Vitamin C is required to generate and mobilize leukocytes to fight cancer. Vitamin C is preferentially toxic to cancer cells, i.e., kills cancer cells without harming normal cells. Research has shown that high-dose vitamin C can increase hydrogen peroxide (H2O2) levels within cancer cells and eradicate the cancer cells. See: www.pnas.org/cgi/content/abstract/102/38/13604.

Studies have shown that intravenous vitamin C (IVC) is the best protocol for administering the amounts of vitamin C necessary to attack the cancer cells.

See: www.internetwks.com/cathcart/Catcart2low.rm

www.doctoryourself.com/cameron.html.

www.brightspot.org.

**Ozone Therapy**

This therapy is administered by holistic, alternative medical doctors in any of the 14 "health freedom" states in America. In Canada it's performed by naturopaths. This is performed routinely in Europe. It involves intravenously inducing ozone into the blood system or by infusion (removing some blood and saturating it with ozone and then replacing the blood into the patient's system.

See: www.antiagingmedicine.com

**Dr. Kelley's Enzyme/Metabolic Therapy**

The fact that cancer cells are indistinguishable from placental cells (trophoblasts) found in pregnancy can be traced back to research dating back to 1900. These trophoblasts secrete a hormone called human chorionic gonadotropin (hCG). This hormone coats the trophoblast cells and the cancer cells and makes them impervious to our immune system. hCG is found in no other human cells. The Navarro Urine Test can detect hCG in the urine. Enzymes, especially trypsin, chymotrypsin and amylase, break down the negatively charged protein coating of trophoblasts.

With this in mind, Dr. Kelly treated over 33,000 cancer patients with a 93% success rate. Pancreatic enzymes are critical for this therapy. Patients were also restricted from pasteurized milk, peanuts, white flour, sugar, chlorinated water and all processed foods. The diets emphasized whole grains, fruits, vegetables, raw juices, sprouts and pancreatic enzymes. Restricted protein, 70% to 80% raw foods and emphasis on whole grains, fruits, vegetables, raw juices were all a part of Dr. Kelley's therapy. Coffee enemas were used to detoxify the body and eliminate toxins from dissolving tumors.

Dr. Kelley's radical views of treating cancer caused a great deal of concern with the AMA. He was relentlessly persecuted by the AMA and the cancer industry. He was even jailed for continuing to help cancer patients. In 1981 Dr. Nicholas Gonzales was sent to investigate Dr. Kelley and his maverick practices. He reviewed Dr. Kelley's records and procedures and found a dramatic success rate. Dr. Gonzales later returned to New York where he used a form of this protocol with a similarly high success rate.

See: www.drkelley.com/CANLIVER55.html
www.dr-gonzalez.com

After combining Dr. Gonzalez's, Dr. Kelley's and several other prominent doctors' protocols, a summarized protocol was established. This is not meant as a prescription or an alternative to standard care. The protocol and diet are as follows:

## PROTOCOL

Review health history with the doctor
Perform an EAV test and take the drops as directed to help re-balance the system.

Detox:
Take a minimum of three colonics or enemas (2 coffee and 1 yogurt).
Mix one part regular coffee to three parts water – detoxifies the colon and liver.
Mix one part plain yogurt to three parts water – detoxifies and replaces good bacteria.
Ionic Foot Baths – at least 4.
Baking Soda bath – 1 ½ cups of baking soda per bath. Reheat every 10-15 minutes.
Repeat for 30-60 minutes. Then shower with a brush to remove toxins from the surface of skin.

Eliminate allergies:
NAET allergy elimination is the easiest, quickest and most lasting way to eliminate allergies.

For skin cancer or lesions mix equal amounts of Frankincense, Tea Tree and Raspberry seed essential oils and rub onto the skin three times daily. This mixture should be mixed with a carrier oil such as coconut oil or olive oil.

## PROPOSED HEALTHY DIET

The following is a diet shown to be successful in eliminating cancer in many cases. It may take a little effort and a little more expense than the "regular" American diet, but it will be well worth it.

1. Eat 70-80% of your diet as raw, organic, non-GMO foods.
2. Restrict protein. Eat very little red meat. Fish is easily digested but high in protein so go lightly with the fish. Chicken and poultry free from hormones, pesticides and herbicides, are good choices for protein. Eat plenty of green leafy vegetables and use sunflower seeds abundantly. Emphasize whole grains, fruits, vegetables, raw juices and sprouts.
3. Use very little salt as it restricts potassium from penetrating the cells.
4. Drink 3 glasses of grape juice (pure concord, not reconstituted) daily. The grape juice can be diluted half and half with distilled water.
5. Eat 10 almonds (raw or unsalted) after breakfast and 10 after lunch. Don't eat any more after 2:30 in the afternoon.
6. All foods should be fresh, organic, and non-GMO (as much as possible). Avoid foods packed in plastic. Food and drink in glass jars is preferred.
7. Avoid or completely eliminate:
   Peanuts
   Alcohol
   Smoking

Sugar
Bleached flour
Milk products
Stress
All processed foods
Chlorinated and fluoridated water

8. Eat more (70%) alkaline foods and less (30%) acidic foods.

9. Take a multi amino acid and a multi enzyme with each meal to assist in digestion. The enzymes should include: Protease, lipase, amylase, trypsin, and chymotrypsin.

10. If indigestion becomes a concern, take Betaine Hydrochloric acid just prior to each meal. An alternative would be one ounce of Bragg's Apple Cider Vinegar. This can be mixed with water or any fruit juice.

11. The following supplements should be taken daily. Be sure to get the highest quality supplements that you can find. Remember, discount vitamins give discount results.

Multiple vitamin and mineral
Vitamin A – 50,000 IU
Vitamin B Complex – 100-250 mg.
Vitamin C – 2,000 mg.
Calcium D-Glucarate
Phosfood (Standard Process) in apple juice – 35 mg.
Magnesium – 300-500 mg. – half in AM and half before retiring at night.
Potassium – 100-300 mg.

12. Other important "supplements:"

Essiac Tea
Vitamin B-17 – seeds rather than pills
Slowly increase up to 30 seeds per day.
Carnivora
Methyljasminate

# Appendix 2
## Blood Analysis

Reading the results of our blood test can be confusing and even depressing. There is nothing mystical about those results. With a little rational thinking and knowing what those readings mean, anyone can get a feel for what's going on in the body and take some positive measures to correct any abnormalities. The following is a brief guide to what those frightening numbers mean. Remember, don't jump to any conclusions based only on those numbers. Other factors must be considered, i.e., history, symptoms, other tests, etc. This does not take the place of a qualified physician interpreting the results. The normal range may vary some from laboratory to laboratory.

### GLUCOSE (85-100) mg/dL
Glucose is our main source of energy. The liver converts glycogen (from carbohydrates) into glucose. Two hormones, insulin and glucagon, regulate blood glucose in the body. Insulin reduces blood glucose levels, while glucagon causes the blood glucose level to rise.

**Increased** (>100)

> Non-Fasting States
> Insulin Resistance 100-127 fasting (most common)
> >127 fasting = diabetes
> Acute Liver Failure

**Decreased** (<85)
>>> Reactive Hypoglycemia (<85) (most common)
>>> Hypoglycemia
>>> Chronic Liver Disease

## CHOLESTEROL (150-200 mg/dL)

Cholesterol is an essential component of many necessary actions in the body including: Bile acid production, adrenal steroids, sex hormones and cell membrane development. It is found in the blood, brain, liver, kidneys and nerve fiber myelin sheaths. Smaller amounts are found throughout the body.

**Increased** (>200 mg/dL)
>> Insulin resistance/Diabetes
>> Hypothyroidism
>> Numerous Pathological Conditions

**Decreased** (<150 mb/dL)
>> Overdose of Statin Drugs
>> Genetics
>> Inflammatory/Oxidative Stress
>> Unknown Etiology

## TRIGLYCERIDES (75-100 mg/dL)

Triglycerides are made up of Glycerol and fatty acids. They are either produced in the liver or consumed in the diet. Elevated triglycerides can be an early indication of insulin insensitivity. Very high levels of triglycerides may cause acute pancreatitis especially in those with alcohol abuse and hypercalcemia.

**Increased**(>100)
>> Non-Fasting States
>> Insulin Resistance/Diabetes
>> Hyperlipidproteinemia Disorders
>> Hypothyroidism
>> Obesity
>> Alcohol consumption
>> Medications

**Decreased**
>Due to decreased animal product consumption or
>fat in the past 24 hours
>Malabsorption Syndromes
>Hyperthyroidism
>Severe Hepatic disorder
>Autoimmune disorders
>Immune hyperactivity

## LOW DENISTY LIPOPROTEIN (LDL) (<120 mg/dL)

Most LDL's are remnants of degraded very low-density lipoproteins (VLDL's). Most serum cholesterol is present in LDL's
whereas the VLDL's are the major carriers of triglycerides.

**Increased** (>120 mg/dl)
>Diet high in saturated fat and cholesterol
>Insulin Resistance/Diabetes mellitus
>Anorexia nervosa
>Lipidprotenemia
>Chronic renal failure
>Porphyria
>Hepatic obstruction
>Numerous Pathological Conditions

**Decreased**(<120 mg/dl)
>Hypolipoproteinemia
>Hyperthyroidism
>Chronic anemias
>Reye's syndrome
>Tangier's disease
>Chronic pulmonary disease
>Acute stress (illness, burns)
>Inflammatory joint disease

## HIGH DENSITY LIPOPROTEIN (HDL) (>55 mg/dL)

HDL, produced by the liver and intestines, helps transport cholesterol from peripheral tissues to the liver. A balance between

LDL and HDL is maintained when, working together, when LDL moves cholesterol into the arteries and HDL removes it from the arteries.

**Elevated** (men >70 mg/dl, women >85 mg/dl)
> Chronic liver disease
> Long term aerobic/vigorous exercise
> Familial hyper-lipoproteinemia

**Decreased** (<55)
> Insulin Resistance/Diabetes
> Inflammatory Responses
> Lack of Physical Activity
> Hypertriglyceridemia
> Premature coronary heart disease
> Chronic renal failure
> Numerous Pathological Conditions

## CHOLESTEROL/HDL Ratio (<3.1)

This number (total cholesterol divided by HDL) is used to assess cardiovascular risk. Numbers above 3.1 indicate an increased risk for cardiovascular disease. The higher the number, the greater the risk.

**Increased**
> Cardiovascular disease
> Diabetes
> Lipidprotenemia
> Numerous Pathological Conditions
> Hypothyroidism

## IRON (85-130 ug/dL)

Iron is mostly synthesized by the liver and is necessary for the production of hemoglobin. The body's ability to deal with infection is demonstrated by high levels of transferrin.

**Increased** (>130)
> Increased Iron Supplementation or Exposure
> Iron overload syndromes

Numerous Pathological Conditions and chronic disease
Hemolytic anemias
Acute hepatitis
Lead poisoning
Transfusions
Acute leukemia

**Decreased** (<85)
Iron deficiency anemia
Chronic disease impacting RBCs
Blood loss
Inadequate absorption of iron
Hemolytic anemia
Third trimester of pregnancy

## TIBC (250-350) (Total Iron Binding Capacity)

As the name implies, this number indicates the body's ability to bind iron.

**Increased** (>350)
Iron Deficiency
Blood Loss
Acute hepatitis
Late pregnancy
Numerous Pathological Conditions

**Decreased** (<250)
Iron Overload Disorders
Non-Iron Anemia
Hemochromatosis
Liver cirrhosis
Nephroses
Numerous Pathological Conditions

## HEMOGLOBIN (Hgb) (F= 13.5-14.5 g/dl, M= 14-15 g/dl)

As the main component of red blood cells, hemoglobin is the vehicle for carrying oxygen and carbon dioxide. It is composed of heme, which is made of iron, the red pigment porphyrine and amino acids that together form a protein called globin.

    **Increased** (F>14.5, M>15)

        Dehydration

        Erthyrocytosis

        Polycythemia

        Congestive heart failure (CHF)

        Chronic obstructive pulmonary disease (COPD)

    **Decreased** (F<13.5, M<14)

        Anemia

## HEMATOCRIT (HCT) (F=37-44, M=40-48)

The hematocrit test is a measure of red blood cell production.

    **Increased** (F>44, M>48)

        Dehydration

        Erthyrocytosis

        Polycythemia

        Shock

        Dehydration

        High altitude

    **Decreased** (F<37, M<40)

        Anemia

        Adrenal insufficiency

        Blood loss

        Leukemias, Hodgkin's disease

        Chronic disease

        Menstruation

## RED BLOOD CELLS (RBC) (F=3.9-4.5, M=4.2-4.9)

The function of red blood cells, also called erythrocytes, is to carry oxygen from the lungs to the body tissues. It also transfers carbon dioxide from the tissues to the lungs.

    **Increased** (F>4.5, M>4.9)

        Dehydration

        Erthyrocytosis

      Polycythemia
      Kidney disease
      Pulmonary disease
      Cardiovascular disease
      High altitude
**Decreased** (F<3.9, M<4.2)
      Anemia
      Multiple myeloma
      Lupus erythematosus
      Addison's disease
      Hodgkin's disease
      Chronic infection
      Hemorrhage

## MEAN CORPUSCULAR VOLUME (MCV) (85-92 cu microns)

MCV is an indicator of the size of the red blood cell. This helps in classifying different types of anemias.

    **Increased** (>92)
      B12 / Folic Acid deficiency
      Pernicious Anemia
      High Altitude
      Homocystinemia
    **Decreased** (<85)
      Iron Anemia
      Anemia due to RBC Destruction
      Intestinal Parasites
      Internal Bleeding
      Free Radical Pathology
      Vitamin B6 deficiency

## MEAN CORPUSCULAR HEMOGLOBIN (MCH) (27-32)

MCH measures the average weight of hemoglobin per red blood cell. This is used mostly in diagnosing severely anemic patients.

    **Increased** (>32)

B12/Folic Acid deficiency
Pernicious Anemia
Macrocytic anemia
**Decreased (<27)**
Iron Anemia
Anemia due to RBC Destruction
Internal Bleeding
Free Radical Pathology
Microcytic anemia

## MEAN CORPUSCULAR HEMOGLOBIN CONCENTRATION (MCHC) (32-35%)

The MCHC measures the concentration of hemoglobin in the red blood cells and hematocrit. This is the most specific measure in monitoring anemia therapy.

**Increased (>35%)**
B12/Folic acid deficiency
Pernicious Anemia
High Altitude
Homocystinemia
**Decreased (<32%)**
Vitamin B6 deficiency
Iron deficiency
Anemia due to RBC Destruction
Intestinal Parasites
Internal Bleeding
Free Radical Pathology

## RED BLOOD CELL DISTRIBUTION WIDTH (RDW) (<13)

The RDW measurement is useful in differentially diagnosing certain anemias and monitoring response to therapy.

**Increased (>13)**
Iron Deficiency
B12/Folate Deficiency
Immune Hemolytic Anemia

Reticulocytosis

## PLATELETS (150,000-450,000)

Platelets are necessary for blood clotting, vascular integrity, vascular constriction and repair of breaks in vessel walls.

**Increased** (>450,000)

Estrogen Replacement Therapy

Iron Anemia

Acute Infections

Leukemia

Splenectomy

Rheumatoid arthritis

Kidney failure

Numerous Pathological Conditions:

Hodgkin's disease, lymphomas, malignancies, pancreatitis, tuberculosis, inflammatory bowel disease

Asphyxiation

**Decreased** (<150,000)

Leukemia

Immune Dysfunction

## WHITE BLOOD CELLS (WBCs) (5.0-8.0)

Variances in white blood cell readings are generally associated with infections or inflammation. White blood cells are made up of Neutrophils, Lymphocytes, Monocytes, Eosinophils and Basophils. In acute inflammatory processes, WBC's are expected to increase. Neutrophils are the first to elevate in an immune response. Generally speaking, neutrophils will increase in an acute bacterial infection, lymphocytes increase in a viral infection, and eosinophils elevate in response to parasites or allergies.

**Increased** (>8.0)

Acute Infection

**Decreased** (<5.0)

Chronic Infection

## NEUTROPHILS (40-60%)

As the most numerous of the WBC's, neutrophils constitute the primary defense against bacterial infection. Through a process called phagocytosis, neutrophils literally eat up the offending bacteria. However, they can also affect good body tissue.

**Increased** (>60%)

Inflammation
Bacterial Infection (more likely)
Viral Infection (less likely)
Immune Dysfunction
Acute hemorrhage
Tissue necrosis
Intoxication

**Decreased** (<40%)

Viral Infection (more likely)
Bacterial Infection (less likely)
Immune Dysfunction
Parasite infection
Radiation
Drugs and chemicals
Toxins
Hormonal disorders
Anaphylactic shock

## LYMPHOCYTES (25-40%)

Lymphocytes, manufactured in the bone marrow, migrate to areas of inflammation. The B-lymphocytes mature in the bone marrow and control the antigen-antibody response specifically to the offending antigen. The T-lymphocytes, also known as killer cells, are the master immune cells.

**Increased** (>40%)

Inflammation
Measles, mumps, mononucleosis, chicken pox
Upper respiratory tract viral infections
Infectious hepatitis

    Crohn's disease
    Hypoadrenalism, Addison's disease
    Toxoplasmosis
    Thyrotoxicosis
    Immune Dysfunction
    Numerous Pathological Diseases

**Decreased** (<25%)
    Inflammation
    Chemotherapy, radiation therapy
    Hodgkin's disease
    Congestive heart failure, renal failure
    Inherited immune disorders
    Advanced tuberculosis
    Immune Dysfunction
    Numerous Pathological Diseases
    Elevated Cortisone/Prednisone Therapy
    Any severe debilitating illness

## MONOCYTES (<7%)

Monocytes are the largest cells of normal blood. They can reverse and become histocytes (large macrophagic phagocytes). Phagocytes remove microorganisms, dead cells, injured cells and insoluble particles from the blood. They act as scavengers for the blood. They also produce the antiviral agent called interferon.

**Increased**
    Inflammation
    Bacterial infections,
    Bacterial endocarditis
    Tuberculosis
    Syphilis
    Monocytic leukemia
    Chronic ulcerative colitis, enteritis, sprue
    Rickets
    Collagen disease and sarcoidosis
    Ovarian or breast cancer

Surgical trauma
Hodgkin's disease
Lymphomas
Numerous Pathological Diseases
### Decreased
HIV
Overwhelming Infections
Leukemia or Serious Immune Compromise
Prednisone Treatment

## EOSINOPHILS (<3%)

Eosinophils have phagocytic capabilities and infest antigen-antibody complexes. They become more active during the later stages of inflammation. Eosinophils respond to allergic and parasitic diseases. One third of the body's histamine is found in the eosinophil granules

### Increased

Parasite Infections
Allergies
Chronic skin diseases
Addison's disease
Polyarteritis nodosa
Many drug reactions
Immunodeficiency disorders
Gastrointestinal diseases, such as ulcerative colitis, Crohn's disease
Hodgkin's disease
Subacute infections
Chronic skin infections (psoriasis, pemphigus, scabies)
Numerous Pathological Diseases

## BASOPHILS (0-1%)

Basophils are phagocytic cells that contain serotonin, histamines and heparin. Basophils found in the tissue are called mast cells. Their main job is to clean up and repair the blood system.

**Increased (>1.0%)**

>    Granulocytic and basophilic leukemia
>    Hodgkin's disease
>    Sinusitis
>    Inflammation
>    Allergy
>    Following radiation or splenectomy
>    Iron deficiency
>    Polycythemia vera
>    Hypothyroidism
>    Chronic hemolytic anemia
>    Numerous Pathological Diseases

**Decreased (<0.5%)**

>    Hyperthyroidism
>    Allergic reactions
>    Acute infection
>    Following prolonged steroid therapy, radiation, chemotherapy
>    Reaction to stress
>    Hereditary absence of basophils

## THYROID STIMULATING HORMONE (TSH) (1.8-3.0 mIU/L)

TSH is the most sensitive blood test for primary hypothyroidism. TSH is produced by the anterior pituitary gland and stimulates the thyroid gland to release and distribute the stored thyroid hormones. The secretion of T3 and T4 is stimulated by TSH while T3 and T4 regulate the secretion of TSH.

**Increased** (>3.0)

>    Primary Hypothyroidism
>    Hashimoto's thyroiditis
>    TSH antibodies

**Decreased** (<1.8)

>    Hyperthyroidism
>    Primary Pituitary Hypofunction

Thyroid Hormone Replacement Overdose

## THYROXINE T4 (6 ug/dl-12ug/dl)

Thyroxine T4 is so called due to its four atoms of iodine attached to a thyroid hormone. The T4 test is commonly done to rule out hyperthyroidism and hypothyroidism.

**Increased** (>12)

Hyperthyroidism

Hepatitis

Thyroxine Replacement

Acute thyroiditis

**Decreased** (<6)

Primary Hypothyroidism

Secondary Hypothyroidism due to Primary Hypopituitary

T3 Treatment

Hypoproteinemia

## TRIIODOTHYRONINE UPTAKE (T3 UPTAKE) (28 md/dl-38md/dl)

**Increased** (>38)

Testosterone Therapy

Polycystic Ovary Syndrome

Heparin Therapy

Large Dose Salicylates

Drugs

**Decreased** (<28)

Estrogen Therapies

Heparin Therapy

Normal pregnancy

Methadone

Drugs

## FREE THYROXINE INDEX (FTI) (1.2-4.9mg/dl)

FTI is the result of a calculation between T4 and TBG to help in the diagnosis of hyperthyroidism and hypothyroidism.

**Increased** (>11)
> Thyroid Hyperfunction

**Decreased** (<6)
> Thyroid Hypofunction
> Selenium insufficiency

## AST / SGOT (10-26 U/L)

In the tissues of high metabolism, i.e., brain, heart, lung, pancreas, spleen, liver, kidney and skeletal muscle, an enzyme called Aspartate transaminase (AST) lies dormant until injury or death of cells occurs in that tissue. The amount of AST in the blood will rise as a result of any injury or disease to the tissue and will elevate according to the amount of injury or length of time since the injury or disease. The elevated AST levels will become apparent from 12 hours to 5 days following severe cell damage.

**Increased** (>26 U/L)
> Liver Dysfunction
> Fatty Liver
> Hepatitis
> Cirrhosis
> Liver necrosis or metastasis
> Carcinoma
> Infectious mononucleosis
> Reye's syndrome
> Acute pancreatitis
> Congestive heart failure
> Traumatic injuries
> Mushroom poisoning
> Gangrene
> Trichinosis
> Polymyositis
> Progressive muscular dystrophy
> Pulmonary emboli
> Hemolytic anemia
> Exhaustion

Heat stroke

Muscle damage

**Decreased (<10 U/L)**

Fatty Liver

B6 Deficiency

Renal Dialysis

## ALT / SGPT (10-26 U/L)

Alanine aminotransferase (ALT) is an enzyme that's highly concentrated in the liver. It rises with liver disease. Relatively low concentrations are found in the heart, kidney and muscle.

**Increased (>26)**

Liver Dysfunction

Fatty Liver

Hepatitis

Cirrhosis

Pancreatitis

Polymyositis

Metastatic liver tumor

Obstructive jaundice

Myocardial infarction

Infectious mononucleosis

Severe burns

Severe shock

Breakdown of tissues that contain SGPT: liver, heart, skeletal muscle and kidney

**Decreased**

Fatty Liver

B6 Deficiency

Renal Dialysis

Malnutrition

GI tract infection

## GGTP (10-26 U/L)

Glutamyl transferase (GGTP) is an enzyme primarily found in

the kidneys but is considered to be produced in the liver. The presence of this enzyme is also found in the pancreas. The results of this test are used to determine liver dysfunction and to detect alcohol induced liver disease. This enzyme is elevated in all forms of liver disease.

### Increased (>26)
Liver Disease
Gall Stones
Alcohol Exposure
Pancreatitis
Hepatitis
Cirrhosis
Infectious mononucleosis
Hyperthyroidism
Carcinomas of the liver, breast, prostate and lung
4 Days after Myocardial Infarction

### Decreased (<10)
Fatty Liver
B6 Deficiency
Renal Dialysis
Hypothyroidism

## LACTIC ACID DEHYDROGENASE (140-180 U/L)

Lactic acid dehydrogenase is an enzyme (comprised of 5 iso-enzymes) found in many tissues of the body. An increase usually indicates leakage and death to the cell. This test should be used in conjunction with other tests to determine the specific organs involved.

### Increased (>180)
36-55 Hours after Myocardial Infarction
Renal infarct
Liver Disease
Breakdown of tissues that contain LDH: liver, heart, skeletal muscle, adrenal, lung, kidney, pancreas, red blood cells.

        Megloblastic Anemias, Hemolytic Anemias
        Sickle Cell Disease
        Lung disease
        Shock
        Hypoxia
        Hyperthermia
        Hypothyroidism
        Cancer, leukemia

**Decreased** (<140)
        Reactive Hypoglycemia
        Positive response to cancer therapy

## ALKALINE PHOSPHATASE (70-90 U/L)

This enzyme originates mainly in the liver, bone and placenta. It functions best in an alkaline environment such as pH 9. Elevated levels, along with other tests, may indicate obstruction of the biliary tract, liver disease, bone healing and bone disease.

    **Increased** (>90)
        Liver disease
        Normal Bone Development in Children
        Pregnancy
        Bone Diseases and Metastasis to Bone
        Numerous Pathological Diseases
        Hepatocellular cirrhosis
        Diabetes mellitus
        Hepatic cholestasis
        Hepatitis
        Infectious mononucleosis
        Paget's disease
        Osteomalacia
        Osteogenic sarcoma
        Sarcoidosis
        Amyloidosis
        Ulcerative colitis
        Hodgkin's disease

Chronic renal failure
Perforation of the bowel
Lung or pancreatic cancer
Myocardial infarction
Pulmonary infarction
Hyperphosphatasial
**Decreased (<70)**
Magnesium and zinc deficiency
Hypothyroidism
Pernicious anemia
Malnutrition
Celiac sprue
Congenital hypophosphatasia
Vitamin C deficiency

## TOTAL BILIRUBIN (0.2-1.2 mg/dL)

Bilirubin is a measurement of the product of red blood cell destruction. It is removed from the blood by the liver. It is excreted into the bile and that's what gives bile its major pigmentation. When there is a major destruction or the liver is unable to excrete the normal amounts of bilirubin, an elevation in serum levels occurs. Two forms of biliruben are found in the body: unconjugated or indirect and conjugated or direct. Direct biliruben is the free-flowing form that elevates whenever there is a blockage or dysfunction of the liver. Elevated unconjugated bilirubin occurs when there is an increase in red blood cell destruction. Total bilirubin is the routinely ordered test, however, if excessively high, a request can be made to differentiate between conjugated and unconjugated.

**Increased (>1.2)**
Gilbert's
Hepatocellular Jaundice
Obstructive Jaundice
Hemolytic jaundice
Liver Dysfunction

Red Blood Cell Disorders
Cirrhosis
Pernicious anemia
Sickle cell anemia
Viral hepatitis
Infectious mononucleosis
After blood transfusions
Erythroblastosis fetalis
Increased unconjugated
Trauma with large hematoma
Hemolytic anemia with large hematoma
Hemorrhagic pulmonary infarcts
Gilbert's disease
Crigler-Najjar syndrome
Increased conjugated
Pancreatic cancer
Dubin-Johnson syndrome
Choledocholithiasis
**Decreased** (<0.2)
No known significance

## TOTAL PROTEIN (6.9-7.4 G/dL)

Total protein in the serum is a combination of albumin plus globulin. Albumin carries many small molecules and is important in maintaining the osmotic pressure of the blood. Osmotic pressure is what keeps the fluid from leaking into the tissues. Total protein is increased during HCL deficiency, amino acid deficiency and protein deficiency.

**Increased** (>7.4)
Increased uric acid
High protein diet
Hypochlorhydria
Gout
**Decreased** (<6.9)
Hypochlorhydria

Protein Malnutrition
Liver disease leading to depressed protein metabo-
lism
Fatty liver congestion
Hepatic insufficiency

## ALBUMIN (4.0-5.0 G/dL)

Albumin is a protein made in the liver. By binding to calcium, some hormones and certain drugs, to keep them in circulation, prevent them from being excreted by the kidneys. Albumin regulates water between tissues and the bloodstream by directing water to areas of higher salt or protein concentrations.

Increased (>5.0)
Dehydration (with slightly elevated HCT, HCB, RBC)
Decreased (<4.0)
Liver Disease
Vitamin C deficiency

## GLOBULIN (2.4-2.8 G/100ml)

Larger in size than albumin, globulins are divided into three main groups: alpha, beta and gamma. Gobulins are enzymes and proteins produced in the lungs and liver. They prevent excretion by the kidneys and are involved in fat and iron transport and blood clotting. They are also involved in the immune system by responding to infections, allergic reactions and organ transplants. Tests can be done to identify which globulin is involved when high.

Increased (>2.8)
Hypochlorhydria
Inflammatory/Free Radical Pathologies
Parasitic infection
Early malignancy
Multiple myeloma
Typhoid fever
Lymphogranuloma venereum

**Decreased** (<2.4)

    Severe Hemorrhage

    Severe Anemias

    Liver dysfunction

    Digestive inflammation

## A/G RATIO (1.5-2.0 Units)

The A/G ratio is arrived at by dividing the total albumin level by the total gobulin level. When abnormal, it usually indicates liver disease.

**Increased** (>2.0)

    Dehydration

**Decreased** (<1.5)

    Infection and Inflammatory Disorders

    Burns

    Congestive heart failure

    Cachexia

    Chronic glomerulonephritis

    Pernicious anemia

    Metastatic carcinoma

    Sarcoidosis

    Viral hepatitis

    Portal Chirrhosis

    Intestinal obstructions

    Peritonitis

    Severe thyrotoxicosis

## SODIUM (135-140 mmol/L)

Sodium (Na+) is utilized by the body to maintain osmotic pressure, maintain the body's acid-base balance and to transmit nerve impulses. Several other systems are used to maintain the acid-base (or acid-alkialine) balance at a slightly alkaline level. Several disorders, including cancer, thrive in an acid environment.

**Increased** (>140 mmol/L)

    Functional Dysglycemia/Functional Adrenal Disorder

Diabetes insipidus
Cushing's Disease
Conn's syndrome
Dehydration
Tracheobronchitis
Coma
Primary aldosteronism
Use of water softeners
Kidney dysfunction
**Decreased** (<135 mmol/L)
Functional Dysglycemia/Functional Adrenal Disorder
Addison's Disease
Hypothyroidism
Congestive heart failure
Excessive fluid loss (severe diarrhea, etc.)
Severely excessive hydration by mouth
Edema
Diabetic acidosis
Diuretic drugs
Malabsorption syndrome
Severe nephritis
Pyloric obstruction
Excessive IV induction of non-electrolyte fluids
(glucose)
Low salt diets
Hypofunctioning adrenals

## POTASSIUM (4.0-4.5 mmol/L)

Approximately 90% of the body's potassium (K+) is concentrated in the cells. The bones and blood contain a small amount. It is the principle electrolyte of intracellular fluid. Potassium is excreted by the kidneys, stools and sweat; but mostly by the kidneys. It is vitally important to the heart. Along with magnesium and calcium, it assists in the rate and force of contraction of the heart and in cardiac output. It assists in maintaining the acid-base balance, osmotic pressure, muscle function and nerve conduction.

**Increased** (>4.5 mmol/L)

Functional Dysglycemia/Functional Adrenal Disorders

Renal Failure

Pseudohypoaldsteronism

Uncontrolled Diabetes

Metabolic acidosis

Dehydration

Cell damage

Addison's disease

Adrenal hypofunction

Tissue destruction

Primary acquired hyperkalemia

Adrenal hypofunction

**Decreased** (<4.0)

Funtional Dysglycemia/Functional Adrenal Disorders

Diuretic or Antibiotic Use

Starvation, Malabsorption, Diarrhea, Vomiting, Sweating

Alcoholism

Severe burns

Draining wounds

Diabetes

Cystic fibrosis

Adrenal hyperfunction

Renal dysfunction

Numerous other pathologic conditions

## CHLORIDE (100-106 mmol/L)

Chloride is a blood electrolyte that exists as a part of hydrochloric acid and sodium chloride. It helps maintain cellular integrity by influencing osmotic pressure, acid-base balance and water balance. Chlorides are lost during excessive urination, diarrhea and vomiting.

**Increased** (>106 mmol/L)

    Excessive salicylate Use

    Dehydration

    Prolonged Diarrhea

    Some kidney disorders

    Hyperventilation

    Hypothalamic damage by head injury

    Diabetes insipidus

    Cushing's syndrome

    Primary hyperparathyroidism

    Numerous Pathological Conditions

    Adrenal hyperfunction

    Excessive salt or aspirin use

**Decreased** (<100 mmol/L)

    Addison's Disease

    Severe Vomiting

    Sodium Losing Diseases

    Burns

    Gastric suction

    Water intoxication (excessive hydration)

    Metabolic acidosis

    Acute intermittent porphyria

    Congestive heart failure

    Renal dysfunction

    Vitamin B-1 deficiency

    Adrenal hypofunction

    Numerous Pathological Conditions

## CARBON DIOXIDE (25-30 mmol/L)

By assessing the carbon dioxide ($CO_2$) levels, doctors can assess lung gases.

**Increased**(>30 mmol/L)

    Emphysema

    Diuretic Usage

    Aldosteronism

Severe Vomiting
Use of mercurial diuretics
Alkalosis
**Decreased** (<25 mmol/L)
Secondary to Functional Dysglycemia (most common)
Excessive salicylate Use
Diuretic Usage (second most common)
Starvation
Severe diarrhea
Acute kidney failure
Use of chlorothiazide diuretics
Acidosis

## ANION GAP (7-12 mmol/L)

The anion gap is determined by finding the differences between the sum of sodium and potassium levels and the sum of chloride and bicarbonate levels.

**Increased** (>12 mmol/L)
Secondary to Functional Dysglycemia
Ketogenic Diets
Thiamine deficiency
Fasting and Starvation
Salicylate Toxicity
Alcoholic and Diabetic Ketoacidosis
Metabolic acidosis
**Decreased** (<7 mmol/L)
Multiple Myeloma
Bromide Ingestion

## BLOOD UREA NITROGEN (13-18 mg/dL)

The BUN test is used to determine kidney function in the production and excretion of urea. Urea, formed in the liver, when combined with carbon dioxide results in the final product of protein metabolism. Diabetes, fevers, increased adrenal gland activity, and dietary protein intake all directly affect the amount of urea excreted.

>**Increased** (>18 mg/dL)
>>Impaired kidney function
>>Salt and water depletion
>>Stress
>>Hypochlorhydria
>>Acute myocardial Infection
>>Urinary tract obstruction
>>Shock
>>Excessive protein intake
>>GI tract hemorrhage
>>Chronic kidney disease

>**Decreased** (<13 mg/dL)
>>Liver dysfunction or failure
>>Impaired absorption (Celiac Disease)
>>Malnutrition
>>Hypochlorhydria
>>Anabolic steroid Use
>>Nephrotic syndrome

## CREATININE (0.7-1.1 mg/dL)

Creatinine is often used to determine kidney function. A by-product in the breakdown of muscle creatinine phosphate and a result of energy metabolism, creatinine is excreted by the kidneys. It is removed from the body at a constant level as long as the muscle mass of the person remains constant. If the kidneys malfunction, blood creatinine levels will elevate because of reduced amounts excreted.

>**Increased** (>1.1 mg/dL)
>>Dehydration
>>Kidney Dysfunction
>>Prostate Hypertrophy
>>Chronic nephritis
>>Muscular dystrophy

Acromegaly
Gigantism
Poliomyelitis
Shock
Urinary tract obstruction
Congestive heart failure
Numerous Pathological Conditions
**Decreased** (<0.7 mg/dL)
Decrease Muscle Mass Stature
Inadequate Dietary Protein
Pregnancy
Severe and Advanced Liver Disease
Small stature

## CALCIUM (9.2-10.1 mg/dL)

Most of the body's calcium (98%-99%) is stored in the skeleton and teeth. As huge reservoirs for maintaining blood calcium levels, the body draws on these reservoirs for muscular contraction, nerve transmissions, blood clotting and cardiac function. Therefore, any variance from the normal range is normally indicative of a pathological condition.

**Increased** (>10.1 mg/dL)
Increased Thyroid Intake or Thyroid Toxicosis
Alcoholism
Paget's disease
Acute pancreatitis
Kidney transplant or failure
Advanced osteomalacia
Hyperparathyroidism
Malabsorption due to celiac disease, sprue
Hodgkin's lymphoma
Cancer – breast, lung, thyroid, kidney, liver, pancreas
Leukemia
Metastatic bone cancer
Bone fractures with prolonged immobilization

Alkalosis
Numerous other pathological conditions
**Decreased** (<9.2 mg/dL)
Secondary to Thyroid Imbalance
Vitamin D and/or Magnesium Deficiency
Multiple organ failure
Toxic shock syndrome
Acute pancreatitis
Hypoparathyroidism
Hyperventilation to control intracranial pressure
Bicarbonate administration to control metabolic acidosis
Numerous other pathological conditions

## MAGNESIUM (2.0-2.5 mg/dL)

Magnesium is found in all cells, including bones and cartilage. Magnesium is important in carbohydrate metabolism, protein synthesis, nucleic acid synthesis and muscular contraction. It is also used as a source of energy.

**Increased** (>2.5 mg/dL)
Hypothyroidism
Hypoadrenia
Severe Diabetic Acidosis
Kidney impairment or failure
Use of antacids containing magnesium
Excessive supplemental magnesium use
Addison's Disease
Dehydration
Adrenalectomy
**Decreased** (<2.0 mg/dL)
Magnesium deficiency
Malabsorption
Excessive loss of body fluids
Hypercalcemia
Pregnancy

    Chronic alcoholism
    Diabetic acidosis
    Hemodialysis
    Hypoparathyroidism
    Numerous other pathological conditions

## PHOSPHORUS (3.5-4.0 mg/dL)

15% of phosphorous lives in the cells of the body while the remaining 85% is combined with calcium in the bones. Phosphorous is important in the storage and transfer of energy, metabolism of glucose and lipids (fats), and for the generation of bone tissue. Glucose carries phosphorus into the red blood cells and lowers in the plasma after ingesting carbohydrates.

**Increased** (>4.0 mg/dL)
- Excessive Intake of Vitamin D
- Kidney Impairment and uremia
- Fractures in the Healing Stage
- Severe Nephritis
- Hypoparathyroidism
- Hypocalcemia
- Excessive Intake of Alkali
- Bone Tumors
- Addison's Disease
- Acromegaly

**Decreased** (<3.5 mg/dL)
- Vitamin D Deficiency
- Hypochlorhydria
- Vomiting and Severe Diarrhea
- Hyperparathyroidism
- Rickets or Osteomalacia
- Hyperinsulinism
- Hypercalcemia
- Diabetic coma
- Acute alcoholism
- Liver disease

Gram-negative septicemia
Protein/amino acid deficiency

## URIC ACID (M=3.7-6.0 mg/dL, F=3.2-5.5 mg/dL)

Uric acid is a waste byproduct of metabolism. Purines are nitrogen containing compounds from meats, seafood and alcoholic beverages that break down to form uric acid. In healthy individuals, uric acid is excreted through the kidneys and intestines. If uric acid builds up in the body and is not removed by the kidneys, it will accumulate in the blood causing too much uric acid for the body to handle (hyperuricemia). In gout the uric acid begins to solidify turning into crystals which tend to accumulate in and around joints, the ears and the kidneys. The result is pain and inflammation. That often leads to other symptoms.

**Increased** (>6.0 male, 5.5 female)

        Gout
        Kidney stones
        Arteriosclerosis
        Rheumatic arthritis
        Insulin Resistance/Diabetes
        Starvation
        Stress
        Alcoholism
        Chemotherapy
        Violent exercise
        Leukemia
        Lymphomas
        Metastatic Cancer
        Multiple Myeloma
        Leukemia
        Multiple myeloma
        Lead Poisoning
        Metabolic Acidosis
        Obesity
        Hyperlipidemia

Liver disease
Lead poisoning
Psoriasis
Down's syndrome
Toxemia of pregnancy
Sickle cell anemia
Hemolytic anemia
**Decreased** (<3.7 male, 3.2 female)
B12/Folic Acid Deficiency
Molybdenum Deficiency
When taking uricosuric drugs
Wilson's disease
Hodgkin's disease
Multiple myeloma
Vitamin B-12 deficiency

## PROSTATE SPECIFIC ANTIGEN (PSA Test)

Prostate specific antigen is a glycoprotein produced by epithelial cells of the prostate gland, the lining of the urethra, and the bulbourethral gland for the purpose of breaking down high weight proteins to smaller polypeptides. This results in the semen becoming more liquid. It is currently the preferred method in the medical world to detect localized prostatic cancer. However, it lacks specificity in that it also is increased in patients with benign prostatic hyperplasia (BPH). The following is a list of conditions that produce an elevated PSA:

Benign prostatic hyperplasia
Acute urinary retention
Prostatitis
Advance age
Prostate cancer

The normal range of PSA is age-dependent. Remember, different labs have different cut-off values.

Age (Years)        PSA Upper Limit Range (ng/mL)

| | |
|---|---|
| <40 | <2.0 |
| 40-49 | < or = 2.0-2.7 |
| 50-59 | < or = 3.5-3.9 |
| 60-69 | < or = 4.5-5.0 |
| 70-79 | < or = 6.5-7.2 |
| <or = 80 | < or = 7.2 |

As you can tell, there is a wide range between values depending on the laboratory. It's sometimes wise to have it checked at different independent labs. Even a test with normal results does not eliminate the possibility of cancer. It's estimated that 25% of men with prostate cancer have or had PSA results in the normal range. And positive results are not always specific for a malignancy. Prostate cancer is one of the slowest growing cancers to deal with. Many doctors today are opting for an alternative approach to prostate cancer rather than surgery, chemotherapy or radiation therapy. It's also estimated that if PSA levels are elevated between 4 and 10, there's only about a 25% chance that it's due to cancer.

The United States Preventative Services Task Force (USPSTF) recently released guidelines recommending against PSA testing in healthy men. Their reasoning, the test can't distinguish between serious causes of elevated PSA levels and other causes. Here are some reasons PSA levels may be high and yet non-cancerous:

Inflamed prostate (Prostatitis)

Certain medical procedures, namely a prostate exam – allow 2-3 weeks between a prostate exam and a PSA test

Benign prostatic hyperplasia (BPH)

Urinary tract infection (UTI)

Advancing age

After sex – allow 2-3 days after ejaculation before taking a PSA test

Prolonged bicycle or horseback riding

**VITAMIN D DEFIECIENCY TEST (25-hydroxy vitamin D test)**

Not long ago anything over 300 IU's per day of vitamin D was considered toxic. Now some people are taking up to 60,000 IU's per day to help with certain conditions. Vitamin D is converted from 25-hydroxy vitamin D to its active form in the kidneys. As we age, our kidneys can't convert vitamin D as it once did. Certain condtions such as Crohn's disease, celiac disease and cystic fibrosis hinders the intestines from absorbing vitamin D. Lack of exposure to the sun and lack of enough vitamin D in our diet are the two primary reasons for vitamin D deficiency.

This test measures how much vitamin D is in the body. It's measured in ng/mL (nanograms/milliter). The normal range varies from lab to lab. However, the accepted normal range should be between 20 ng/mL and 50 ng/mL. A level less than 12 ng/mL is considered a vitamin D deficiency.

## A1C test

The A1C test is a form of feedback to help control diabetes and improve diabetes care habits. This test measures the average blood glucose, especially for the last month, but up to 2-3 months before that.

The normal range (for those without diabetes) is 4-6%. For those with diabetes (A1C of 6-6.5% depending upon the authority), the lower the number above the normal range, the better the control of diabetes they have and less risk of developing complications. A person with diabetes should have for an A1C goal of less than 7%. Generally, 6-7% is considered prediabetes.

The following is a chart of A1C levels and corresponding average blood sugar levels:
5% - 97 mg/dL – Normal
6% - 126 mg/dL – above is considered prediabetic
7% - 154 mg/dL – above is considered diabetic
8% - 183 mg/dL
9% - 212 mg/dL
10% - 240 mg/dL

# Appendix 3
## Urinalysis

Urine reveals a great deal of information about a body's elimination process and therefore its overall health status. Changes in the appearance and fragrance can be indicative of a serious condition or what was eaten last night.

A strong ammonia odor could be due to an infection, urinary stones, dehydration, or consumption of high protein foods such as meat and eggs. Urine can smell sickeningly sweet because of a condition known as Maple Syrup Urine disease. This condition is almost always misdiagnosed as diabetes when, in fact, it is simply the missing of two amino acids. Some foods such as asparagus can give a foul, eggy or cabbagy stench. A sulfur compound called methyl mercaptan, also found in skunk and garlic, is responsible for the aroma. A sweet or fruity smell can be detected from those who have uncontrolled diabetes. Urinary tract infections, medications and some supplements can give off distinctive odors.

The kidneys filter excess water, waste and toxins from the blood. By being aware of what is "normal," then what appears or smells "abnormal" will help us determine the cause of the "abnormality." Normal urine is clear (95% water) and has a straw yellow color caused by a bile pigment called urobilin. Urine changes color depending on the time of day, how much water consumed, exercise, supplements, medications and food consumed.

The following is a list of colors and the possible cause of the variation from "normal."

## Yellow/Gold

This is the typical or "normal" color of urine, generally indicative of a healthy urinary tract. The yellow color may brightly intensify by taking certain vitamins, especially B vitamins.

## Fluorescent Yellow

Occasionally you'll notice that the urine will appear a brilliant or fluorescent yellow in color. Sometimes it's enough to cause a double take and create a fear that something is wrong. Vitamin B2, whether taken separately or in a multivitamin, will cause excess B vitamins to "spill" over into the kidneys to be excreted. Sometimes when treating a condition with B vitamins, seeing that fluorescent yellow color can be reassurance that the body is maintaining a high level of B vitamins.

## Red/Pink

This may indicate fresh blood in the urine (hematuria). Possible causes include: Urinary tract infection (UTI), kidney stones, eating red foods such as beets, blueberries, red food dyes, rhubarb; iron supplements; Pepto-Bismol, Maalox, and several other drugs. A "port wine" color may indicate a genetic disorder called porphyria. If blood in the urine is suspected, a physician should be contacted soon.

## White/Colorless

Usually drinking excessive amounts of liquids, i.e. water, coffee, etc. will dilute urine and remove most, if not all, of the golden color.

## Orange

Dehydration or holding your bladder too long are common causes of orange urine. Other causes include: Following strenuous exercise, consuming orange foods (carrots, squash, or foods with orange or red dyes), taking some drugs, liver or pituitary problems. Drinking more water and frequent urination should alleviate the problem. However, if the problem persists, consult a natural physician.

### Amber

Amber urine is similar to orange except more concentrated and of more concern. Some causes might include: Severe dehydration related to strenuous exercise or heat, excess caffeine or salt, blood in the urine, decreased urine production (oliguria or anuria), a problem with the pituitary gland (ADH, or antidiuretic hormone), or a metabolic problem. A natural doctor should be consulted should the condition persist after adequate hydration.

### Brown

The possible causes for brown urine include: A very dense urine concentration often from extreme dehydration from lack of fluid intake, intensive exercise, or heat; excessive particles in the urine (melanuria); urinary tract infection (UTI); kidney stone; consumption of fava beans; kidney tumor or blood clot; Addison's disease; pituitary problem (antidiuretic hormone, ADH); proteinuria; glycosuria; renal artery stenosis. If the condition persists even after adequate hydration, and especially if accompanied by pale stools or yellow skin or eyes a physician should be consulted.

### Black

This very rare genetic disorder called Alkaptonuria is a disorder of phenylalanine and tyrosine metabolism marked by an accumulation of homogentisic acid in the blood. This can also be caused by poisoning. If this occurs, contact a physician soon.

### Green

Another rare site is green urine. Most commonly it is from eating certain foods such as asparagus. Occasionally unusual urinary tract infections can cause this condition. This condition is generally benign and self limiting. However, if the condition persists, along with pain or burning (dysuria) and/or frequent urination (polyuria), a natural physician should be contacted. These may be signs of a urinary tract infection (UTI).

## Blue

Another rare condition is blue urine. This usually occurs as a result of taking certain medications, drugs or foods with artificial coloring. This condition is generally benign but very concerning if the color is not expected. A natural physician should be contacted especially if the same symptoms occur as in the green urine above.

## Cloudy

A urinary tract infection or kidney problem is the most common reason for cloudy urine. However, some metabolic problems, lymph fluid in the urine (chyluria), phosphate crystals in the urine (phosphaturia), or pituitary problems may also lead to cloudy urine. The same precautions should be taken as in the green urine and blue urine as described above.

## Sediment

Sediment in the urine can be from the same causes as described above concerning cloudy urine. However, a urinary tract infection, kidney stones, protein particles (proteinuria) or albumin (albuminuria) can also cause cloudy urine. In this case, a natural physician should be contacted.

## Foamy

Diabetes, high blood pressure (hypertension) and proteinuria are the most common causes of foamy urine. A natural physician should be contacted in any case.

It's one thing to have a blood test or a urinalysis test done. But what does it mean? The following is a brief overview of what some of the urinalysis tests mean. This is not meant to diagnose or imply a certain condition. It is simply a list of what these values might indicate. Your doctor can use these, along with other tests and history, to determine what indicators are present at the time the tests were made.

## COLOR

One of the urinalysis values that is noted on a lab report is the color of the patient's urine. Normal urine is yellow, with concentration increasing the more yellow a sample is. Some medications can cause a change in urine color, which can alter the urinalysis values and change the way urinalysis interpretation is done by a physician or other health care personnel. Tea colored urine is due to blood in the urine. Bright yellow urine may be secondary to vitamin intake. Colorless urine may be due to excessive liquid intake. Normally the urine should be clear. If the urine is turbid, cloudy or hazy, it may be due to amorphous phosphates or amorphous urates in the urine – a sign of mineral imbalance in the body.

## SPECIFIC GRAVITY

This test is used in the evaluation of kidney function and can aid in the diagnosis of various renal diseases.

**Normal Range:** 1.002 to 1.028 g/ml.

**Increases:** dehydration, diarrhea, emesis, excessive sweating, glucosuria, renal artery stenosis, hepatorenal syndrome, decreased blood flow to the kidney, and hormonal imbalance.

**Decreases:** renal failre, pyelonephritis, diabetes insipidus, necrosis, kidney inflammation, and excessive fluid intake.

## pH
This is an indicator of the body's acid/alkaline level. The higher the pH, the more alkaline the body is. Increased amounts of sodium or animal protein increases the acidity. Citrus fruits and vege-

tables increase the alkalinity.

Ideally, urine should be neutral or slightly acidic (pH 5.8 – pH 7). Urine below 5.5 is considered very acidic and encourages infection. If an infection is established, it gives rise to alkaline urine (pH 7.5 or higher). This alkaline urine causes stinging and burning. Testing one's one urine can be done anytime throughout the day. It's best not to test urine first thing in the morning. Cranberry juice is used to lower the pH while vitamin C will raise it.

**Average pH:** 6

**Acid urine (less than 7)** is found in acidosis, uncontrolled diabetes, pulmonary emphysema, diarrhea, starvation, dehydration.

**Alkaline urine (above 7)** is found in urinary tract infections, pyloric obstruction, salicylate intoxications, renal tubular acidosis, chronic renal failure, and certain respiratory diseases involving hyperventilation and loss of $CO_2$.

## LEUKOCYTES

Leukocytes are white blood cells in the urine that may indicate an inflammatory condition.

**Normal value:** Negative

**Increase:** Bacterial infection, inflammation or infection.

## NITRITE

Bacteria reduces nitrates to nitrites by using an enzyme. Therefore, nitrites are usually present due to bacterial activity.

**Normal value:** Negative

**Increase:** Urinary tract infection, bacterial infection.

## PROTEIN

Protein should not be found in the urine. If it appears in the urine, it is usually due to a kidney disorder.

**Normal value:** Negative

**Increase:** Kidney dysfunction, systemic lupus erythematosus, congestive heart failure.

## GLUCOSE

Glucose should not be found in the urine normally. The threshold of blood glucose is 250 mg percent. When glucose exceeds this number, sugar overflows into the urine.

**Normal value:** Negative

**Increase:** Diabetes

## KETONES

Ketones are compounds that are produced as by-products when fatty acids are broken down for energy. Keytone bodies help supply energy to the heart and brain.

**Normal value:** Negative

**Increase:** High fat diet and a low carbohydrate diet, fever, anorexia, diarrhea, fasting, starvation, prolonged vomiting, following anesthesis, acute illnesses, certain drugs, ketoacidosis, fever, fasting.

## UROBILINOGEN

Urobilinogen is formed in the intestines by the reduction of biliruben. Small amounts may be normal in the urine.

**Normal:** 125-250 Erlich units/24 hr.

**Increase:** Liver disease, congestive heart failure, anemias, hepatitis A, biliary disease, cirrhosis, hemolytic anemia.

**Decrease:** Cholelithiasis (gallstones) and renal insufficiency.

## BILIRUBIN

Bilirubin is a bile pigment, a breakdown product of blood cells.

**Normal:** None should be found in the urine.

**Increase:** Liver dysfunction, early signs of jaundice, biliary stasis.

## BLOOD

**Normal:** None should be found in the urine.

**Increase:** Lower urinary tract infection, Lupus erythematosis, polyarteritis, hypertension, bacterial endocarditis, heavy smokers, certain drugs, trauma, kidney damage.

Over the years, many scientists weren't satisfied with just the above urinalysis tests. They continued to research. Further tests were developed that could actually detect certain conditions before they developed into symptoms. The following are tests that have developed from some of those studies. Some are not based on urinalysis, but are listed here because they are usually performed along with the following functional urinalysis tests.

## Oxidata Urine Test

Oxidized cell lipid membrane material converts to MDA (malondilaldehyde). MDA in the urine reacts with a reagent. This test measures actual cell damage.

**Increase:** low available adrenaline, sympathetic nervous system stress, increased insulin, petrochemicals, heavy metals, medications, radiation, malabsorption, low HCL, low enzymes, low exercise, high exercise, poor rest and relaxation.

## Adrenal Stress Test

Symptoms may appear as allergies, osteoporosis, hypoglycemia, infections, hyperlipidemia, loss of lean tissue, obesity, edema, lower tolerance to alcohol.

## Malabsorption Test

Malabsorption is associated with IBS, celiac disease, hypochlorhydria, gastric ulcer, diverticulosis, scleroderma, pancreatic insufficiency, diminished peristalsis, intestinal obstruction, biliary obstruction, allergies, auto-immune conditions, parasite proliferation, yeast overgrowth, arthritis, dermatitis, chronic respiratory infections, fibromyalgia, lower abdominal pain/cramping, constipation, diarrhea, flatulence, feeling of incomplete bowel emptying, rectal pain or cramps and hemorrhoids.

## Zinc Test

Some of the functions of zinc include: HCl production, enhances cell membranes, stronger, more vibrant teeth, bones, hair, nails and skin, reduces radiation risk, increases O2 use, fights obesity, enhances thymus, testes, pituitary, thyroid and adrenal function, aids fetal growth, antagonistic to calcium, copper, mercury and cadmium.

## Vitamin C Test

Vitamin C functions in collagen production, connective tissue function, vessels, bones, joints, organs, muscles, eyes, teeth, ligaments, skin, wbc's & interferon, inhibits LDL, oxidation, adrenal hormones, tryptophan to serotonin, reduces cancer risk in stomach, esophagus, colon, lung, larynx, reduces cataract risk, reduces histamines, protects skin, minimizes gallstones, stabilizes Vitamin E.

## Calcium Urine Test

Calcium absorption is increased by: protein intake, fat intake, Vitamin D, pregnancy & nursing, exercise, growth, EFA's, parathyroid activity.

Calcium absorption is decreased by: excess protein, excess fat, low exercise, excess phosphorus, excess grains, excess oxalic acid, stress, low HCl, low thyroid function.

## Electrolytes

Abnormalities are noted in acidosis, high salt diet, low fluid levels, excess mineral corticoids, some prescriptions, low HCl, malabsorption, kidney stress, low exercise, tap water, poor excretion, environmental stress.

## Total Sugars

Abnormalities are noted in adrenal stress, adrenal fatigue, high carb diet, sympathetic nervous system stress, infection, prescription medications, alcohol, addictive drugs, low enzymes, pancreas dysfunction, liver dysfunction, low exercise.

## Hydration Index

This test displays the body's ability to retain fluids.

## Lipids

Lipids affect cholesterol and triglyceride levels.

## HCl

Conditions associated with low HCl (hydrochloric acid) include: small bowel bacterial overgrowth, chronic candidiasis, parasite infections, bacterial infections, Addison's disease, alcoholism, pernicious anemia, rheumatoid arthritis, asthma, auto-immune disorders, stomach carcinoma, celiac disease, depression, dermatitis, diabetes mellitus, diabetic neuropathies, eczema, flatulent dyspepsia, gallbladder disease, gastric polyps, hepatitis, hyperthyroidism, lupus, myasthenia gravis, osteoporosis, psoriasis, rosacea, Sjorgren's disease, thyrotoxicosis, ulcerative colitis, urticaria, vitiligo.

## Ammonia

Abnormalities are noted in stress acidosis, excess protein, malabsorption, bacteria, cellular dysfunction, kidney dysfunction, liver dysfunction.

## Nitrate

Abnormalities are noted in poor excretion, adrenaline shifts, inflammation, infection, allergies, insulin shifts, alcohol, prescription medications, toxic exposure, tap water, low HCl, low exercise.

## Saliva pH Acid Challenge

Special litmus paper can be purchased at health food stores and pharmacies. By placing a strip of paper on your tongue and comparing it to an accompanying reference chart, one can determine the pH of the saliva. The reference chart will show response colors according to the pH. It will also designate the normal pH.

## Iodine Skin Test

Iodine should be absorbed through the skin within a specified period of time. Abnormalities occur if there is a presence of thyroid dysfunction. A drop of iodine is placed on the forearm and observed for 24 hours. Evidence of the iodine should be present for 18 hours. If not, consider further thyroid tests.

# Appendix 4
## Barnes Temperature Test

Dr. Broda Barnes, M.D. was for many years the leading authority on the thyroid gland. His books and articles remain the foundation of our knowledge of the thyroid gland as well as its influence on the heart and other glands. He was for many years the head of the University of Colorado Medical School Endocrinology department. He was not a fan of the standard thyroid blood tests claiming that there were too many false positives and false negatives. He did, however, have other tests that he felt were more accurate in disclosing the actual state of the thyroid. One of these tests was coined the Barnes Temperature Test. The following are the instructions that I give my patients based on Barnes' protocol.

**Barnes Temperature Test**
1. Upon waking up in the morning, with the least amount of movement as possible, place a thermometer in the left axilla (arm pit).
2. Do not move or talk for 5-10 minutes.
3. Remove the thermometer and record the reading.

The temperature should be 97.8 - 98.2. If it is above 98.2, there's a strong possibility that you are experiencing a hyperthyroid condition. Below 97.8 is indicative of a hypothyroid condition or low thyroid.

# Appendix 5
## Adrenal Tests

**1. Ragland Test:**
Lie down for 10 minutes
Take blood pressure
Stand up quickly and take blood pressure
Pressure should rise 10-20 mmHg
    If BP falls, you feel weak, shaky or dizzy, sign of adrenal fatigue

**2. Flashlight Test:**
Stand in front of a mirror in a dark room
Shine a flashlight across your eyes
Pupils should immediately contract
    If pupils contract then dilate it's a sign of adrenal fatigue
    Dilation will last 30-40 seconds then return to normal

**3. The White Line Test**
Stroke the skin on your abdomen or forearm with a fork or end of ball point pen
Stroke for approximately 4 inches
If the mark is white initially then turns red – that's normal
If the mark stays white for about 2 minutes then turns red – it's possibly adrenal fatigue

# Appendix 6
## The Meridian Clock

There are 12 major meridians in the body. These flow up and down the entire body and provide energy (or chi) to every organ of the body. Each meridian is linked to a specific part of the body. They are also linked together as Yin (receiving energy) and Yang (expressing energy). Every two hours one meridian will be stronger than the others. That dominance will last for two hours then to be taken over by another meridian. These strong periods correspond to specific times of the day. According to acupuncture, there are five elements that influence each meridian. Those elements are: Fire, wood, water, metal and earth. To fully explain the merdian clock and the five elements would be too exhaustive for this appendix. Suffice it to say that a basic understanding of these meridians and the times of greatest strength and weaknesses may help answer why some things happen frequently at certain times. Please note that correlating a symptom with an organ on the meridian clock does not necessarily mean that there is a problem with that organ. However, it is helpful in guiding a person to the possible cause of a problem.

The following is a general overview of meridians of the meridian clock, their associated times and some possible symptoms that might be experienced in that time frame. All of these areas can demonstrate pain along the meridian.

**Gallbladder** (yang) 11pm – 1am Ear and ear conditions, dizziness, low back and hip conditions

**Liver** (yin) 1 am – 3am Liver conditions, lower abdominal pain, vomiting, urinary conditions

**Lung** (yin) 3am – 5am Shoulder pain, respiratory conditions, colds, sore throat

**Large Intestine** (yang) 5am – 7am Elimination problems, diarrhea, constipation, abdominal pain, lower gum pain, sore throat, nasal conditions including discharge and bleeding

**Stomach** (yang) 7am – 9am Abdominal pain, stomach conditions, sore throat, abdominal distension, edema, vomiting, upper gum pain, sore throat, facial paralysis

**Spleen** (yin) 9am – 11am Abdominal distension, pain, swelling, vomiting, jaundice, pancreas and spleen conditions.

**Heart** (yin) 11am – 1pm Dryiness and/or horseness of the throat, heart conditions

**Small Intestine** (yang) 1pm – 3pm Lower abdominal pain, facial swelling, facial paralysis, sore/raspy throat, loss of hearing

**Bladder** (yang) 3pm – 5pm Pain in the neck, low back and/or sciatic pain, headache, eye conditions, bladder conditions

**Kidney** (yin) 5pm – 7pm Kidney and lung conditions, low back pain, constipation and/or diarrhea, dry tongue, swelling

**Pericardium** (yin) 7pm – 9pm Chest pain (angina), heart palpitations, decreased circulation, agitation, irritability, personality changes, conditions of the sex glands and organs

**Triple Warmer** (yang) 9pm – 11pm Adrenal and thyroid conditions, sore throat, ear conditions, swelling of the abdomen and cheeks

# Index

## Y

## Z

CPSIA information can be obtained
at www.ICGtesting.com
Printed in the USA
BVHW061022130620
581303BV00004B/76